Contents

Child Mental Health in Primary Care

Quentin Spender, Niki Salt, Judith Dawkins, Tony Kendrick and Peter Hill

Forewords by
David Hall

Professor of Community Paediatrics

Institute of General Practice and Community Health Trust

Sheffield

and

Jackie Carnell

Director

Community Practitioners' and

Health Visitors' Association

Radcliffe Medical Press

Radcliffe Medical Press Ltd
18 Marcham Road, Abingdon, Oxon OX14 1AA

British Library Cataloguing in Publication Data

A catalogue record for this book is available from the British Library.

ISBN 1 85775 262 7

Typeset by Advance Typesetting Ltd, Oxfordshire
Printed and bound by TJ International Ltd, Padstow, Cornwall

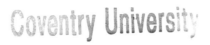

Foreword

I saw my first child psychiatry case as a second year medical student. A mother brought her three-year-old son to the clinic, with the apparently trivial complaint that he was taking things out of her handbag. It took the psychiatrist just a few moments to ascertain that his father was in Wandsworth gaol for burglary, and his mother was convinced that the boy was already embarking on a life of crime. I was deeply impressed. I know now that few cases are so purely psychological and that few are so easily solved, but most paediatric problems have a psychological dimension. Unless these are addressed, the consultation will fail to satisfy either parents or the child.

Every primary care physician and every paediatrician must be familiar with the psychological problems and psychosomatic disorders of childhood. This knowledge is not an optional extra, but an essential part of everyday practice. Without it, many opportunities will be lost to relieve anxiety, intervene promptly for serious problems, and avoid unnecessary investigations for non-existent organic disease.

I have over the years accumulated a large collection of books on child psychiatry and psychology, but until now I had never found one that I could confidently recommend to our junior doctors training for general practice or paediatrics. I wanted one that offered a theoretical basis for its approach, without being too abstruse; a common sense approach that recognised the realities of clinical consultations; some guidance as to what is or is not suitable for the non-specialist to tackle without referral; and short snappy chapters that could be accessed quickly. At last, here is a book that matches that specification.

The Audit Commission recently reviewed services for child mental health problems across the country and revealed some very disturbing facts. Most striking was the remarkable disparity between districts in the provision made for these children. There is an obvious need for greater investment in this area. But part of the reason for the inadequacy of services and the long waiting lists is the tendency to refer every problem straight to the child psychiatry team, without considering if there might be a solution that could be applied by the non-specialist. If general practitioners and general paediatricians equip themselves with the basic skills and knowledge outlined in this book, the rate of referral will go down, parents and children will be more satisfied, and the specialist teams will be able to concentrate on those more complex, baffling or intractable cases that really need their skills.

Every trainee in general practice and in paediatrics should buy this book, read it, and read it again. And those whose job it is to teach them will need a copy as well.

David Hall
Professor of Community Paediatrics
Institute of General Practice and Community Health Trust
Sheffield
November 2000

Foreword

The recent strong emphasis by government ministers on the importance of primary care, as outlined in the NHS Plan and the White Paper *Saving Lives, Our Healthier Nation*, provides the perfect backdrop for this excellent book *Child Mental Health in Primary Care*.

Having read this book with great interest, I am convinced that it will quickly become a standard text for health visitors, school nurses and community practitioners because of the wide and embracing scope adopted by the distinguished band of contributors and through the excellent use of case studies.

Having had more than 20 years' experience in this field, both as a health visitor and now as a manager, I know that child mental health issues are ones on which primary care professionals spend much time and energy. And it is by tackling these issues in a sensitive way that many long-term problems affecting the child and family can be overcome.

Children develop at a bewilderingly fast rate. The contributors cover the problems that may arise in the early years, through to the school-age years when, for example, bullying may occur, and on to the emotional minefield of 'being a teenager', when depression, substance abuse and eating disorders could come to the fore. With the aid of case studies, the book lays out strategies that could be adopted to resolve the child's distress and provide support structures for the family as a whole. It also approaches cultural and ethnic issues, appropriate for a multi-cultural society.

The book's common sense and straightforward direction can only inspire confidence in the health professional, many of whom are hard-pressed with giant caseloads to deal with. It will contribute to greater understanding and this in turn will facilitate smoother team work within the primary care setting. The more that health visitors are able to understand the complexity of child mental health issues, the fewer the families that will need to be referred to the specialist services.

I know, remembering my days as a health visitor, that I would have greatly appreciated and benefited from having a book such as this on my desk. It is comprehensive, easy-to-read and thankfully free from the liberal use of jargon that sometimes bedevils such publications.

The excellence of this book, however, can't disguise the fact that the campaign for enough resources to sustain and develop work in this field must continue. Under the NHS Plan, more money and more staff are promised and this is to be greatly welcomed. But there will be the inevitable struggle by competing priorities for their share of additional resources, and those of us working in primary care must be conscious of this.

I was pleased to have been asked to write this foreword as the subject goes to the very core of what we, at the Community Practitioners' and Health Visitors' Association, believe in and promote on a daily basis. Every health professional working in primary care is well advised to study this book at some stage, preferably sooner rather than later. It will increase their circle of knowledge.

Jackie Carnell
Director
Community Practitioners' and
Health Visitors' Association
November 2000

Preface

This book aims to help general practitioners, health visitors and other professionals working in primary care settings to assess, manage and refer children and adolescents with mental health problems. Recent reorganisations in the health service in the UK have encouraged the provision of services at the primary care level, rather than exclusively within specialist services. Some parts of the book may also be useful for school medical officers, social workers and educational psychologists, many of whom are in the front line of mental health provision for children and young people.

The book is composed mainly of chapters with a uniform structure that is designed to emphasise what can realistically be done in primary care. Each of these chapters starts with an introduction, including definitions, and then proceeds to an outline of assessment, followed by management options, and finally indications for referral. The introductory chapters give an overview of general themes. Illustrative case examples are included in almost all chapters, and most of these examples are based on real individual cases, or amalgams of several cases.

We often use the terms 'child or 'children' to refer to both children and adolescents. In most places we refer to the child as 'he', except when the condition in question is more common in girls. A single parent is usually referred to as 'she', but the comments should be taken to include single fathers.

We are grateful to a number of colleagues who have advised us about the content of some of the chapters. These include Professor David Candy, Deborah Fulford, Dr Pat Hughes, Ann Kimber, Karen King, Dr Rebecca Park, Dr Josephine Richards, Julia Robb, Dr Andrew Singleton, Dr Jean Sherrington and Dr Jeremy Turk.

QS, NS, JD, TK, PH
November 2000

List of contributors

Judith Dawkins MB BS BSc MRCPSYCH
Senior Lecturer in Child and Adolescent
 Psychiatry
St George's Hospital Medical School
London, UK

Consultant in Child and Adolescent
 Psychiatry
Surrey Hampshire Borders NHS Trust
Guildford, UK

Peter Hill MA FRCP FRCPSYCH FRCPCH
Professor of Child and Adolescent
 Psychiatry
Hospital for Sick Children
Great Ormond Street
London, UK

Tony Kendrick BSc MD MRCPSYCH FRCGP
Professor of Primary Medical Care
Medical School, University of
 Southampton
Southampton, UK

Sangeeta Patel MRCGP MA
General Practitioner
Balham, London, UK

Clinical Lecturer
Department of General Practice and
 Primary Care
St George's Hospital Medical School
London, UK

Niki Salt MB BS DCH MRCP (PAEDIATRICS) MRCGP
General Practitioner
Thurleigh Road Group Practice
London, UK

Quentin Spender MB BS DCH MRCP
 (PAEDIATRICS) MRCPSYCH
Senior Lecturer in Child and Adolescent
 Psychiatry
St George's Hospital Medical School
London, UK

Consultant in Child and Adolescent
 Psychiatry
Sussex Weald and Downs NHS Trust
Chichester, UK

PART 1

Introduction

CHAPTER ONE

Assessment in child mental health

Introduction

Definition of child mental health

Mental health in children and young people has been defined as:[1]

- a capacity to enter into and sustain mutually satisfying personal relationships
- a continuing progression of psychological development
- an ability to play and to learn so that attainments are appropriate for age and intellectual level
- a developing moral sense of right and wrong
- the degree of psychological distress and maladaptive behaviour being within normal limits for the child's age and context.

Child mental health problems are therefore difficulties or disabilities in these areas that may arise from any number of congenital, constitutional, environmental, family or illness factors. Such problems have two components. First, the presenting features are outside the normal range for the child's age, intellectual level and culture, and secondly, the child or others in contact with them are suffering from the dysfunction.

Prevalence

In UK studies, 2–5% of children seen in primary care settings are presented by their parents with mental health problems as the main complaint. Hyperactivity, anxiety or behavioural problems are the principal concerns.[2] Interviews conducted with children and parents attending primary care services suggest that about 25% of all children who are seen by members of the primary care team have psychological difficulties associated with physical problems[3] of a degree sufficient to be defined as a mental health disturbance.[4] This is higher than the rate in the general population of 7–20% (varies with age, gender and locality). It is not always easy to tell whether the psychological symptoms are a consequence of the physical disorder, or whether the physical symptoms are a somatic presentation of a mental health problem (or both). The distinction is not always helpful, and it may be more valuable to view childhood illnesses as existing on a continuum from purely somatic to purely psychological (*see* Box 1.1).[5]

Box 1.1:   The spectrum of childhood illness

Completely   Completely

somatic   psychological

The implication of these epidemiological findings is that many more children attend primary care settings who have disorders of child mental health than present with these, just as there are many children with mental health problems who do not present to primary care at all. It would not be appropriate to refer all such children to specialist settings, and in any case many parents and children do not want this. Children who are particularly likely to suffer from mental health problems are those with one or more of the risk factors shown in Box 1.2.

Box 1.2:   Risk factors for psychological disturbance in children

Chronic physical illness
Low intelligence
Damaged brain
Parental psychiatric disorder
Family disruption
Angry, bitter family relationships
Rejection by parents
Rejection by peers

Assessment

The three most important parts of a child mental health assessment are the *history of the presenting complaint*, the *developmental history* and the *family and social history*.

The *history of the presenting complaint* includes what is bringing the family to the health centre, who is most worried about it, what it is they are most concerned about, what they think could be done about the problem, and why they are presenting now.

Case study 1.1

Tom, a previously healthy 9-year-old, was brought by his mother Sue to a fit-in appointment at the end of Monday morning surgery. Sue told the doctor that Tom had been suffering from stomach pains from time to time over the past few weeks, and had missed several days off school as a result. The pains were poorly localised and were not associated with any bowel or urinary symptoms, or with headaches. Tom was eating well and was as physically active as usual. The doctor examined him and could find no abnormality – indeed he seemed very well. She arranged for a urine specimen to be sent to the laboratory to exclude infection, and she advised Sue to give Tom some paracetamol and send him back to school.

Two weeks later Tom was again brought to a fit-in appointment, this time at the end of Monday evening surgery, with the same complaint. The pains were not being helped by paracetamol, and he had missed a few more days off school. Again, he appeared very healthy on examination. The urine specimen had tested negative for infection. The doctor asked whether everything was all right at school, and was told that there was no problem as far as Tom's mother and teachers could tell. Tom did not always want to go to school, but Sue always made him go unless he was ill, when she felt she could not force him. She asked whether a blood test could be done, and the doctor agreed to send off a sample for a blood count, as she hoped that a negative result would reassure Tom's mother that nothing too serious was going on.

At the follow-up consultation 10 days later the doctor assured Sue that the blood test was normal. However, Tom had missed several more days of school. The doctor asked if she could have a few words with Tom alone, and while his mother waited outside she asked Tom whether he was enjoying school, and about his friends. Tom was not very communicative, but denied that anything was wrong at home or at school, and told the doctor he was not afraid of anyone bullying him. The doctor informed Sue that stomach pains were quite common in children of Tom's age, usually coming and going for a few months but then clearing up completely with time. Sue wanted to know the cause, and the doctor had to admit to uncertainty, but she explained that sometimes stomach pains were the first sign of migraine in a child. The doctor sensed that Sue was not reassured by this explanation, and offered to refer Tom for a specialist opinion. Tom's mother then explained that she was satisfied with the doctor's explanation, but that her husband John was worried that something serious was wrong. John insisted that if Tom was too ill to go to school he had to see the doctor the same day, so that Sue could tell John what the problem was when he came home from work that evening. John's sister had died the previous year, at only 36 years of age, from cancer which had involved the liver, and Sue agreed that this might have made the whole family more concerned about the possible meaning of Tom's pains. Sue felt that she should be more firm about making Tom go to school despite his pains, but that her husband would not support her in this course of action. The doctor agreed to see Tom with Sue again, but at an evening appointment when John could come along, too.

A *clear description of what the child does* can help enormously in understanding the nature of a problem. It is also illuminating to work out when the problem occurs, what triggers it, and how others respond to it. This may help to determine the perpetuating or maintaining causes that are keeping the problem at a troublesome level. It may be useful to ask parents to fill in an 'ABC' diary (*see* Box 1.3).

Box 1.3:   An example of an ABC diary

Date, time, place	*Antecedents*	*Behaviour*	*Consequences*
Tesco's checkout, Friday, 11.00 a.m.	Being bored; seeing the sweets on the rack	Screaming, shouting, kicking	I was embarrassed – everyone was watching. I had to give in; then the screaming stopped

---

Asking *how and when the problem developed* may help to shed light on the precipitating causes, although perpetuating causes may be more important. It is useful to bear in mind the three-part question 'Why have *this* family come with *this* problem at *this* time?'[6] A recently developed problem, or a chronic problem that has recently taken a turn for the worse, may provide a partial answer. In addition, it is worth enquiring about what shift in perception may have led the family to ask for help *now*. This may provide a clue as to how ready they are to change the way in which they currently cope with the problem.

The purpose of the *developmental history* is to find out whether there are any factors in the pregnancy or early years of childhood that might contribute to the current problem. It also helps to build a picture of whether attachment is secure or insecure. Some of this information may already be available in the primary care notes. Relevant factors include the following:

- medical difficulties in the pregnancy that might affect the mother's attitude to the newborn child
- prematurity or being small for dates
- a period in the special-care baby unit
- maternal depression during the first year of the baby's life
- difficulties with feeding, sleeping or excessive crying during the first year of life, which are usually synonymous with a difficult temperament
- developmental milestones – age of walking and progress in speech seem to be the easiest for parents to remember
- relationship difficulties between the parents during the first few years of the child's life
- separation of the child from their primary caregiver
- excessive clinging
- integration into play group, nursery school and first full-time school

- any major losses for the child, such as death of a close relative, a parent leaving, or moving house.

The *family and social history* may be unnecessary if the family is well known to the practice, but there is always more to find out, and it can provide a good opportunity to involve the child. Information about who is living at home and what they do may be less important than the attitudes of different family members to the presenting problem, and the way in which it affects their lives. Additional questions that may be useful when taking the family history include the following.

- What makes this different from the other children?
- Does he remind you of anyone?
- What sort of things were you doing when you were his age?

From whom should you obtain the history?

The history is usually taken from the parents, but it is helpful if the child can contribute. The normal method used in paediatrics is to start taking the history from the parent or parents present, and then to involve the child once he is used to you. This technique can be equally useful in child mental health, but:

- it may be unpleasant for the child to hear a litany of negative comments about him. Ways around this include seeing the parents alone, or keeping the history of the presenting complaint very brief
- older children may prefer to be seen alone.

Interviewing the parents

If both parents can attend, this results in a more complete account, allows you a glimpse of the different parental perspectives, and provides an opportunity to see how the parents work together. However, it is nearly always mothers who bring children to see general practitioners, and fathers are often out at work when health visitors call, so there is little opportunity in primary care to practise interviewing two parents at once, or to reap the advantages of this.

Interviewing pre-adolescent children

The style and content of any interview with a child will depend on the reason for that interview. This may be:

- to discover facts that only the child knows

- to ascertain the child's emotional state
- to observe the child's language, social or cognitive functioning.

Question-and-answer interviews are quite adequate for children aged six years or over. The use of drawings and play as a means of interviewing should probably be left to specialists. Nevertheless, it is helpful to have felt-tip pens, paper, and imaginative toys available, and to observe a child's drawings or play as a substitute for interview, particularly in the case of pre-school children. Do not read too much into these without confirmation from the child. The most useful types of observations are of the child's interactions with their siblings or parents. These are more likely to be natural if the child is relaxed as a result of being pleasurably occupied.

If you decide to conduct an interview, it is crucial to take into account how children's differences from adults are likely to affect the interview. First, *children think in a completely different way from adults*, and do not have the capacity for abstract conceptualisation that comes naturally to an adult professional. Instead, they are of necessity bound to the specific, concrete, and particular. Second, *they have little concept of therapeutic contracts and doctor–patient relationships*. Therefore they may well not understand why you are asking particular questions, or what types of answers they are supposed to supply.

For these reasons, it is necessary to support the child's attempts to communicate. Be friendly. Either sit down or position yourself at the same level as the child. It cannot be very encouraging for the child to have an adult towering over him and talking at him. Try to talk *with* rather than *at* the child, use simple words and ideas, check that the child understands your questions, exaggerate your facial expressions and tone of voice, and show an interest in his responses. Beware of teasing or jokes that may be misunderstood.

If you decide that it is necessary to see the child on their own, explain to their parent or parents that this is your normal practice and ask them to wait outside for a few minutes. Tell the child that you are going to have a private talk with them and that you are not going to give them any injections or ask them to undress. It is not usually necessary to go into details of confidentiality. Often it is wise to tell the child what you do and do not know, as children often assume that doctors already know all about their problem.

There are several things that can be done in an individual interview with a child. The fact that you are conducting such an interview at all indicates that you are taking the child seriously. The answers to questions may provide important information that could not be obtained in any other way.

An interview to discover facts that only the child knows

- Explain what you are going to ask about:
  'I want to know something about the pain in your tummy.'
  'Let's talk about what made you cross last time you had a temper.'
- Start with neutral topics in order to establish a conversation. You can then move on to more loaded topics later. If you sense that the child's anxiety or embarrassment is inhibiting him, move back to a more neutral topic.

- Ask very specific questions that do not require any generalisations:
'The very last time you took something that wasn't yours ... tell me when it was and what happened' is preferable to asking 'How often do you steal?'
'What is the name of your best friend?' is better than asking 'Do you have lots of friends?'

An interview to ascertain the child's emotional state

- Explain that you want to know something about the child's thoughts and feelings, and that you are going to ask questions about them.
- Start with a relatively neutral area. If this is school, ask the questions
'Which school do you go to? What year are you in? What's the name of your teacher?'
in order to set the scene. Then say 'Most children have things they like about school and things they don't like. What do you like about your school? What's your favourite subject? What are you best at? What things don't you like? Is there anyone you don't like?'
The idea is to allow the child to practise talking about their own responses and feelings.
- Give legitimacy to feelings by prefacing some questions with remarks such as
'Many children have ...' or 'A girl I once knew ...'. For instance, it might be appropriate to proceed as follows: 'A lot of children feel very cross with their brothers when they do some things, and feel very nice towards them when they do other things. What sort of things does your brother do? How do you feel about that?'
- Because most children of primary school age have rather poor vocabularies with which to describe their feelings and relationships, it may be appropriate to present questions in a multiple-choice format, in order to indicate to the child the range of possible responses expected and the words that might be used. For example, you could ask 'When your father left home and went away, I wonder how you felt?' Pause to see if a reply is forthcoming. 'You might have felt pleased or you might have felt sad. Some boys would have felt frightened or cross or had some different sort of feeling. How about you?' Note the use of the phrase 'some different sort of feeling' to cover the possibility of an unexpected emotional response. If some open choice such as this is not included, the child may feel that there are some thoughts and feelings that he is not allowed to express.

An interview to observe language, social or cognitive functioning.

- During the interview, clinical observations about the form rather than the content of the child's responses can provide information about language development, capacity to relate to adults, level of intelligence and, if a drawing or a piece of writing is requested, fine motor co-ordination.

Case study 1.2

A 7-year-old girl, Lucy, is brought to you by her mother. The school complains that she is very withdrawn in class, but her mother claims that there is very little wrong at home. The mother does not want a psychiatric referral. You ask the mother to leave you alone for ten minutes, and you then explain to Lucy that her mother says people at school are worried about her, and you want to know what she thinks. Initially she seems very shy, so you provide her with some felt-tip pens and paper, and you both sit on the floor. You ask her to draw the people who are at home, and she immediately tells you how much she misses her father, who left three months ago ...

Interviewing adolescents

Interviewing 12- to 18-year-olds can be achieved by means of conversation. However, there are various hurdles to bear in mind.

- *The adolescent is often brought to see you, rather than coming of his own accord.* This means that he may not know why he is seeing you, or he may be resentful about being brought. Engagement may be easier if you offer to see him on his own at an early stage, as soon as possible after the presenting problem has been described. Explain that you would like to hear how things are from his point of view, and ask the parents to wait outside. If he refuses to see you on his own, do not insist upon this, but leave it until later, or another occasion. If he agrees to see you on his own, ask him whose idea it was for him to come, in order to acknowledge if he is there under protest.
- An adolescent may assume that you know everything about him already, and *may not understand why you need to ask so many questions.* For this reason it may be worth explaining how discussing something may help you to understand it, and then you may have some ideas about what to do about it, or it may help just to talk about it.
- Whether or not you should promise *confidentiality* is something of a dilemma. The problem is that it is easy to think of areas for which you would have to break confidentiality, such as sexual abuse, and you do not really want to get involved in a long discussion of these at the beginning of the interview. One way out of this difficulty is to address it before you see the adolescent's parents again, by asking him what is acceptable to tell his parents, or whether there is anything he does not want them to know. If, at this stage, something emerges that you feel you have to tell social services, tell him you have to do this. It may not be his wish, but he needs to know before you go ahead.
- Most adolescents have *a limited capacity for abstract thought.* On the whole, they will not have the same facility for conceptual thought as a doctor would have had in his own adolescence. It is very easy to talk over their heads, and they are unlikely to understand metaphor or abstract generalisations, or the types of concepts that

doctors talk about all the time. It is wise to keep language simple, and to check that they understand what you mean (or will admit to you if they do not).

- Some adolescents respond by *clamming up* or providing a string of 'I don't know's'. In such cases, try changing tack and asking simple closed questions on neutral topics, such as the latest football scores, to re-establish the flow of conversation. You can then edge towards a hot topic or back away from it accordingly.

A useful conversation-starter is to *draw a family tree*. If you move your position so that you are sitting almost next to the adolescent, he is more likely to get involved in this approach. You can then ask with whom he gets on best, who is the kindest family member, who is the angriest, and so on.

Particularly when interviewing boys, who often seem to be more wary of authority than girls, you should try to keep the tone of your voice light. There is no point whatsoever in telling a teenager off; this will certainly already have been done. It is equally dangerous to ingratiate yourself, although it is usually appropriate to find some common external object of amusement. The aim is to make the adolescent feel that you understand his point of view, while still respecting that of his parents. However, this is not always possible.

Be careful about self-disclosure, which can easily sound patronising or irrelevant to a contemporary adolescent who may see little common ground between himself and you. The use of the phrase 'I remember when I was your age ...' is best avoided.

The interview will probably be easier if you do not make notes at the time. However, if you have to do this, it is probably best to make it clear what you are writing, either by allowing the notes to be read, or by explaining them. You can always add your own observations and any suspicions later. Some teenagers may otherwise be distracted from your questions by trying to read your notes upside down.

Interviewing families

This should be different from interviewing the parents in the presence of the child, in that the child or children present should be actively involved in the conversation. Parents often do not see the point of involving siblings of the affected child, but they can be a valuable source of new information.

Why bother?

The aims of a family interview are as follows:

- to assess the impact of the presenting problem on different family members
- to investigate the interactions between family members
- to clarify shared beliefs and attitudes
- to find out whether the problem is serving the family a useful function. For instance, a scapegoated child can be useful for every other family member in that this situation allows their behaviour to continue unchecked.

Techniques you can use

- Introduce yourself to each family member. Adopt a child-appropriate stance suitable for each child's age.
- Provide toys and drawing materials and tell small children that they can play with these. It is reasonable to ask children of five years or over to listen while playing. Most of them will do so.
- Bring the level of language down to that of the youngest children involved in the conversation.
- Ask who is worried about what, and who wants what to change. The '*miracle question*' can come in useful: 'If you woke up tomorrow morning and found everything was all right, how would things be different?'
- Find out what has worked, and what are the occasions when the problem has not been present. This can lead to ideas about what can be done to improve the situation.
- Ask questions that involve more than one family member. For instance, 'Who do you think is more worried about that, your mum or your dad?'.
- Construct a family tree using a child to help, particularly with parents' ages.
- Try to provide opportunities for everyone to talk. Address questions specifically to silent members.
- Try to maintain neutrality and not to take sides.
- Watch how small children's play or actions interlink with the topics under discussion. For instance, they may divert the conversation from a difficult subject – thus protecting their parents – by misbehaving or by asking to go to the toilet.
- If children disrupt the meeting, insist that the parents should quieten them. This provides very useful information about how effective the parents can be, and how well they work together.
- *Reframing* means describing things in a way that can alter attitudes. For instance, if the parents are describing how annoying a particular child is, you could point out what an expert he is at winding people up, or in the case of a child who is not responding to parental control, you might point out how helpful he is being in showing what the problem is like at home. The idea is to cast the situation in a more positive light, or to introduce a new perspective that may help the parents to adopt a new perspective.

Making sense of it

You should organise the information that you obtain into three areas:

- the here and now – this includes the current family structure, power balance, alliances, communication and emotional atmosphere
- the development of this family as a unit – this information may overlap with the developmental history
- important influences from previous generations.

If you achieve your aims, you should have a clearer understanding of the way in which family interactions and relationships maintain the problem, and how different family members view it.

Case study 1.3

A 12-year-old boy, Alex, has asthma, which is mild enough to be managed in primary care. Whenever he is wheezy in the morning, his mother keeps him away from school. At the insistence of the educational welfare officer, you have referred him to the local child psychiatry service, but the parents have been once and refuse to go back. In desperation, you persuade the whole family to come and see you. You try to explore how each family member reacts when Alex is wheezy, and what their anxieties are based upon. Towards the end of your first interview, it emerges that the mother's younger brother died of asthma, something that neither you nor the child psychiatrist were told before. Your impression is that the father always gives in to the mother, and that the mother always gives in to Alex ...

Reports from other sources

It is important to check with other members of the primary care team about their involvement with the case. Often a telephone call to the child's school may be necessary in order to clarify what it is the school is worried about, or any reports of bullying. In other situations, a telephone conversation with the child's social worker may be invaluable.

Box 1.4:   Practice points for assessment in child and adolescent mental health

Three aspects of the history worth considering:
- the history of the presenting complaint
- the developmental history
- the family history.

Three questions about the presenting symptom:
- why this symptom?
- why this family member?
- why now?

Alternatives to taking the history from the mother in the presence of the child:
- see the child or young person alone briefly
- see the parents together on a separate occasion
- see the parents and children together.

References

1   Williams R, Richardson G, Kurtz Z *et al.* (1995) The definition, epidemiology and nature of child and adolescent mental health problems and disorders. In: Health Advisory Service (ed.) *Child and Adolescent Mental Health Services: Together We Stand.* HMSO, London.

2   Garralda ME (1994) Primary care psychiatry. In: M Rutter, E Taylor and L Hersov (eds) *Child and Adolescent Psychiatry.* Blackwell Science, Oxford.

3   Bailey V, Graham P and Boniface D (1978) How much child psychiatry does a general practitioner do? *J R Coll Gen Pract.* **28**: 621–6.

4   Garralda ME and Bailey D (1986) Children with psychiatric disorders in primary care. *J Child Psychol Psychiatry.* **27**: 611–24.

5   Lask B and Fosson A (1989) *Childhood Illness: The Psychosomatic Approach.* John Wiley & Sons, Chichester.

6   Balint M (1968) *The Doctor, his Patient and the Illness.* Pitman, London.

CHAPTER TWO

Referral, consent and confidentiality

The pattern of services

Children's mental health needs, in the broadest sense, are met by a multitude of people – first, and most obviously, by their parents, other relatives and friends, but also by a variety of professionals, ranging from teachers and health visitors to child psychiatrists and child psychologists. This way of thinking is the basis for the Health Advisory Service Report *Together We Stand*,[1] which has provided the blueprint for much service development in child mental health in recent years. The report views the variety of children's mental health needs as being met initially by themselves, then by their parents, and then if necessary by professionals.

The traditional threefold division is into primary care, which refers to secondary or specialist care, which in turn refers to tertiary, even more specialist teaching hospital care. The authors of the report[2.1] instead proposed a fourfold division of the providers for children's mental health, which some have found confusing. The other confusing element is that the same professional may function at different tiers in different contexts. Between each tier there is a filter through which clients are referred. As a blueprint for organising services, this idea conceives of child mental health provision in a new light, recognising that child mental health needs are met not just by the health service, but also by many other services. Hence the move away from the 'general practitioner – district hospital – teaching hospital' model. This new way of thinking also suggests that children's mental health needs should be met at the lowest tier possible. The ideas presented in this book can be seen as part of this general trend.

Those ideas are summarised in Figure 2.1, which gives examples at each tier. *Tier 1* is the 'front line' of services, involving professionals who are not primarily child mental health workers but who nevertheless deal with many child mental health problems very effectively. *Tier 2* is defined as including any child mental health professional *when they are working in isolation*. The same individuals may also work in specialist teams, which are defined as *tier 3*, and usually cover only a limited geographical area. By contrast, *tier 4* consists of specialised services taking referrals from a large geographical area. Currently,

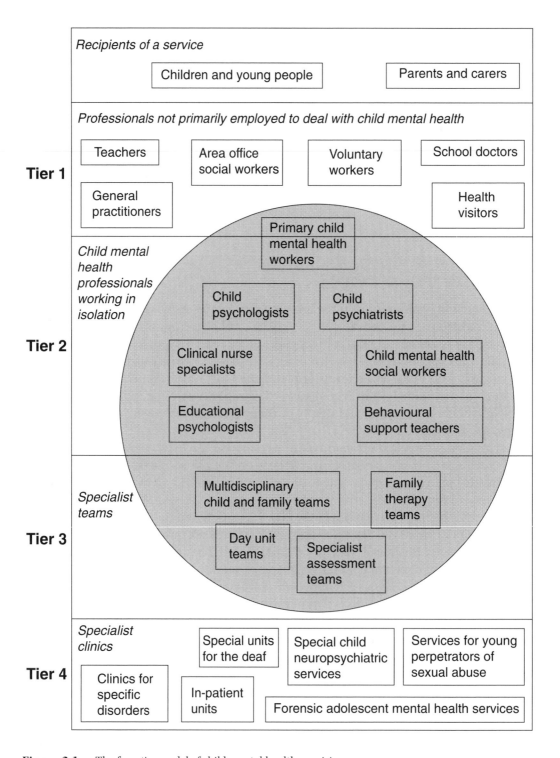

Figure 2.1:   The four-tier model of child mental health provision.

some district services are organised principally as tier 2 (different disciplines working separately), and some are organised principally as tier 3 (different disciplines working together in a multidisciplinary team).

The multidisciplinary team

A specialist child and adolescent mental health service, represented in Figure 2.1 by the oval shaded in grey, may include professionals who for part of the time work within a specialist team, and at other times work in isolation. For instance, a consultant child psychiatrist or child psychologist who conducts sessions alone in a health centre or community clinic is working in tier 2, but if she involves other members of a team in the care of a child, this then becomes a tier 3 service.

The idea behind multidisciplinary working dates back to the child guidance movement of the 1920s. Different specialties each have their own training, skills and background of experience. Originally, the teams might have consisted of a child psychiatrist, an educational psychologist, a psychiatric social worker and possibly a child psychotherapist. In recent decades, educational psychologists have been withdrawn from the teams to work solely in schools, and psychiatric social workers have been replaced by generic social workers, who are increasingly being withdrawn to local area Social Services teams. Contemporary teams therefore vary widely, but may include some or all of the following:

- someone with a basic medical training and specialist training in psychiatry as applied to young people (a child psychiatrist)
- someone with a psychology degree and subsequent clinical training (a clinical psychologist)
- someone with mental health nursing training and specialist training in child mental health nursing (a clinical nurse specialist)
- someone who supports families and highlights child protection issues (a psychiatric social worker)
- someone who treats families and adopts a systemic perspective (a family therapist)
- someone who treats children individually (a child psychotherapist, play therapist or art therapist).

There is no research evidence to prove that multidisciplinary working has a better outcome than unidisciplinary working, but clinical experience suggests that straightforward cases can be helped effectively by a skilled worker from almost any relevant background, whereas more complex cases require the input of more than one discipline.

Case study 2.1

Daniel, aged 8 years, was brought to his general practitioner by his parents, who told the doctor they were concerned that he was about to be expelled from school, apparently because of his persistent disruptive behaviour. Daniel's headteacher had told them that there was a long waiting-list to see the educational psychologist, and had suggested they should ask their doctor for a referral to the local child and family mental health service. Both the school and the parents wanted to know whether Daniel was hyperactive. The general practitioner observed that Daniel was apparently very restless, picking up and examining all of the items on the doctor's desk before moving over to the shelves and then turning the taps on in the sink. The doctor agreed to the referral, and also took the opportunity to discuss the family with the practice health visitor the next day.

Despite repeated requests for an urgent appointment, Daniel was not seen by the mental health service until after he had been permanently excluded from school. His parents came to see the general practitioner and reported that they had been seen by a social worker at the mental health service, who had asked a lot of questions about the family background that the parents thought were irrelevant. She had seen Daniel on his own and, after discussion with other team members at the clinic, had told his parents that she thought he ought to have full testing and medical assessment for possible hyperactivity disorder.

The general practitioner saw the family again two months later, at which time they reported that Daniel had been assessed by a clinical psychologist and found to be dyslexic, but of average intelligence. The child psychiatry assessment confirmed that he had attention-deficit hyperactivity disorder. The parents gave the general practitioner a letter from the child psychiatrist requesting that the general practitioner should prescribe methylphenidate. The general practitioner looked up the drug and discussed its effects and side-effects with the parents who, although dubious initially, agreed to give the treatment a try.

One week later, Daniel's mother came back to report a dramatic improvement in his behaviour during the day. He seemed calmer and more able to concentrate. A clinical nurse specialist had also visited the family and advised them about handling some of his behavioural difficulties at home.

At the start of the next school term Daniel was allowed to join another mainstream school nearby, and was provided with extra support for his literacy difficulties after a report had been sent to the school by the mental health service psychologist. The general practitioner continued to see Daniel on a monthly basis to review his methylphenidate prescription. Daniel's mother reported that, although his behaviour was still challenging at times, the class teacher had found it possible to control him, having attended a training course on the management of children with attention-deficit hyperactivity disorder.

This case illustrates that the difficulties experienced by some children cannot be regarded as purely behavioural, emotional or biological, but may have components of all three. Without the thorough assessment that was made possible by access to different professionals, Daniel's parents would have been assumed to be the source of his bad behaviour, or would at least have felt that they were.

Clinical responsibility

One of the difficulties in making multidisciplinary teams work is the potential for power struggles within them, and the diffusion of clinical responsibility. General practitioners prefer to be able to refer directly to a consultant, thus ensuring that they know who is taking over medico-legal responsibility for the patient. Most services accept this and acknowledge that the consultant will oversee those patients seen only by other members of the team. Each of the different professionals is supervised, so that clinical responsibility is either shared or passed up a chain. If a multidisciplinary team seems to be unclear as to who has ultimate responsibility for cases, then it behoves the referring primary care groups to demand clear lines of accountability.

The concept of the primary child mental health worker

To link the development of child mental health provision in tier 1 settings with existing tier 2 and tier 3 provision, the Health Advisory Service proposed the new job title of 'primary child mental health worker'. It was not intended that this would be a new discipline. On the contrary, professionals filling this role could include clinical nurse specialists, child psychologists and any other child mental health professionals with sufficient training to work as generalists in a primary care setting. Their role could include not only direct assessment and treatment, but also consultation and advising other members of the primary care team (thus building up skills within tier 1), and referral when necessary to the local tier 3 service.

This idea has been slower to catch on than the notion of tiered services as a whole, as it involves extra funding. However, some community trusts in the UK have developed this idea in various ways. The primary child mental health worker is a tier 2 worker functioning in a tier 1 setting. To ensure professional support and supervision, she should have close links with a local tier 3 service, and ideally work within a specialist team for part of the week. She would then be both part of the tier 1 team *and* part of the tier 3 team. Future developments may include the funding of such posts by primary care trusts.

Guidance for purchasers and providers

Child mental health is mainly a non-acute, out-patient service, and thus commands a smaller budget than many overlapping services such as adult psychiatry and acute paediatrics. Both purchasers and providers therefore tend not to focus on the development of child and adolescent mental health services, and children continue to be a disenfranchised group. More enlightened planners perceive that children may one day become adults, and that early intervention may reduce costs later on. They may need to be informed not only about the prevalence of children's mental health needs (which will be dealt with throughout the rest of this book), but also about desirable components of provision.

Box 2.1 shows some generally agreed characteristics of an effective tier 3 service. Most services will be able to develop only some aspects of this, and some services may be highly developed in some ways but not in others. Primary care groups may be in a position as purchasers to insist that providers use this as a blueprint.

Box 2.1:   Components of a good child and adolescent mental health service

1   An effective multidisciplinary team (tier 3):
   • this should include a variety of professionals
   • a range of assessment and treatment models should be available, and these should be chosen according to research findings on treatment outcome
   • team members should have the option of working separately or together on each case
   • clinical issues should be discussed in team meetings in order to enable the key worker to benefit from the experience and thinking of other team members.

2   A response to referrals that acknowledges the needs of the child or young person, the family and the referrer:
   • referrals should be accepted from a range of other professionals who deal with children
   • self-referrals by the young person or their family should be considered
   • referrals should be prioritised to enable urgent or needy cases to be seen before non-urgent cases
   • careful thought should be given to the nature of referrals, particularly in complex cases, to ensure that the most helpful response is made. In some cases, a different service may need to be involved in order to best meet the child's needs. Further discussion with the referrer may be needed before a decision is made.

3   Access to the service should be as convenient as possible, given the need to centralise resources:
   • outreach clinics (tier 2) should be held in as many community sites as possible
   • there should be close links between the tier 3 service and counselling within schools.

4   Some members of the team should also be primary child mental health workers, meaning that they function as tier 2 professionals within the primary care setting as well as tier 3 professionals within the multidisciplinary team. This enables closer collaboration with health visitors and general practitioners than is possible from a central site.

5   There should be close working relationships with other relevant services, such as primary care, Social Services, education, community paediatrics, hospital paediatrics, adult psychiatry and youth court services.

6   There should be an emergency on-call service to ensure a prompt response for young people who take overdoses or attempt suicide by other methods. Such a service needs to work in close co-operation with acute paediatric services and accident and emergency departments.

continued opposite

---

7   There should be an adolescent service for young people in the age range 15–19 years, and it should have the following components:
    • flexible access, such as self-referral, drop-in clinics and easy availability
    • clearly defined confidentiality for the young person
    • the possibility of day-patient care
    • the possibility of in-patient care.
8   There should be an established referral network to tier 4 (specialised) services.

How to make a referral

One common reason for a referral failing to achieve its objective is due to it being inadequately thought through. In each of the chapters in this book we try to consider the clinical reasons for opting to refer. However, there are other important considerations, too. In particular, does the child, young person or family (or someone else) *want* a referral? Do they have a clear idea of what this can and cannot achieve? For instance, if a parent merely wants the child to receive a good telling off, and the young person can see no value in the referral, then it will be difficult to engage them in any meaningful process of change.

It is an essential part of referring to a child and adolescent mental health service to ask the following questions.

• Who wants the referral?
• What do they want?
• Can the service provide them with something that they want?
• Does it matter if the service that they want is not provided?
• What should be included in the referral letter?

Who wants the referral?

If no one in the family wants the referral, then it is unlikely to achieve much. Could it be that someone else wants the referral? For instance, a class teacher or headteacher will often put pressure on a parent to ask the general practitioner for help from a child mental health service. Unless the parent can acknowledge that there is something *they* want to change (and not just the school), there is little point in making the referral. It may be necessary to contact the school in order to ask exactly what they would like the referral to achieve, or to ask the parent to renegotiate with the school a shared perception of the problem and what needs to be changed. You may have to put pressure on the school to make sure that the child is seen by an educational psychologist. Sending any available letters from the school will help. If the parents are articulate, it can be helpful to ask them to write a letter explaining what they would like to be achieved by the referral, and include this with your own referral letter.

Children often say that they dislike family meetings (i.e. meetings with a professional that involve several family members). This may be partly because professionals do not pay them enough attention.[2] It may also be due to their not being involved in decisions about referral. The older the child, the more important this issue becomes. Referring a teenager without some type of negotiation about the purpose of the referral is a sure recipe for an unproductive clinic visit.

What do they want?

The school may want the child to behave better. You may want the family to work on relationships that you know all too well are unsatisfactory. However, the parents may just want a different child. This mismatch of expectations can make it difficult for the family to make use of what most clinics have to offer. It is part of the referrer's job to clarify what different family members want, and to decide whether this is something that might be achieved by going to the clinic.

In some families, the child who is presented as having problems is *scapegoated*. Both parents seem to believe that this child is much more difficult than any of the other children in the family, and sometimes it seems to the professional that the child can do nothing right. The belief is often very difficult for anyone to shift. As mentioned earlier, positive ways of describing the situation, such as 'So he's very skilled at winding everyone up' may help a little. Sometimes the finding of an 'organic' problem in the child, such as a specific learning difficulty, dyspraxia or attention-deficit hyperactivity disorder, can dramatically transform the situation. The child then has an excuse for being so 'difficult', the parents feel believed, they are suddenly sympathetic to the child, and they join forces with the school in helping the child to overcome the identified difficulty. The implication of this is that looking for such a problem may be a good reason for referral, but not necessarily to a child and adolescent mental health service. An educational psychologist or paediatrician may be more appropriate, at least in the first instance.

Can the service provide them with something that they want?

There is tremendous variation in the availability and quality of child mental health services nationally. One specific area of variability is the provision (or lack of provision) of services for adolescents, whose needs are often lost in the gap between services for children and families and services for adults. Conceiving adolescence broadly, those in the age range 15–25 years require a flexible response to their needs, easy access to services, and workers who will listen, preferably in confidence and without asking intrusive questions.[3] A general practitioner may frequently be a key individual for such an adolescent,[4] but the voluntary sector often provides the best service. Voluntary agencies that meet the mental health and counselling needs of adolescents may be viewed as entirely separate to family services, and may offer drop-in clinics, evening access and

24-hour helplines. However, because of funding difficulties, geographical coverage is patchy and serendipitous, with no central planning.

It is important to be familiar with your local service. What is the range of services provided? How are these delivered? What are the strengths and weaknesses of any local clinics? For example, there is little point in sending parents who can see no reason for talking about a problem to a clinic where the main therapeutic options are exclusively psychological. Giving family members clear expectations of what is likely to happen during the clinic visit will help to adjust their expectations and thus increase the likelihood of a successful therapeutic engagement.

Does it matter if the service that they want is not provided?

This is a matter of clinical judgement. If there is no service available to see a suicidally depressed teenager, then this clearly matters, whereas if there is no service for a five-year-old with nocturnal enuresis or a six-year-old with a behavioural feeding problem and normal growth, then this may not matter very much. These problems can generally be managed in primary care in any case. The parent may feel that specialist input is necessary, but you can explain the reasons why the condition would not be regarded as a priority. (In the case of enuresis, the condition improves with time, whereas food fads are unlikely to improve until the child is old enough to want to eat a more varied diet.) If, as a referrer, you feel that it is essential to obtain a service for your patient, then you may have to refer to alternative services, or lobby your purchasing organisation to insist that adequate services are provided.

Box 2.2:   What should be included in the referral letter?

Essential: a clear description of the problem, who wants it to change, and how the decision to involve the clinic was made; background information needed to understand the problem.

Optional: other background information (e.g. family composition and structure, developmental history, school performance, medical history, medication, and past involvement with child mental health).

The waiting-list

Some tier 2 and tier 3 services operate without a waiting-list, while others impose a long waiting time for non-urgent cases between referral and the first appointment. It is simplistic to assume that waiting times depend on the ratio between referrals received and staff available. Many other factors are involved, including the productivity of staff, the models of treatment used, the average length of treatment, and the way in which the waiting-list is managed administratively. For instance, an opt-in appointment system can reduce the number of appointment slots wasted by non-attendance, and brief therapy may speed up turnover.[5] Some services are selective about which categories of referral they will take, while others pass on a proportion of referrals to other services.

In a resource-limited environment it is not usually possible to guarantee an immediate service for everyone, and priorities need to be set. If you are dissatisfied with the service that your clients are receiving, then your primary care group should be negotiating with your provider to make improvements based on mutually agreed priorities.

The thorny problem of consent

The issue of consent is complex and is not always easy to unravel. Culturally, children are accorded a low priority in UK society. They tend not to be included in making decisions that affect their lives, and they may not be given developmentally appropriate information about issues that concern them, such as the death of a close relative, or their own illness. For a child to give informed consent to referral, assessment or treatment, the information that is given needs to be adapted to the child's cognitive level and emotional maturity.

Historically, children have been given increasing rights by legislation within recent decades, including the UK government's adoption of the United Nations Convention on the Rights of the Child.[6] This emphasises the following:

*   the need to put the child's best interests first
*   children's right to be heard
*   that children deprived of a family environment are entitled to special protection from the State
*   that the State has an obligation to prevent all forms of abuse
*   that disabled children have the right to special treatment, education and care.

The so-called 'Gillick principle' evolved out of a dispute between a mother and her daughter about whether a girl under 16 years of age could be prescribed the oral contraceptive pill without her parents' knowledge or consent. The legal dispute ascended to the House of Lords, who found in the daughter's favour.

The *Gillick principle* is defined as follows:

A person under the age of 16 years shall have legal capacity to consent to any surgical, medical or dental procedure or treatment where, in the opinion of a qualified medical practitioner attending him, he is capable of understanding the nature and possible consequences of the procedure or treatment.

The principle was subsequently enshrined in a much larger body of law, namely the Children Act, 1989. There it is effectively summed up in the phrase 'sufficient age and understanding'.

In practical terms, a girl under 16 years of age who comes to a health centre asking for contraception can be given it without her parents' knowledge or consent. There are four preconditions for this:[7]

- that the girl will understand the contraceptive advice
- that the general practitioner cannot persuade her to inform her parents or allow him to inform her parents
- that she is very likely to begin or continue having sexual intercourse with or without contraceptive treatment
- that unless she receives contraceptive treatment, her physical or mental health or both are likely to suffer *or* that her best interests require contraceptive treatment.

As 20% of teenage girls have had full sexual intercourse before their sixteenth birthday,[8] and may use unsatisfactory methods of contraception (if any), such as condoms or the morning-after pill,[9] these four criteria are frequently met. A survey of 1500 secondary school pupils aged 13–18 years revealed self-reported vaginal intercourse in 12% of 13-year-olds, 17% of 14-year-olds and 28% of 15-year-olds, and oral sex in 8%, 10% and 14%, respectively. Younger teenagers were less likely to use contraception than older teenagers.[8]

There is a high rate of teenage pregnancy in the UK, and clinical practice suggests that teenagers feel uncomfortable about asking for contraception from their family doctor, whom they regard as allied to their parents. Not being aware of the Gillick principle, they suspect that their parents will be told. (For such teenagers, family planning clinics would be preferable, but many young people are not familiar with these, or find them difficult to access.)

The same *general principles* apply to any form of assessment or treatment. The young person has the right to consent on their own behalf, if they are of sufficient age and understanding in relation to the issues involved. It is important to emphasise that competence in the Gillick sense is specific to the matter in question. For instance, a nine-year-old whose parents have separated and entered into a legal battle over custody and access may be competent to express his wishes as to whether or not he wants to see his father (and he is entitled to his own free legal representation to negotiate this), whereas a 15-year-old may need help in deciding whether to consent to a limb amputation for osteosarcoma. If the consent of the young person in isolation is needed, then the above four conditions should be appropriately modified. In most cases, it is sufficient to explain the procedure to the young person and their parents, and to obtain consent from at least one person with parental responsibility (*see* next section).

Emergency medical treatment can be performed without consent. Emergency psychiatric treatment for life-threatening mental illness can be sanctioned if necessary by invoking the Mental Health Act (for which there is no minimum age). The capacity to understand may be significantly impaired by mental illness, so that the young person may not be Gillick competent. (In practice, enforcing the wishes of the parents of a young person under 16 years of age may obviate use of the Mental Health Act).

In non-urgent cases, it is wise to allow time for children and their families to think things through, once they have been given (and have absorbed) sufficient information. It may be helpful for the parents to obtain advice from others, such as neighbours, friends or grandparents, and for the child to talk to friends and teachers. It is here that the relationship between the doctor and individual family members is crucial, as is the relationship between the child and his parents. Does the child have as much trust in the doctor as the parents do? Is the child still guided by the parents, or has his general opposition to his parents' wishes contributed to any difficulties in obtaining consent?

Legally, the consent of someone with parental responsibility can authorise procedures that a competent child has refused, except in Scotland.[10] In contrast, the Children Act states that young people whose medical or psychiatric assessment is ordered by the court as part of child protection proceedings may withhold consent provided that they are of sufficient age or understanding.[11] By way of resolving these two apparently contradictory pieces of legislation, the courts have become used to overriding the refusal of medical or psychiatric intervention by a young person when the indications are sufficiently clear.[12]

In practice, it is very difficult to conduct more than a partial psychiatric assessment without a young person's consent, so every effort should be made to obtain this as well as parental consent. If a young person (of sufficient age and understanding) cannot agree to a referral to an adolescent mental health service, then this referral should not be made, unless the sole aim is to assess the parents' point of view and to provide them with professional support.

Parental responsibility

This is a term that was introduced by the Children Act 1989. It is defined as 'all the rights, duties, powers, responsibilities and authority that by law the parent of a child has in relation to the child and his property'. The child's mother automatically has parental responsibility, and she can only lose this if the child is adopted or freed for adoption. The child's father only has this responsibility if married to the child's mother at the time of birth. Otherwise, he can obtain it either by making a parental responsibility agreement with the mother, or by applying to a court. Anyone who is given a residence order by the court (often a grandparent or other family member) automatically obtains parental responsibility. A legally appointed guardian also assumes parental responsibility. For a child on a care order or interim care order, parental responsibility lies with Social Services, and is exercised by the allocated social worker.

The relevance of this is that if parental consent (to referral, assessment or treatment) is necessary, this must be given by someone with parental responsibility. Only one consent is necessary. If the child is accommodated (i.e. lodged with an adult, or in a children's home, by agreement between a parent and Social Services), then consent from the foster-carer or relative with whom the child is living is *not* sufficient. The natural parent's consent must be obtained before a referral is made. If the child is on a care order (or an interim care order), then the consent of the social worker should be obtained.

Dilemmas

What is the youngest age at which it is ethical to treat a child without informing the parents? This hinges on whether the professional judges the child to have sufficient age and understanding. To take an extreme case, most practitioners would probably consider that a sexual relationship between an 11-year-old girl and a 17-year-old boy would justify a breach of confidentiality (informing the parents and possibly Social Services). However, if a physically and emotionally mature 13-year-old girl was in a relationship with a 15-year-old boy, there would be scope for differences of opinion.

The same issues apply to referral to a mental health service. It is generally accepted that 18-year-olds can be referred and seen without any reference to their parents, unless they have severe mental illness or learning difficulties. For those between 16 and 18 years of age, parental consent is not required, but it is preferable. For those under 16 years, parental consent is usually required, but can be dispensed with if there is good reason (e.g. abuse, or relationship difficulties with the parents). The young person must be of sufficient age and understanding to give consent herself.

It is essential that the referral letter makes it clear whether the parents are aware of the referral, and if the young person does *not* want her parents to be informed. It may be necessary to give an alternative address or contact telephone number (e.g. at school) in order to avoid the parents inadvertently seeing the appointment letter.

Informing parents

If the parents are to be informed, there is room for debate about *who* should be informed. In general, it should be the parent with whom the young person is living. However, if this is a foster parent or a relative, then she may not have parental responsibility. Moreover, absent fathers (and mothers) sometimes object, after the event, to a child being referred without their knowledge. There can be no firm guidelines about this – whether the absent parent needs to be informed depends on their degree of involvement – but it would be prudent for referrers always to enquire who has parental responsibility, and whether the absent parent needs to know about the referral before it takes place. If it is clear that they do not know, then this should be stated in the referral letter.

Conclusions

Consent to being seen in a child and adolescent mental health service is not as straightforward as it might appear. It is important for the referrer to get things started on the right footing, otherwise the clinic may encounter problems later and be subject to justified complaints (e.g. as a result of unwittingly seeing a child without parental consent).

Children and young people should be kept as fully informed as possible, and should be involved as much as their cognitive and emotional maturity will allow, in accordance with the United Nations Convention on the Rights of The Child.[13] It is no longer acceptable for healthcare professionals to leave it up to parents to tell their child what they think the child needs to know. Such information is often woefully inadequate, and the parents may need advice on how to explain things.

Box 2.3:   Check-list for a child's consent to referral, assessment or treatment[14]

1   What is the child's level of understanding:
    • about the problems discussed with the parents?
    • about what the proposed intervention involves?
2   Is the child generally likely to agree with parental wishes?
3   Does the child trust the general practitioner or regard him as an ally of the parents?
4   Whose opinion might influence the child (friends, teachers, grandparents ...) and how?
5   What is the risk/benefit balance for intervention or non-intervention?
6   Is the young person's problem potentially life-threatening?
7   Is the young person mentally ill?

Case study 2.2

A mother comes without her 15-year-old son to complain that he is on the verge of expulsion from school for aggressive behaviour. He is also truanting. She cannot manage him at home, and he is not coming home on time. Systematic questioning reveals no evidence of a mood disorder. The general practitioner asks her to try to get him to come for an appointment. The mother returns in three weeks to say that he has refused to come. Again there is nothing to suggest mental illness, although there are suspicions of social drug use. The general practitioner explains that there is nothing he can do to help the boy. If he is expelled from school, the mother will need to discuss with the education department how he is to be educated.

Case study 2.3

A mother brings her 15-year-old daughter to the general practitioner, complaining that she has been eating less and less over the last six months. Plotting height and weight on a growth chart shows a height on the 75th centile and a weight on the 9th centile. Although no previous weights are immediately available, this shows that the girl's weight is 75% of its expected value for her age and height (*see* Chapter 35 on eating disorders). The girl says that she sees nothing wrong with dieting, and simply wants to be as thin as her friends. She thinks that she is still too fat. She turns down the suggestion of referral to an adolescent psychiatrist, and her mother acquiesces to this. The general practitioner arranges to see the mother on her own the following week. He persuades her to agree to the appointment, even though her daughter will resist going, and he discusses ways in which the daughter could be persuaded to go. He stresses the medical severity of the daughter's probable anorexia nervosa, and its life-threatening potential. He mentions the possible use of the Mental Health Act if weight loss continues, but explains that it should normally be possible to avoid this approach. Eventually it is agreed that the general practitioner will request an urgent appointment, and the mother will persuade the girl's father to take time off work, and ensure that the girl goes, too.

It is not difficult to think of cases intermediate between these two extremes, for which the answers might be less clear-cut.

Confidentiality

The legal position with regard to confidentiality is much clearer than that for the mine-field of consent.[15] Guidance with regard to good practice is also more generally agreed upon.

The general practitioner owes a *duty of confidentiality* to all of his patients. Although in principle young people should be informed of this, they are unlikely to believe it until they have tested it out (e.g. by admitting that they have used street drugs or had sexual intercourse about which they don't wish their parents to know) and it is difficult to give a concise explanation in practice. Not only is there an obvious time constraint, but it would be dangerous on the one hand to promise unconditional confidentiality, and on the other to go into detail about what circumstances would prompt a breach of confidentiality. A reassuring comment such as 'I won't need to tell anyone else what you say unless I think someone could come to harm' is a possibility, but is still not entirely satisfactory.

The main indication for breaching confidentiality is the *disclosure of abuse*. If a child discloses to any professional that they have been abused – physically, emotionally or sexually – then it is the professional's duty to inform a statutory agency (Social Services, the National Society for the Prevention of Cruelty to Children or the police). However, there is no legal obligation to do this. In the USA, failure to report abuse can result in a charge of professional misconduct by the relevant professional regulatory agency. In the UK, it is merely government guidance to work closely with other agencies for the protection of children;[16] there are no sanctions for not doing so. The Children Act makes it clear that health professionals have a duty to assist Social Services in carrying out their investigations,[17] except in circumstances where 'not doing so would be unreasonable in all the circumstances of the case'. In practice, it may be more difficult for a general practitioner to breach confidentiality than for a specialist to do so, because of the loyalty he feels towards the family as a whole, and the need to maintain working relationships with them.

The need to breach confidentiality raises the following issues (also *see* Chapter 11 on child abuse):

- *The child's interests are paramount.* This is a central tenet of the Children Act. If a child is being abused, it is in their interests for this abuse to stop. This consideration overrides any scruples about the emotional needs of the parents. It may be difficult for a general practitioner who has got to know a parent much better than her child to put her feelings second to those of her child, but this has to be done. If there is any reason to believe that other children may be suffering abuse, then the interests of all the children need to be considered.

- *The risk of abuse must reach a certain threshold.* This is encompassed by the phrase '*significant harm*'. The implication of these two words is that the level of harm justifies intervention. To justify a breach of confidentiality, a child must either have experienced significant harm, be currently suffering from ongoing significant harm, or be at risk of significant harm in the future. If the risk is in the present or future, this clearly gives more urgency to the need to involve agencies that can prevent further harm from occurring. Even if the reported risk is only a past one, other children may still be at risk from the alleged perpetrator(s) of the abuse.

- *What should you say to the child?* It is good practice to inform the child of what you will be saying to other people before you do so. Otherwise you run the risk of losing not only the child's confidence in yourself, but also their trust in other professionals. This means that if you decide you need to break confidentiality after the end of an appointment, you will need to see the child again before informing another agency (preferably not on a Friday afternoon!). Attempts should be made to obtain the child's consent to any breach of confidentiality. In the absence of this, you can explain that you *have to inform agencies*, because of your professional duty to children in general, as well as to that child in particular. Most children seem to accept this. You should explain the consequences of your telling other professionals – it is amazing how much emotional trauma children can withstand if they are prepared for it. One common concern of abused children is the consequence of threats made by the perpetrator. It may be necessary to discuss how the child can be kept safe at the same time as you discuss the consequences of involving other agencies.

- *Is the child's consent necessary for you to breach confidentiality?* It is clear that, for younger children, their consent is not necessary. For young people over the age of

16 years, it is generally accepted that their consent is necessary if the risk is only to them and is not life-threatening. Allegations of extreme violence or ongoing sexual abuse of a younger child would justify informing agencies without the young person's consent, although most young people over the age of 16 years could be persuaded to give their consent in these circumstances, once they have reached the stage of disclosing. Others will only disclose a small step at a time, and need to rehearse the consequences of disclosure before doing so. For these children, knowing that Social Services and the police do not have to be informed may help them to come to terms with disclosure. What about children below the age of 16 years? Can they be considered to have sufficient understanding of the issues involved to withhold consent to their allegations of abuse being shared? This judgement has to be made by the professional who is seeing the child, and they must weigh the best interests of the young person against her wishes. Where there is a conflict between the two, the young person's best interests may be more important, and this may justify acting without her consent.

- *Should the parents be informed?* In general it would be advisable for general practitioners to keep the parents informed in advance of a notification to Social Services, in order to preserve the trusting relationship which it may have taken many years to establish. There are two provisos to this. First, if possible the child should give consent to her parents being informed. Since they will have to be told by Social Services in any case, and you should be warning the child of this, it is not usually a problem. Secondly (and this gives rise to more differences of opinion), Social Services departments and the police often prefer that the parents are not told in advance. Social Services will be concerned that the child may come to harm before they can intervene. This is a real risk in cases of physical abuse, particularly impulsive violence, and it most commonly involves children under 5 years of age. The police will be concerned that, if they are given advance warning, the parents may tamper with evidence, agree upon a common false story, or make threats to the child in order to force her to retract her story. This is also a real concern. It is in the child's interests for the full story to emerge and for justice to be done, although many children do not want their parents to be punished by the police, but just want the abuse to stop. It is up to the general practitioner, using his knowledge of the family, to decide where the priorities lie. It is not necessary to do everything that the police and Social Services want, although obviously professional relationships will be improved if you do so.

Requests to see notes

Another common circumstance in which confidentiality comes into question is a request to see notes. This can arise from a number of different sources.

- *The police.* There is no duty to disclose to the police that a child (or adult) has committed a criminal offence. If a child discloses such an offence, this should be kept confidential (unless it is the type of offence that puts other children at risk, such as perpetration of sexual abuse). Health records are protected from seizure by the police, and can only be obtained by specific order from a judge – a power that is rarely used.

- *Social Services* rely on the co-operation of other services to fulfil their role in child protection. For instance, child protection case conferences cannot function if important information is withheld from them. Background knowledge of parents may be essential to investigations of child abuse, particularly emotional abuse or Munchausen by proxy. In such circumstances, it may not be appropriate to ask for consent from the parents first. Confidential information relating to the child should only be released if it directly relates to the child protection issue under investigation. As before, prior consent from the child, particularly if they are Gillick-competent, is preferable.

- *Employers* may request confidential information about a young person who is applying for a job. No confidential information should be disclosed without the express consent of the young person concerned.

- *Parents* may request to see their child's records, but they cannot do so without their child's consent if the child was Gillick-competent at the time when the records were made. Even if the child was not Gillick-competent, their consent is still advisable if they are Gillick-competent at the time of the request.

- *Young people themselves* may wish to look at their own records. In general, the record-holder has to accede to this request, provided that the young person understands what they are asking. Some young people may need help to understand what is written in the notes. Parts of the notes that apply to third parties are confidential in relation to them, and should be excluded unless those parties have given consent. There are two other caveats. First, the notes need not be shown if the record-holder considers that this will adversely affect the young person's emotional condition or mental health. Secondly, documents in a health record that originate from other agencies should not be shown without the consent of those agencies. For instance, a case conference report in a health record should only be shown if Social Services have given consent, and a teacher's report should only be revealed if the teacher or the school gives consent to this. Although all of these considerations may involve considerable effort, it can be very beneficial for a young person to see what professionals have written about them, and how concerned they have been – this may lead to greater understanding and insight.

Box 2.4:   Check-list for confidentiality

Who needs to know the information?
Is it in the child's best interests for them to know this information?
Whose consent is required?
Do the parents need to be informed?
Is there a conflict between the child's interests and wishes?
Is there a conflict between the child's interests and the parents' wishes?

Case study 2.4

Tina, a 12-year-old girl, attended the doctor's Monday morning surgery as an extra at the end of his list, together with a school-friend of the same age. She asked the doctor for the morning-after pill, and on enquiry revealed that an 18-year-old boy had forced her to have sexual intercourse in the local park late on Saturday night. She had been drunk at the time and powerless to resist. She had suffered some bruising of her arms and legs.

The doctor agreed to prescribe the pill and explained carefully how to take it. He then telephoned the girl's mother to ask her to come down to the surgery, explaining to the girl that he was obliged to involve the police in a case of rape. The doctor saw the mother together with Tina and advised them gently that a medical examination by a police doctor would be required, but that this would need both Tina's consent and the consent of her mother.

One week later the girl's mother came to see the doctor to disclose that Tina had told her mother that she had witnessed her father sexually abusing her half-sister on several occasions when they had shared a bedroom at her father's house three years previously. She had pretended to be asleep and had told nobody about this until after the incident in which she had been raped. The doctor agreed to report the incident to Social Services and the police, on the mother's behalf.

Two weeks later, the doctor received a note from the girl's mother informing him that Tina's father and half-sister had both denied the allegations against them, so no further action could be taken. When the alleged rape came to court six months later, the young man pleaded guilty to unlawful sexual intercourse, but claimed that the girl had consented. He was cleared of rape, apparently on the grounds that the girl should not have allowed herself to get drunk.

Notes

2.1   The authors included Peter Hill, Richard Williams, Zarina Kurtz, Peter Wilson and William Parry-Jones.

References

1   Health Advisory Service (1995) *Together We Stand: the Commissioning, Role and Management of Child and Adolescent Mental Health Services*. HMSO, London.

2   Spender Q (1998) Clinical audit of outcomes in out-patient child psychiatry using problem rating scales. In: E Hardman and C Joughin (eds) *Focus on Clinical Audit in Child and Adolescent Mental Health Services*. Royal College of Psychiatrists, London.

3   The Mental Health Foundation (1999) *Bright Futures*. The Mental Health Foundation, London.

4   Jacobson LD and Wilkinson CE (1994) Review of teenage health: time for a new direction. *Br J Gen Pract*. **44**: 420–4.

5   Stallard P and Sayers J (1998) An opt-in appointment system and brief therapy: perspectives on a waiting-list initiative. *Clin Child Psychol Psychiatry.* **3**: 199–212.

6   United Nations General Assembly (1989) *The United Nations Convention on the Rights of the Child*; http://www.unicef.org/crc/conven.htm

7   White R, Williams R, Harbour A and Bingley W (1996) *Safeguards for Young Minds: Young People and Protective Legislation.* Royal College of Psychiatrists and the Health Advisory Service, London.

8   Burack R (1999) Teenage sexual behaviour: attitudes towards and declared sexual activity. *Br J Fam Plan.* **24**: 145–8.

9   Kosunen E, Vikat A, Rimpelä M, Rimpelä A and Huhtala H (1999) Questionnaire study of the use of emergency contraception amongst teenagers. *BMJ.* **319**: 91.

10   General Medical Council (1999) Seeking patients' consent: the ethical considerations. General Medical Council, London.

11   White R, Williams R, Harbour A and Bingley W (1996) *Safeguards for Young Minds: Young People and Protective Legislation.* Royal College of Psychiatrists and the Health Advisory Service, London.

12   Bailey S and Harbour A (1999) The law and a child's consent to treatment. *Child Psychol Psychiatry Rev.* **4**: 30–5.

13   Bulford R (1997) Personal view: children have rights, too. *BMJ.* **314**: 1421–2.

14   Pearce J (1994) Consent to treatment during childhood. *Br J Psychiatry.* **165**: 713–16.

15   Hamilton C and Hopegood L (1998) *Offering Children Confidentiality: Law and Guidance.* Children's Legal Centre, University of Essex.

16   Department of Health (1995) *Child Protection: Medical Responsibilities.* HMSO, London.

17   *Children Act 1989.* Section 47(9)–(11).

CHAPTER THREE

Cultural and ethnic issues

Sangeeta Patel

Introduction

'Cultural and ethnic issues' have been a source of concern among health workers, who may assume that the categories which they use are neutral, but then find themselves having to deal with a negative response from clients or patients. This is because 'culture' and 'ethnicity' are also part of a complex social discourse linked with notions of agency, power, discrimination and oppression.

Such discourse contributes to the collective consciousness, affecting the interactions between health workers and their clients or patients. This is particularly pertinent in child psychiatry, where patients' perspectives are key factors in assessment, and enlisting family support is vital in treatment. This chapter, by focusing on the interpretations of a consultation in general practice, aims to outline some of the issues that make this a potentially sensitive arena for health workers.

Case study 3.1

Scene: A doctor's consulting-room. The doctor, a smart man in his forties, stands up, checks the time, leaves and returns followed by a dark woman in her twenties wearing a sari and carrying an infant.
Doctor: Come in, Mrs Patel, have a seat.
The woman sits down, and she then stands the infant on the floor. He wanders towards the box of toys.
Mrs Patel: Hello doctor, how are you?
Doctor: I am fine, and you?
Mrs Patel: Fine, and your family?

continued overleaf

Doctor: (*hurried*) Fine – what can I do for you?
Mrs Patel: (*agitated*) Doctor, it is Sunil; he's not well. He's crying, crying, crying for the whole night. He's scratching, scratching; his skin is all red ... and bleeding even! And so much sweating – he gets so hot. I give yoghurt and rice and he just vomits, then starts coughing, coughing, coughing – he can't sleep. One minute too hot, sweating, scratching, then next minute too cold, shivering, coughing. The whole family has no sleep, and is exhausted. (*She wipes away tears*) I gave Calpol, it works for an hour only. The Indian doctor, in Leicester, gave me very good treatment for everyone – made diarrhoea – but I can't go to see him. Can you give anything? The yellow medicine, Amoxil? It is very good. Gives diarrhoea. It helps the fever and cough, so we can all sleep.[3.1]

This scene can be used to demonstrate the different ways in which both doctor and patient made sense of this scenario. For each of them, the words signify aspects of different socially constructed paradigms. The emphasis in this chapter is upon biomedical paradigms as they apply to everyday interactions between health workers and *other* 'cultural and ethnic' groups, from the perspective of two questions that face health workers, namely: 'What is *really* going on?' and 'How can I deal with this?'.

What is 'really' going on? The general practitioner's interpretation

The patient's 'otherness'

Scene: A doctor's consulting-room. The doctor, a smart man in his forties, stands up, checks the **time**, *leaves and returns followed by a* **dark woman** *in her* **twenties** *wearing a* **sari** *and carrying an* **infant**.

Before this patient has even spoken, the general practitioner has registered various features, here highlighted in bold type. He is aware of the time and of the constraint it imposes on making his assessment. The fact that the patient is dark, young and dressed in a sari has a significance to him that will depend upon his own experience and knowledge of the cultural and ethnic groups that these characteristics represent. Each general practitioner's experience and knowledge will be different, although all will have been influenced by longstanding assumptions of the European collective consciousness. These include the belief that people whose appearance or behaviour suggests that their origins are not in the European middle or upper classes are in some way culturally or intellectually inferior.[3.2] Thus although this general practitioner may have considered himself to have been completely neutral and objective, this could not be so in reality. The process of becoming a biomedical doctor emphasises classification based on physical characteristics and morbidity, so that 'ethnic minority' status is considered to be a risk factor for morbidity. In this scenario, unless the doctor's personal experience has suggested otherwise, a 'dark woman in her twenties wearing a sari' may thus evoke an image of someone ignorant of (and possibly resistant to) health issues, particularly psychological health. Hence this general practitioner was already primed to notice characteristics that would support that viewpoint.

The mother's understanding of the child's illness

> *The woman sits down, and she then stands the infant on the floor. He* **wanders** *towards the box of toys.*

When the general practitioner sees that the infant is capable of wandering off he may be more sceptical of the mother's descriptions of the severity of his illness. When he then perceives that she is not getting to the point (*his* point),[3.3] he may adopt a firmer approach that is focused more on clinical features.

> *Mrs Patel:* (**agitated**) Doctor, it is Sunil; he's not well. He's crying, crying, crying for the whole night. He's **scratching**, scratching; his skin is all red ... and bleeding even! And so much sweating – he gets so **hot**. I give yoghurt and rice and he just **vomits**, then starts **coughing**, coughing, coughing – he can't sleep. One minute **too hot**, sweating, scratching, then next minute **too cold**, shivering, coughing. The whole family has no sleep, and is exhausted. (*She wipes away* **tears**) I gave **Calpol, it works** for an hour only. The **Indian doctor**, in Leicester, gave me very good treatment for everyone – made **diarrhoea** – but I can't go to see him. Can you give anything? The yellow medicine, **Amoxil?** It is very good. **Gives diarrhoea**. It helps the fever and cough, so we can all sleep.

The general practitioner's priority would be to distil out those features that indicate disease. For him, 'scratching' suggests eczema, particularly when he is 'coughing, coughing', which may indicate asthma, and the two are often associated. 'Too hot' and 'too cold' suggests a swinging pyrexia characteristic of an infection, but perhaps one that is not too serious because 'Calpol, it works'. The 'Indian doctor' can again evoke a whole range of images, depending upon this general practitioner's previous experience, but again the notions of 'otherness' and 'inferiority' in the European collective consciousness may prime the general practitioner to be suspicious of that doctor's knowledge, integrity or orthodoxy (in biomedicine). 'Amoxil' currently strikes a chord with general practitioners, who are under pressure from the government to resist prescribing antibiotics for viral illnesses. For this general practitioner the fact that Amoxil 'gives diarrhoea' would be viewed as a 'side-effect' to consider as a further reason not to give antibiotics. It may also lead the general practitioner to question whether the mother is indeed giving the child's health priority over her own (implied in 'so we can all sleep'), or he may view the situation more sympathetically, particularly in conjunction with her 'tears' as a symptom of her desperation, or possible depression.

This reductionist process is fundamental to the biomedical model, which relies upon this general practitioner's expertise to enable him to 'see through' Mrs Patel's interpretations as if to 'uncover' the real disease, whether it be biological or psychological. The process is made meaningful to the doctor by his knowledge of the biomedical system, underpinned by the assumption that diseases exist as separate entities (in this case eczema, asthma and infection) found in individual bodies – as separate uniform physical beings – producing characteristic symptoms and signs. For the doctor, the other information that this mother provides is at best irrelevant and at worst troublesome. The general practitioner's role is made easier if his patients share this conception and present their symptoms bearing this in mind. However, patients with different cultural backgrounds may present their symptoms with a different conception of health. For the doctor, that cultural background may feel like an impediment to his diagnostic process.

However, he may still take note of some of the mother's interpretations. Those interpretations are important in helping him to make an assessment of the patient's mental state, to decide whether (and when) to explore it further, and to help him to negotiate a management plan. This process seems logical to both the doctor and the reader because it is based on the socially constructed view of the patient's body as an 'object' and on the categorical distinction between 'normal' and 'abnormal'. These categories overlap with 'healthy'/'unhealthy', and less directly with 'body'/'mind' and 'physical'/'mental' dichotomies that have become commonplace in the European collective consciousness.[3,4] Imposing these dichotomies on the patient's body thus involves moral connotations – 'normal', 'healthy' and 'physical disease' do not have the same associations of inferiority and lack of capability as 'abnormal', 'unhealthy' and 'mental illness'.

In this scenario, if the general practitioner has been primed by his presuppositions to question Mrs Patel's ability to make a rational judgement, he may try to make sense of her distress about an infant who appears to be well, by assuming that it is the mother who is either 'abnormal' or 'unhealthy' – a 'somatiser' (by proxy in this case) or depressed. To a middle-class European, this general practitioner's train of thought makes perfect sense, as the biomedical viewpoint itself is based on European cultural assumptions. However, Mrs Patel did not share those assumptions. For *her*, the doctor's interpretation did *not* make sense.

What is *really* going on? The mother's interpretation

Mrs Patel entered this scenario with a different history. I shall now illustrate some of the features that made the doctor's interpretation seem so alien to her.

> *Scene*: *A **doctor's consulting-room**. The doctor, a **smart man** in his **forties**, stands up, **checks the time**, leaves and returns followed by a dark woman in her twenties wearing a sari and carrying an infant.*

For Mrs Patel, the doctor is a professional man with knowledge and expertise, and this is demonstrated by his surroundings, his age and his appearance. However, her recent experience had not born this out. Shortly after she had moved to London from India to be with her husband, her daughter Anna developed a fever and became ill. She consulted her previous general practitioner, who understood Gujarati. He told her that Anna had a 'virus' and did not need any treatment. Anna's fever rose further, and she had a fit and was taken to hospital to be treated. Three weeks later, the same thing happened, and again Mrs Patel's general practitioner told her not to worry, although this time the fit and unconsciousness lasted longer. Mrs Patel began to doubt her general practitioner's expertise, so she registered with another practice, even though they only spoke English. Her younger son, Sunil, then began to develop a fever that even showed in his skin. She consulted a female doctor in the practice, hoping that she would be more approachable and sympathetic, but instead she found her impatient and dismissive. Although she had often encountered this attitude among professionals in this country, she had no alternative but to consult them, so she approached the present scenario feeling hesitant and tentative.

> *Doctor*: Come in, Mrs Patel, have a seat.
> *The woman sits down, and she then stands the infant on the floor. He wanders towards the box of toys.*
> *Mrs Patel*: Hello doctor, how are you?
> *Doctor*: I am fine, and you?
> *Mrs Patel*: Fine, and your family?
> *Doctor*: (***hurried***) **Fine – what can I do for you?**

This doctor also seemed too hurried to observe the most basic of social conventions. Rather than explaining the whole story, Mrs Patel struggled to keep her explanation concise, limiting her description to the immediate problems.

> *Mrs Patel*: (*agitated*) Doctor, it is **Sunil; he's not well**. He's **crying, crying, crying for the whole night**. He's **scratching, scratching; his skin is all red ... and bleeding** even! And so **much sweating** – he gets **so hot**. I give **yoghurt and rice** and **he just vomits, then starts coughing, coughing, coughing – he can't sleep. One minute too hot, sweating, scratching, then next minute too cold, shivering, coughing. The whole**
>
> *continued overleaf*

> **family has no sleep, and is exhausted.** (*She wipes away tears*) I gave **Calpol; it works for an hour only.** The **Indian doctor, in Leicester**, gave me **very good treatment for everyone – made diarrhoea – but I can't go** to see him. **Can you give anything? The yellow medicine, Amoxil? It is very good.** Gives **diarrhoea**. It **helps the fever and cough**, so we can **all** sleep.

For Mrs Patel, all of these features are significant. With a little more background, and a short narrative of this illness, the significance of these symptoms becomes clearer. The constant crying was not only a sign of Sunil's deep distress and the severity of his illness, but it unbalanced the whole family by preventing their sleep and compromising their functioning. His heat and scratching, which was so severe that he was bleeding, was evidence of a dangerous excess of heat, just as it had been with Anna previously. When Mrs Patel consulted the previous doctor, she did not appear to make any assessment of Sunil's energy balance, and she seemed unable to advise Mrs Patel on what to do, except to apply superficial creams (which did not work). As Sunil's condition worsened, Mrs Patel noted the similarity to Anna's illness so, in desperation, she gave him the 'Amoxil' that she still had left over from the hospital. It purged him and he began to improve. When the Amoxil ran out, she returned to the doctor for more, but the doctor seemed annoyed about this and insisted that it would not help. When Mrs Patel began to get upset, the doctor responded with embarrassing and intrusive questions about her mood and her ability to cope. On returning home she asked friends and family for sources of more appropriate advice directed at the cause of Sunil's illness. She turned to an Ayurvedic doctor in Leicester, who provided her with medicine, and lifestyle and dietary advice, involving cooling foods to be taken by the whole family in order to help to restore the imbalance. Anna stopped having fits and Sunil's skin improved. Unfortunately, the treatment appeared to be over-cooling him, and he developed an imbalance of phlegm, resulting in an excess, which made him cough. Mrs Patel stopped all the cooling treatments, and Sunil's skin became hot and itchy in addition to the by now incessant coughing. Mrs Patel no longer knew what to do for the best, she had run out of 'Amoxil' and so, in desperation, she came to consult another general practitioner in the practice (which is the point at which this scenario began).

Thus there is rather a difference between 'what is *really* going on' for the patient and for the doctor. For doctors to give the patient's interpretation the same credence and respect as the general practitioner's interpretation requires empathy, humility and self-awareness. Not only would the doctor need to be willing to listen to the mother's perspective and withhold judgement, but he would also need to afford her conception of health (and another medical system) equal respect. Both the biomedical system and the Ayurvedic system upon which Mrs Patel's knowledge is loosely based are social constructions, and most doctors are only familiar with one of them, namely the biomedical system.

How can I deal with this?

So far I have used a scenario involving stereotypes of patient and general practitioner from different cultures. However, in practice consultations are rarely so simplistic, and stereotypes by their very nature point to a generality which rarely exists in reality. Just as not all general practitioners would frame their ideas or behaviour in the ways I have described, neither would all Mrs Patels.

With the existence of such heterogeneity within cultural and ethnic groups, as well as among doctors, there cannot be a single right answer as to how each health worker can most effectively deal with patients from one group or another. Consultation models and guidance on communication skills are widely available, but all too often they are based on temporally and socially constructed notions of autonomy and roles. Furthermore, much of what goes on during consultations is affected by the general practitioner's personality, so that superficial mores or codes of behaviour that seem natural to one general practitioner will appear artificial to another. That said, in the remainder of this chapter I shall offer suggestions for more general directions, describing some of the options available to health workers when dealing with their patients from different cultural backgrounds.

Tackling perceived constraints

Lack of time is the reason often given for not exploring individual perspectives during consultations, or reflecting upon them later. It assumes that the doctor's time is one of the most important factors in assessing the outcome of the consultation, whereas many would refute that view.[3,5] Complaints about lack of time are used by so many individuals to justify their priorities that they can sound like a lame excuse, particularly coming from professionals who are expected by the public to have the autonomy to be able to manage their time appropriately and make suitable organisational changes.[3,6] In this scenario, Mrs Patel did not appreciate the preoccupation of the various doctors with time. She therefore rationalised their impatience by interpreting it as a personal disinterest or antipathy (of which there were indeed other indications), whereas in fact the general practitioners did not feel that they had enough time to attend to her needs because they had a waiting-room full of patients. Rather than accepting that situation without question and directing their frustration at her, they could attempt to change the situation by exploring their appointment system, or offering more appointments. As organisational issues so often reflect doctors' priorities rather than their patients' needs, it can seem both defeatist not to challenge those structural constraints and unkind to blame patients for not adhering to them.

Nevertheless, many general practitioners do feel too constrained by time to attempt what they may consider to be too detailed an analysis of each patient's problem, and instead they adopt a pragmatic approach to the task in hand. In this scenario, the general practitioner's priorities were culturally framed – he faced the dilemmas of whether or not to spend time exploring Mrs Patel's mental state, and whether or not to give antibiotics (and so risk reinforcing what he felt to be 'inappropriate' patient behaviour). In other scenarios, where the mental health or functioning of the child or family is more obviously disturbed, the general practitioner may have to give it a higher priority. In situations of greater uncertainty, general practitioners may feel more comfortable considering such biomedical concerns rather than attending to the meaning or significance of the symptoms for the patient. Time spent attending to their own needs will leave them less capable of skilfully weaving a way through the differences in cultural constructions to provide an explanation and treatment that are meaningful to the patient as well as to the doctor. Furthermore, as was demonstrated in the above scenario, the general practitioner's impatience may lead patients to voice the bare minimum of facts, thus giving the doctor less opportunity to make a culturally sensitive assessment.

Becoming aware of one's own position

A basic appreciation of the cultural insensitivity of the biomedical model and the social constructions on which it is based will help the general practitioner to understand the limitations of his own model. For example, an appreciation of the reduction characteristic of the biomedical diagnostic process would have led this general practitioner to view Mrs Patel's description more sympathetically, rather than being irritated by the information that she provided, but which he considered to be extraneous.

Similarly, if this general practitioner (and the one whom Mrs Patel had previously encountered) had understood that the associations he was making were based on European constructions of normality and health, he might have handled the situation more sensitively, rather than behaving as though his view was the 'truth' and her views were based on mistaken 'beliefs', for which she needed education – an approach that she found both patronising and inappropriate. However, she had to 'comply' as she felt bound by the rules of social deference that affect patients who may not agree with the doctor's management, but who feel that they have little alternative but to accept it. Social deference, although it will vary between individuals and cultures, is nevertheless influenced by the collective consciousness which places those of 'non-white' ethnic origin at a disadvantage.[3.7] They in turn may attach significance to particular characteristics of the general practitioner, so that the doctor's appearance, dress, gender, confidence or manner may be perceived as symbols of expertise or authority. These perceived relative power differences between the patient and the doctor may have the effect of inhibiting the patient, preventing her from expressing her needs. This may be the reason why, in this scenario, Mrs Patel did not feel able to question or challenge her doctors until she was desperate.[3.8]

However, the very characteristics that for some individuals represent expertise or authority, can to others be symbols of oppression, and consequently patients, and indeed doctors, may adopt defensive positions against the values that they associate with those characteristics. Patients may feel more confident with and able to challenge doctors who share their ethnic origin. Those very doctors may in turn consider that they have no alternative but to ally themselves fiercely with the biomedical model and be more critical of those patients who do not 'comply' with biomedical systems, as was the case with the first Gujarati-speaking doctor whom Mrs Patel consulted.

The doctor's origin is rarely referred to in biomedical discourse. It is usually the patients who are the object of investigation, whereas doctors are more commonly the subjects and are considered to be professional, neutral and unaffected by their own 'ethnicity'. Nevertheless, 'ethnicity' is one of the factors that influences the complex power relationships between doctors and patients, but it is usually only invoked when it is not 'white'.[3.9] Although it will be impossible for health workers to be able to change their own physical characteristics to make patients feel comfortable, an awareness of the factors that may make them seem inaccessible, and compensatory efforts to redress the effects of the historical associations of their characteristics, would make individuals more comfortable. In this scenario, the general practitioner could do nothing about his colour and the fact that he was male and in his forties, but he could have made an effort not to look hurried before Mrs Patel had started to speak, but rather to appear attentive to her concerns. In mental health, which relies upon discourse and behaviour for assessment, enabling patients to talk openly and comfortably is especially important, so doctors need to be particularly aware of the influence that they have on patients.

Awareness and respect for others

Heterogeneity within cultures can make the individual situation facing a general practitioner seem far removed from textbook descriptions of those cultures. There are many descriptions of 'other' cultures, ethnic groups and medical systems that tend to emphasise their differences from the implicit 'white' norm. This categorisation of the 'other' can very easily lead to the creation of stereotypes, and such descriptions should be approached with a degree of critical awareness, particularly if they draw the reader into thinking in terms of 'ethnic' or 'racial' stereotypes. These stereotypes can distract the focus of health professionals away from the specific needs of individuals. However, the emphasis of biomedical discourse on classification and generalisations can make it difficult to note individual rather than group characteristics. In the above scenario I have grouped together a few characteristics to invoke a stereotype in an attempt to engage the reader. It is not my intention that readers should use this scenario to confirm their notion of young Asian women, but to show that they need to beware of much of the biomedical literature which can encourage readers to do just that.

When assessing and managing the mental health of children and their families, it is particularly important that doctors are not constrained by stereotypes. They will be best able to make an assessment if they can enable their patients to feel empowered enough to vocalise their perspectives. Those perspectives are crucial, not only to a doctor's understanding of the meaning of the symptoms, but also to negotiating a way forward. For example, in the scenario described above, the general practitioner would have better understood Mrs Patel's position by encouraging her, with a tone and manner that accepted her expertise without compromising his own, to describe the background and significance of her son's symptoms. Listening to and respecting culturally different perspectives and reading literature that comes from those perspectives is often more helpful for health workers than reading about superficial descriptions of 'other' cultures or ethnic groups.

Box 3.1:   Practice points relating to culture and ethnicity

Health care professionals should remember that:
- biomedical approach to illness is predominantly European and may well be foreign to others
- *ethnicity* is composed of *race* and *culture*, and should not be judged from a patient's race alone
- patients interpret and present any symptom in accordance with their own personal history and ethnic background
- these patients are vulnerable not only because of illness, but also because they may not know what is expected of them as patients
- it is the health professional's responsibility to familiarise themselves with their patient's approach to medical treatment, and to adjust their practice accordingly.

Acknowledgements

The author would like to thank Andrew Singleton, research scientist in the Department of General Practice and Primary Care, St George's Hospital Medical School, London, for his comments on an earlier draft of this chapter.

Notes

3.1   This is loosely based upon a consulation in practice, although the names and some features of the characters have been changed in order to preserve confidentiality.

3.2   Historically, race was considered to be a reasonable way of discriminating against people. There are many examples where biomedical discourse (originally anatomy, but more recently behavioural psychology and psychiatry) has used the language of objectivity and neutrality when reporting research that has been utilised to confirm the inferiority of 'non-white' peoples. Race has since been discredited as a term of distinction based on biological differences (as the genetic and phenotypic differences between different 'racial' groups are smaller than the differences within groups, demonstrating the arbitrariness of the categorical distinctions). Ethnicity is a term that has been developed to incorporate the notions of belonging as perceived by any member of that group, so it should enable some contextual appreciation. However, when the choices of ethnic group are broadly based upon racial lines, then their context is not acknowledged, the result being that ethnicity can often be used in the same way as race. Although physicians may assume that it is a neutral term, the social discourse still carries all the layers of meaning that have been applied to race.

3.3   Perhaps confirmed by her spending longer on the social graces than he thought necessary:
Mrs Patel: Hello doctor, how are you?
Doctor: I am fine, and you?
Mrs Patel: **Fine, and your family?**
Doctor: (*hurried*) Fine – **what can I do for you?**

3.4   Furthermore, within those categories, the categories that separate mental health from ill health are based on European constructions. For example, the individualistic notion of personal guilt as evidence of depression does not carry the same weight across all other cultural groups.

3.5   Improving patients' health in the longer term would be more important to some than saving time in the shorter term. Even if time is the most important factor, an understanding of the patient's perspective may save the general practitioner's time later on by avoiding the need for repeated consultations.

3.6   The extent of fatalism among health workers about the systems in which they work (and are in a position to change) can make their criticism of fatalism among their patients about the systems in which they live (and are often not in a position to change) appear rather foolish.

3.7   Historically, all those of a lower social class or 'other' ethnic group have been disadvantaged by not being given access to the tools that enable them to be accorded equal respect and credibility by those in positions of authority. More recently, access to information and consumer rights organisations have empowered some to resist that role of social deference.

3.8   So while an English general practitioner as a patient in this situation may be able to approach her doctor and present her scenario in such a way as to ensure that she gets her own way (that is, to subtly prevent her own general practitioner from exploring her own mental state, and to persuade them to provide her with antibiotics), Mrs Patel could not do so.

3.9   In biomedical categorisations of 'ethnicity', 'white' also does not take into account culture and context, because it is assumed to be the norm. A doctor behaving as 'normal' would be assumed to be 'white' unless it was stated otherwise. In this scenario, I have not stated the doctor's race or ethnic origin, and most readers will have assumed that he is 'white'.

Suggested further reading

Banton M (1987) *Racial Theories*. Cambridge University Press, Cambridge. Gives a clear outline to the development of the historical constructions of 'race'.

Fernando S (1993) *Mental Health, Race and Culture*. Palgrave, formally Macmillan Press. Looks critically at the ethnocentric biomedical interpretations of mental health.

Foucault M (1973) *The Birth of the Clinic. An Archaeology of Medical Perception*. Routledge, London.

Gilman S (1985) *Difference and Pathology: Stereotypes of Sexuality, Race and Madness*. Cornell University Press. Describes the development of stereotypes in biomedicine and their link to categories of 'otherness'.

Good B (1994) *Medicine, Rationality and Experience: An Anthropological Perspective*. Cambridge University Press, Cambridge. Provides an excellent account of the construction of medical knowledge.

Hahn R and Gaines A (1985) *Physicians of Western Medicine: Anthropological Approaches to Theory and Practice*. Reidel Publishing Co., Lancaster.

Helman C (2000) *Culture, Health and Illness: An Introduction for Health Professionals* (2e). Arnold, London. Provides a basic introduction to the constructs described in this chapter.

Inden R (1990) *Imagining India*. Basil Blackwell, Oxford.

Kleinman A (1980) *Patients and Healers in the Context of Culture: An Exploration of the Borderland Between Anthropology, Medicine and Psychiatry*. University of California Press, London.

Kleinman A (1987) Anthropology and psychiatry: the role of culture in cross-cultural research on illness. *Br J Psychiatry*. **151**: 447–54.

Last M (1981) The importance of knowing about not knowing. *Soc Sci Med*. **158**: 387–92.

Littlewood R (1990) From categories to contexts: a decade of the 'new cross-cultural psychiatry'. *Br J Psychiatry*. **156**: 308–27.

Littlewood R and Lipsedge M (1989) *Aliens and Alienists: Ethnic Minorities in Psychiatry*. Unwin Hyman, London.

Overing J (1985) *Reason and Morality*. Tavistock, London.

Rack P (1982) *Race, Culture and Mental Disorder*. Routledge, London.

Rattansi I (1994) 'Western' racisms, ethnicities and identities in a 'postmodern' frame. In: A Rattansi and S Westwood (eds) *Racism, Modernity and Identity on the Western Front*. Polity Press, Cambridge.

Roberts G and Holmes J (1999) *Healing Stories: Narrative in Psychiatry and Psychotherapy*. Oxford University Press, Oxford. Provides fascinating accounts of how narrative approaches can be used to help patients to make sense of their experiences.

Said E (1994) *Culture and Imperialism*. Vintage, London.

Schiebinger L (1994) *Nature's Body*. Pandora, London.

Whorf BL (1956) An American Indian model of the Universe: 1936. In: JB Carroll (ed.) *Language, Thought and Reality: Selected Writings of Benjamin Lee Whorf*. Massachusetts Institute of Technology.

Young A (1981) The creation of medical knowledge: some problems of interpretation. *Soc Sci Med*. **158**: 379–86.

PART 2

Problems that may present at any age

CHAPTER FOUR

Temperament and resilience

Definition of temperament

Children have individual styles of behaviour. A child's characteristic behavioural style is not *just* the consequence of everything that has happened to them since birth. These characteristics are usually referred to as the child's *temperament* or constitution. The term 'temperament' describes the 'how' of behaviour, rather than the 'what' or the 'why'. For instance, siblings may differ widely in the way in which they respond to events, despite sharing the same family environment. Part of this may be due to ordinal position – a first child will have very different developmental pressures from a middle or last child. In addition, genetic factors make a contribution to temperamental differences.

The concept of temperament suggests qualities that endure over time. In fact, styles of behaviour tend to be stable from early childhood into adolescence in both sexes, although behavioural style may be less stable in infancy. Temperamental differences affect the child's environment, including the way in which others respond to that child or adolescent.

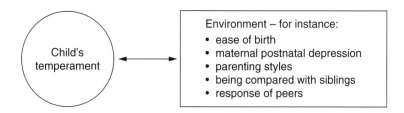

Figure 4.1: Interaction between the child's temperament and his environment.

Assessment of temperament

There are many ways of categorising temperament. One approach is to use three domains, namely emotionality, activity and sociability – the mnemonic is EAS. These domains can be described along an easy/difficult dimension, as shown in Table 4.1, and different temperamental features will appear at different ages.

Table 4.1:   A grid categorisation of temperamental attributes

Domain	Easy	Difficult
Emotionality	A baby who never cries except when hungry Enthusiasm for new situations Placid or phlegmatic Mainly positive moods – being of a 'sunny disposition'	A baby who cries constantly and gets upset easily Resistance to imposed change or novelty; slow to adapt to new situations Having high-intensity emotional responses, such as screaming loudly or over-reacting emotionally Mainly negative moods – a tendency to whinge or grizzle Easily frightened
Activity	A baby who sleeps all night A baby who feeds to contentment A child who prefers quiet games A baby or toddler who readily fits into the structure imposed by their parents	A baby who will not sleep A child who likes to be crawling/running as soon as he wakes up A child who cannot stay still long A child who is always on the go A baby or toddler who cannot be fitted into a routine for sleeping, eating or elimination
Sociability	A baby who likes to be with others A child who makes friends easily A child who tends to be independent	A baby who will not feed A child who tends to be shy A child who prefers to play by himself rather than with others

We have often heard parents say 'If our second child had been born first, we wouldn't have *had* a second one'. These parents can see that the problem is not their fault, because the first child was easy. If the difficult child comes first, parents inevitably feel that they are doing something wrong (and the child's awkward nature makes it difficult for them to be the good parents they wish to be).

The concept of resilience

Some children seem to cope with the same life events much more effectively than others. The protective factors that enable such children to manage better include the following:[1,2]

* *easy temperament*
* *higher intelligence*. As well as predisposing to higher self-esteem, this enables a child to learn problem-solving skills and develop a capacity to reflect. Good communication

skills, including the ability to describe experiences and their emotional impact, also promote resilience

- *support from parents*. Support in this context includes emotional warmth, praise and attentive listening. Specific parenting qualities include supervision and an authoritative style of discipline. A secure attachment to at least one parent is protective
- *support from peers*
- *humour* – this seems to be an important factor in its own right
- *positive experiences at school* – including protection from bullying, receiving praise at all possible opportunities and having support from key teachers. Non-academic opportunities are as important to the development of self-esteem as academic success (e.g. the encouragement of sporting, musical and social activities, and the fostering of responsibility)
- *support from other adults outside the immediate family* – this may include grandparents or adult friends of the family. Adult males who can serve as role models are particularly important for boys whose fathers have left home. It is an interesting observation that some children, despite being disturbed behaviourally or emotionally, elicit positive responses from those about them, whereas others do not. This may be due to positive temperamental features, or to something less easy to define
- *religious faith* – this may help either by encouraging family cohesion and community support, or by providing a framework in which to understand adversity
- *a tendency to plan life decisions and take control of one's life rather than making impulsive choices or leaving things to chance*. Examples include the regular use of contraception, or trying new substances in the company of trustworthy friends rather than strangers
- *some positive experiences may neutralise the effects of adverse factors*. Examples include a warm, close relationship with one parent, which can protect a child against the effects of marital conflict, and positive school experiences, which can give a child a sense of self-efficacy when he does not receive this from his carers
- *some experiences may have a 'steeling' effect*. An example is the effect on an adolescent girl of having to take care of younger siblings when her mother is at work – this can enhance self-efficacy and develop a sense of responsibility. In a pre-adolescent girl, it might have negative effects, particularly if she misses out on the parenting she requires for herself
- *cognitive processing of experiences* – this is an important element in the development or non-development of psychiatric disorder. Children who are able to add meaning to experiences and learn from them are likely to remain healthy, in contrast to those who persist in ruminations or negative attributions about themselves or their surroundings.

Management

Parents of a child with a *difficult temperament* may be enormously helped by professional recognition of this as a constitutional problem rather than the consequence of inadequate parenting. About 10% of small children can be categorised as difficult according to the characteristics listed in the right-hand column of Table 4.1. It is immediately apparent that such a child will be difficult to live with and unrewarding to parent. Given that most parents believe that their child's characteristics are the product of their parenting, they will blame themselves and become demoralised. This will reduce their ability to persist with appropriate child-rearing, because they can see no gains and they believe that they are doing something wrong. They therefore change tactics and expose their child to just the type of inconsistency he resents. Such parents are typically exposed to a welter of advice that implicitly (or explicitly) undermines their confidence in themselves and their ability to parent. Eventually they may take sides against the child and become critical or punitive in an attempt to impose their will. The child will in turn react to harsh handling and his sense of parental rejection with anger, and his attempts either to improve the situation or to alleviate his unhappiness usually make matters worse.

Professional labelling of the child as *'difficult to manage'* in his own right by virtue of nature rather than personal motive can be very helpful. The most helpful initial intervention for the general practitioner or health visitor in these circumstances may be to sympathise about how difficult the child is to manage. They should then explain that this is a problem that some children are born with, rather than immediately giving advice on handling, which may only reinforce the sense of blame. Difficult temperament is a risk factor for emotional and behavioural disorder in childhood, but many children with such temperamental styles do not develop problems. Sensible parents can be told that they may have to work harder to be positive and consistent, and to apply standard behavioural techniques that work much more readily with easier children (*see* Chapter 38). A useful analogy here is that if you have a gene for obesity, you have to work that much harder to be thin – but this is by no means impossible. With less sensible parents, there is a risk that the child will be regarded as the source of all the family's difficulties. The use of the 'difficult to manage' label can backfire, and the child may then become the family *scapegoat*. If he becomes the person in the family who is blamed for everything, the disastrous effects on his self-esteem and frustration tolerance will confirm the parents' negative expectations. Since this is likely to be one way in which the parents deal with feeling blamed themselves, any means of reducing their self-accusation is likely to help the child.

Several different agencies may provide opportunities for *promoting children's resilience.*[1] Primary care initiatives may often be a matter of common sense. Examples include helping an isolated mother to develop contacts with other mothers who are in a similar situation, finding an appropriate nursery school for a vulnerable child, advising parents to find after-school activities for their child, and encouraging a mother to talk through a stressful event with her son.

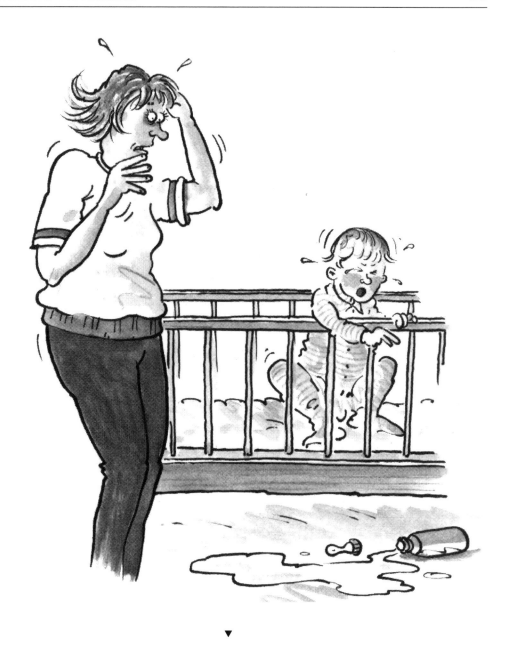

Referral

In general, it should not be necessary to refer children with temperamental difficulties, unless these lead to emotional and behavioural difficulties that require referral in their own right. However, referral for specialist assessment may be indicated if there is a suspicion of *organic reasons* why one child is more difficult than the others in a family.

Examples include dyslexia, attention-deficit hyperactivity disorder and Asperger's syndrome (*see* Chapters 5, 22 and 23).

Case study 4.1

Kyle was the result of his mother Alice's second pregnancy. The labour was long, the second stage was painful, and rotation forceps were used, which Alice found unpleasant. Kyle did not breastfeed as well as her first child – a girl called Samantha. He also had considerably greater difficulty in sleeping, and woke several times a night for most nights during the first year. His father found his evening colic very difficult to manage, felt that his wife was preoccupied with the children and unavailable for him, and left to live with someone else when Kyle was six months old. Alice then became depressed.

The health visitor recognised a multitude of risk factors for the relationship between Kyle and his mother, and decided to make him one of her high-priority cases. Initially, she visited fortnightly and involved the general practitioner in managing Alice's depression. Alice continued to find Kyle very much more difficult than Samantha. She also saw in him many of the personality traits of his father, with whom she was now furious. The health visitor visited every month for three years, and she worked with Alice on a variety of behavioural problems, including Kyle's sleeping difficulties, his faddy eating and his temper tantrums. She framed his being difficult as the way he was born, and as possibly inherited from his father. She developed a sufficiently close relationship with Alice to be able to discuss the fact that she was blaming Kyle for the breakup of the marriage, and her guilt about feeling this way, and about having given birth to the child who drove his father away. The health visitor also arranged for Alice to go to a mother-and-toddler group, and she subsequently helped her to find an appropriate nursery for Kyle, where the staff were particularly good at developing self-confidence and social skills. Gradually Alice was able to re-establish communication on a practical level with Kyle's father, who was able to play a regular part in Kyle's parenting. By the time of school entry, Alice still regarded Kyle as a difficult child, but she felt much more confident about her ability to deal with his challenging behaviour than she had done when he was a baby and she was depressed.

Box 4.1: Practice points – how the idea of temperament can help

- Acknowledging a child's difficult temperament can help parents to deal with this without becoming paralysed by blame.
- A child may be born difficult.
- If parents allow themselves to be overwhelmed by the experience of trying to bring up a difficult child, the result may be scapegoating of the child, which is unlikely to be in his best interests.
- This can be prevented.
- Finding an organic explanation for the child's difficult temperament may help, but it is not always possible.

Box 4.2: Practice points – how the idea of resilience can help

- Looking for protective factors can lead to a more positive mind-set than looking for risk factors.
- During the course of a child's development, there are numerous opportunities to encourage the development of resilience.

References

1 Mental Health Foundation (1999) *Bright Futures: Promoting Children and Young People's Mental Health*. Mental Health Foundation, London.

2 Rutter M (1999) Resilience concepts and findings. *J Fam Therapy*. **21**: 119–44.

CHAPTER FIVE

Disorders of language and social development

Definitions and relevance

Basics

Speech disorders affect speech production (e.g. by lips, tongue and larynx). Examples include dysarthria due to cerebral palsy and hypernasality due to cleft palate, neither of which are common in children attending primary care.

Language disorders affect the central processing of verbal ideas and communication.

Delays of development, in which the normal sequence of events does occur, but later than expected, can be contrasted with *disorders*, in which there is an abnormal sequence of development. These can be categorised in a variety of ways. Figure 5.1 shows a classification of the disorders of development of speech and language that are commonly encountered clinically. There are traditionally four components to language.[1]

- *Phonology* refers to the ability to produce and identify the specific sounds of a given language.
- *Grammar* refers to the underlying rules that organise any specific language. It can be divided into *morphology*, the 'within-word' structure, and *syntax*, the 'between-word' structure.
- *Semantics* refers to meanings. Part of this is *vocabulary*, which is relatively easy to assess informally. By 24 months of age, the average child knows 50 words. A young child can acquire up to ten new words per day. Vocabulary size is the best known predictor of school success. It is heavily dependent on heard words (spoken or read). Thus encouraging parents to speak and read to their child at every available opportunity is likely to help the child's overall development.
- *Pragmatics* refers to the development of skill in communicating. Conversation has implicit rules, such as turn-taking, topic maintenance and conversational repair. There are also unspoken rules about politeness, story-telling, talking for a long time, and signalling what one intends to say.

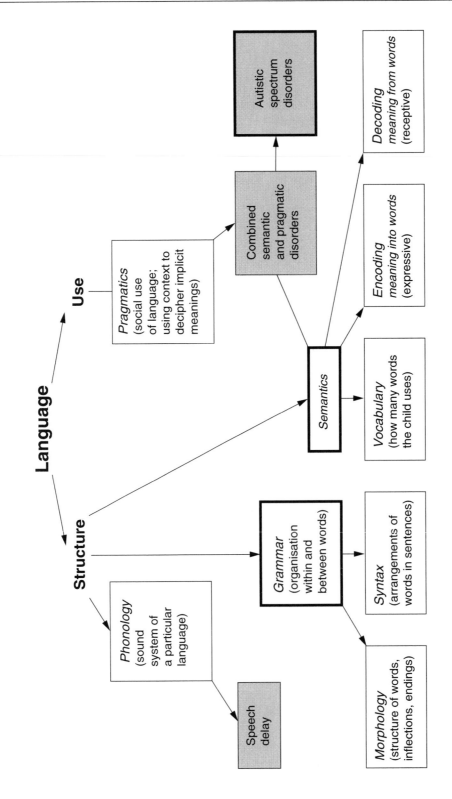

Figure 5.1:   The components of language as a way of classifying language disorders.

Normal development

A number of stages can be identified in normal language development (*see* Table 5.1). However, there is a wide range of variability.

Table 5.1: Population-based norms in language development

Stage	Age
Babbling	6–10 months
Word comprehension	8–10 months
Word production	12–13 months
Word combinations:	14–24 months
telegraphic speech first (e.g. 'daddy car' instead of 'daddy's car')	
Grammatical development	24–30 months
Basic morphology and syntax	By 3 years

Abnormal development

The term '*speech delay*' should in theory be applied only to difficulties at the level of speech production. In practice, the term is used to describe a delay in phonology development. Speech sounds usually normalise by the age of nine years, and residual errors persist after the age of nine years in approximately 5% of the population. There may be a family history. Speech delay linked to glue ear is usually associated with receptive language problems – both are due to fluctuating hearing loss.

Developmental language disorder, also referred to as *specific language impairment, developmental dysphasia* or *aphasia*, refers to a delay or disorder of grammar and vocabulary. This may be mainly expressive, mainly receptive, or both. In six- to seven-year-olds, it is reported to occur in 6% of girls and 8% of boys.[2]

Deficits in the development of *pragmatic* skills are common in autistic disorders (discussed below). They are often combined with semantic difficulties, particularly the misunderstanding of contextual meaning (e.g. taking the command to 'pull your socks up' literally). The term '*semantic-pragmatic disorder*' was coined to describe those children who have these problems but without autism. There is continuing (and perhaps fruitless) debate as to whether or not such children should be regarded as fitting on the autistic spectrum.

A separate category to all the above concerns *problems of fluency*. These range from normal non-fluency to an established *stammer*. Children whose maturity of thought outstrips their maturity of speech production may repeat themselves or trip over words as they try to articulate their thoughts. Some children may become anxious about this, which can then lead to an established problem. This is usually called stammering in the UK, or stuttering in North America and Australia. It is a good example of interplay between emotional and developmental factors.

Relevance to child mental health

What is the link between language disorders and child mental health problems? As with many other aetiological questions, there are three possibilities, namely that A causes B, B causes A, or C causes A and B, and whether the problem is seen as A or as B depends on who is looking at it.

- *A causes B.* Common sense suggests that children who cannot say what they are thinking will become frustrated, and children who cannot understand what adults are saying cannot do what they are told and therefore also become frustrated. Frustration in young children may be expressed as an emotional disorder (withdrawal or anxiety) or in the form of externalising (antisocial) behaviour. It is difficult to see how a child with inadequate language could express frustration directly – he is hardly likely to say 'I am frustrated'.
- *B causes A.* Emotional difficulties may be manifested by not taking things in (receptive difficulties), remaining in a baby-like state (immature expression), or being unable to understand the speaker's point of view (pragmatic difficulties).
- *C causes A and B.* Brain disorders may cause both a language disorder and a child mental health problem.
- *Different perspectives.* A disorder of social communication may be regarded as a language disorder by a speech and language therapist and as a psychiatric problem by a child psychiatrist. The timber merchant, the botanist and the artist do not see the same tree.

Autistic disorders

Autism is a behavioural syndrome, arising from abnormalities in central nervous system development at an early stage, probably in the fetus. It is characterised by multiple qualitative impairments of the following:

- social functioning and interaction, which may be poor or non-existent
- language and non-verbal communication, which by definition is always impaired
- play, which tends to be unimaginative, repetitive, ritualistic or obsessional.

Autism is often associated with moderate or severe generalised learning difficulties. Mild versions of autism, without significant language disorder or learning disability, are often referred to as '*Asperger's disorder*' (after the Austrian paediatrician Hans Asperger, who first described the condition in 1944). Autism represents the severe end of a spectrum, and Asperger's disorder represents a milder disorder within a group of conditions that are known in medical jargon as the '*pervasive developmental disorders*'. We have found this terminology very unhelpful in discussions with parents, and so prefer the more user-friendly and common-sense term '*autistic spectrum disorders*'. This broad category includes children with classical autism, those with high-functioning autism (average or above-average IQ), those with Asperger's syndrome and those with a variety of poorly defined intermediate conditions. In medical jargon, these difficult-to-label children are categorised as having 'pervasive developmental disorder not otherwise specified'. It is considerably easier to inform parents that their child fits on the autistic spectrum. To add to the potential confusion, the term '*social communication disorder*' is often used as an inclusive term for autistic spectrum disorders and semantic pragmatic disorders.

There is clearly a genetic component to autism and Asperger's syndrome. There is often a family history of eccentric relatives or language disorder. Some parents of children with diagnosed autistic spectrum disorders can be seen to have undiagnosed Asperger's disorder or at least autistic traits. There is also an increased prevalence of conditions that affect central nervous system development, such as fragile X, tuberous sclerosis, congenital rubella, infantile spasms and head injury. There is *no* evidence to support aetiological theories based on 'refrigerator parent' models or attachment problems, but all of these conditions are responsible for impaired attachment.

Recent surveys suggest a prevalence rate for all autistic spectrum disorders combined of 1% of the general population.[3] Boys are more often affected than girls. Asperger's syndrome is considerably more common than autism. On an average general practitioner's list there will be about 20 individuals with autistic spectrum disorder. Many of these are undiagnosed adults, mainly with Asperger's syndrome, and most of them can cope without any help. The prototype is the local eccentric who lives in isolation and enjoys engaging in one particular activity, for which he may or may not be paid.

Childhood diagnosis is becoming more common. It is unclear whether this is because of an increased incidence or because of changing diagnostic fashions and improved recognition. Clinical experience suggests that these children encounter many difficulties at school, which can be substantially ameliorated once a diagnosis has been made and the teaching environment suitably adapted.

Most parents like to have some explanation of their child's disability. A recent scapegoat has become the mumps, measles and rubella immunisation. Current expert opinion suggests there is no reason to suspect that the link is causal. Many children with autistic disorders first show symptoms at about the time of the immunisation.

Assessment and referral

Assessment of *language delay or disorder* must include a hearing test. A distraction hearing test may sometimes miss hearing loss, so when in doubt, always refer to the local audiology service.[4] Another common and treatable cause of language delay is under-stimulation (*see* Chapter 11 on neglect).

If it is not clear whether the child merely has delay or actually has a disorder, referral to a speech and language therapist for further assessment should be the next step. A full assessment of possible autistic spectrum disorders is not expected in primary care. Suspected autism should probably be referred as soon as suspicions arise. Milder autistic spectrum disorders, particularly Asperger's syndrome, often benefit from waiting. This gives the parents time to consider whether the diagnosis makes sense to them, and it allows evidence from school and other sources to accumulate. Attempts to diagnose such milder conditions too early may lead to errors.[5]

Table 5.2 provides details of the differences between the conditions described above, and is intended merely as a guide to the implications of the diagnostic terms used in letters received from a speech and language therapist or other specialist. Unfortunately, these terms are used in different ways, and there is no universal agreement on definitions, but the descriptions given are in line with majority practice. In functional terms, there is little difference between high-functioning autism and Asperger's syndrome.

Management

Although a child with *delay in language development* is likely to catch up, this process can be accelerated by appropriate help. The parents should be advised to model the correct way for the child to say things, rather than to correct errors constantly. For instance, a child with normal hearing and otherwise normal development who says 'gog' for 'dog' will pick up the correct pronunciation after hearing it often enough. Similarly, if the structure of sentences is delayed, speaking to the child in slightly longer sentences will enable them to absorb and reproduce the structures. Delayed comprehension can be managed by parents simplifying the way in which they speak to the child, and introducing new concepts by linking them to what they are about, rather than testing the child with questions. In such cases, parental stimulation can help the child to develop age-appropriate language, and speech and language therapy may not be needed.

In contrast, a child with *disordered language development* should be seen by a speech and language therapist. If assessment suggests that adequate treatment can be given by parents and teachers, she is the best person to advise on this. Some children may require frequent direct therapy.

Parents of a child with a *stammer* should avoid laughing at him, making him self-conscious, or increasing his anxiety in other ways. This will give the child time for his language skills to catch up with his thinking. If the problem is clearly more than transient, or simple advice along these lines is ineffective, early referral to a speech and language therapist is advisable, in order to avoid the anxiety becoming so established that it leads to a persistent problem. A chronic stammer may also be an index of other anxieties, or the expression of emotional difficulties, which may need help in their own right.

There is no proven cure for *autism* itself, or for its variants. Treatment fashions come and go, usually with a flush of enthusiasm when the treatment is first publicised, followed gradually by recognition that the responses were few and exaggerated. *Holding* and *facilitated communication* have both been through this cycle of popularity. A recent development is the use of *secretin*, a gut hormone that is also a neurotransmitter. The results of trials are awaited before the anecdotal reports of dramatic improvements can be assessed reliably.

Psychological treatment programmes can be helpful in modifying child behaviour, enabling the parents to cope with the specific difficulties presented by the child, and

Table 5.2: Differential diagnosis and prognosis of language and social communication disorders

	Language delay/ disorder	Autism	High-functioning autism	Asperger's disorder	Autistic spectrum disorder (and none of the others)
Age at which symptoms begin	May become apparent as less than usual child–parent interaction during the first year, or when language milestones are not achieved	Onset before 3 years	Onset of social aloofness or marked rituals before 3 years	There are usually features in the developmental history that make the child appear different, but suspicions may not arise until primary or secondary school, if ever	Symptoms become apparent after 3 years
Age at diagnosis	Usually picked up at pre-school age. Language disorder should be diagnosed by the early years of primary school, but is occasionally missed	Usually diagnosed pre-school	Diagnosis is usually before or just after school entry	Average age of diagnosis is 11 years. May never be diagnosed, as adults with the condition often have insufficient difficulties to justify any diagnosis	Varies
Diagnostic features	Skills deficit in one or several areas of linguistic competence (see Figure 5.1)	Disinterest or disability in communication, social interaction and imagination. Obsessions and/or rituals	Autism diagnostic criteria are satisfied, with early aloofness. Intellectual abilities compensate. Often has a particular skill	Difficulties with social interaction (e.g. subtleties of language, empathy) and routine dependence, repetitive activities or obsessional interests. May have an area of particular skill. Often clumsy	A mixed picture. Most commonly, features of autism falling short of the diagnosis, with too much learning disability and language disorder to fit Asperger's syndrome

Table 5.2: Continued

	Language delay/ disorder	Autism	High-functioning autism	Asperger's disorder	Autistic spectrum disorder (and none of the others)
Schooling and prognosis	Children with delayed language development usually catch up by the early years of primary school. Management under the guidance of a therapist may accelerate this. Children with language disorders may require support in school, or even placement in a language unit. A minority will continue to need help in secondary school	Children usually require special schooling in a school either for autistic children or for children with learning difficulties. About 10% of affected adults work, often in semi-sheltered settings. Many live at home, some attending adult training centres. Others live in supervised residential communities	Can often be integrated into mainstream school, but not always. Secondary school may need to make considerable allowances. Depression may develop in more insightful adolescents due to increasing awareness of loneliness and differences from others	Mainstream primary school should be adequate for most. Secondary school may be much more difficult, and some may require more support than can be given in a mainstream school. After secondary school, life becomes easier, especially if a skill niche can be found	Usually require special schooling. May present management difficulties as children or adults (e.g. with disruptive or aggressive behaviour)

ensuring optimal schooling. Advice to parents can helpfully be based on the adage that it is more effective to adapt the environment around an autistic spectrum child than to attempt to change the child.

The National Autistic Society[5.1] and local support groups may help to provide parents with much needed support from other parents who are facing (or have learned to cope with) similar problems. They may also be able to organise lobbying for facilities such as specialist schools. The disability living allowance may provide much needed financial assistance, as having to care for an autistic child very often prevents one of the parents from going out to work.

Case study 5.1

Joseph's parents became concerned about him when he was 9 years old because of his lack of friends and his increasing difficulties in achieving what was expected of him at school. He seemed unable to understand homework tasks, and in the classroom he often appeared to be in a world of his own. He loved doing word-search puzzles, and was good at mathematics, but was reluctant to make an effort in other subjects, such as English. His parents had seen a television programme about Asperger's syndrome, and thought that many of the descriptions fitted him. In fact, they realised that he had seemed a little different from other children from as early on as nursery school.

Joseph was referred to a specialist at his parents' request. The specialist discussed his situation with members of the school staff, and agreed that the diagnosis fitted. The parents were disappointed that no specific treatment was offered. However, the special needs co-ordinator at the school went to a conference about Asperger's syndrome, which enabled her to advise the other teachers on how best to handle Joseph. This resulted in substantial improvements in his co-operation. At the same time, the school agreed to apply for a statement of educational needs. As a result of reports from the specialist and a speech and language therapist, the statement was granted. This did not make a large difference at primary school, but when the time came for secondary school transfer, Joseph benefited from the resulting special treatment. For instance, he was disapplied from French, and instead had extra help for his English.

In due course, Joseph achieved good grades in science subjects at GCSE level. He went on to a sixth-form college, where the teachers found it difficult to understand his needs. The general practitioner asked the same specialist to review Joseph. This resulted in a meeting with the teachers at the sixth-form college, who then learned much more about the condition for themselves.

Joseph obtained good A-level grades and went to university. The same specialist was again asked to help. He could no longer see Joseph, who was by now too old to be referred to him, but he wrote to the university pastoral care officers recommending that single accommodation should be provided. He also arranged for Joseph to be seen by an adult psychologist with an interest in Asperger's disorder. Joseph eventually became a computer programmer at a chemical engineering works.

Thus Joseph received minimal psychiatric input throughout his educational career, but he benefited from the efforts his teachers had made at various stages to understand the implications of his condition.

Box 5.1:   Practice points for disorders of language and social development

- Refer any case of suspected *language disorder* to a speech and language therapist.
- Refer any case of suspected *autistic spectrum disorder* to a local specialist clinic.
- In cases of *language delay*, encourage the parents to provide as much appropriate stimulation as possible. This includes stretching the child's vocabulary by speaking and reading to them. Some parents may benefit from referral to a speech and language therapist for further advice.

Acknowledgements

The authors are indebted to Deborah Fulford, speech and language therapist at the Maudsley Children's Hospital, and Julia Robb, Speech and Language Therapy Manager for the Sussex Weald and Downs' NHS Trust, for their contribution to this chapter.

Notes

5.1   The umbrella organisation for many parent support groups is the National Autistic Society (tel 020 7833 2299; website http://www.oneworld.org/autism_uk/).

References

1   Toppelberg CO and Shapiro T (2000) Language disorders: a ten-year research update review. *J Am Acad Child Adolesc Psychiatry.* **39**: 143–52.

2   Tomblin JB, Records NL, Buckwalter P, Zhang X, Smith E and O'Brien M (1997) Prevalence of specific language impairment in kindergarten children. *J Speech Lang Hearing Res.* **40**: 1245–60.

3   Wing L (1997) The autistic spectrum. *Lancet.* **350**: 1761–66.

4   Hall D, Hill P and Elliman D (1999) *The Child Surveillance Handbook* (2e). Radcliffe Medical Press, Oxford.

5   Cox A, Klein K, Charman T et al. (1999) Early diagnosis of autistic spectrum disorders. *J Child Psychol Psychiatry.* **40**: 719–32.

Further information

A particularly good website (among many) is http://info.med.yale.edu/chldstdy/autism/.

CHAPTER SIX

Behaviour problems

Overview

Parents complain when their children do not behave as they expect. This may be because the child displays behaviour that does not fall within the norm, or because the parents' expectations are unrealistic. Behaviour problems are the *bête noire* of child psychiatry, at any level of service provision, as they are such a common presenting complaint, and they may appear to defy easy remedies. This is often because simple behavioural techniques are poorly implemented.

Common complaints about children's behaviour include the following:

- 'he's on the go all the time'
- 'he won't do what he's told'
- 'he answers back'
- 'he hits other children'
- 'he goes into one' (meaning a tantrum).

Key questions

The first point to determine when confronted with such a complaint is whether the behaviour can be considered *normal* or *abnormal* for the child's age and stage of development. Pre-school children of 3–5 years of age are expected to be active and boisterous, and to test imposed limits. They are likely to experience difficulties in occupying themselves, and to need more adult attention than some parents are prepared to give. This means that they are likely to discover ways of obtaining adult attention, such as being naughty, resisting instructions, or persisting in making demands. A child of this age who does *not* have tantrums could be regarded as abnormal.

Persistence of such behaviour beyond school entry is also common, but they should subside with age. The key question to consider is whether the behaviour results in *dysfunction*. Examples of adverse consequences of oppositional or defiant behaviour include escalations of conflict within the home, management difficulties for the schoolteacher, and friendship difficulties. Behaviour problems that are serious enough to cause some dysfunction are common, affecting approximately 5% of children and 10% of adolescents. They are more common in urban than rural areas.

Parents of under-fives often bring their complaints to the health visitor, who is in an excellent position to intervene effectively with potentially long-lasting benefits. Parents of school-aged children may be reluctant to go to their general practitioner about their child's behaviour problems, fearing that they will merely be told it is all their fault, and often they will only go because they are pressurised by the child's school. Parents of delinquent teenagers have often given up – an attitude that is shared by many professionals.

Theory

There are clear continuities in behaviour. For instance, aggression is remarkably persistent over time. Pre-school behaviour problems (e.g. oppositionality, defiance and tantrums) above the norm are likely to continue into middle childhood and adolescence, taking a slightly different form at each stage. The pre-schooler who tantrums and refuses to comply may become the disruptive primary school child with academic failure, the teenager whose behaviour breaks the law (i.e. a delinquent), and the adult with an antisocial personality and continuing criminal behaviour. In contrast, antisocial behaviour that arises for the first time in adolescence is more likely to subside. Because of this clear developmental trajectory, it is dangerous to say of difficult pre-schoolers 'He'll grow out of it'. Some will, but usually only because their parents find effective ways of coping with the behaviour.

Parents may obtain help with their child's behaviour from a variety of sources, including neighbours, relatives and books, but if they come to the health service for help, that service should either provide such help or direct them to a source where it is available. At any stage there are opportunities for professionals to intervene, but the best opportunity is in children under the age of eight years, who have not yet developed ingrained habits of antisocial behaviour or joined a deviant peer group.

Conduct disorder is a psychiatric term that simply implies having more than three of the behaviours shown in Box 6.1.[1] A milder and earlier form is called *oppositional-defiant disorder*, for which there should be at least four of the features shown in Box 6.2.[6.1] It is not necessary to make these diagnoses in primary care in order to be able to help, but it is important to distinguish between those children who are healthily naughty, and those whose behaviours are causing dysfunction within their families, at school or within their friendship networks. Such children are regarded as having a psychiatric disorder but not a mental illness. It is most helpful to view disruptive behaviour disorders (oppositional defiant disorder, conduct disorder and attention-deficit hyperactivity disorder) as existing along a continuum. The greater the number of features in the boxes that a child displays, the more worrying the situation.

Box 6.1: Behaviours seen in conduct disorder

Excessive fighting, with frequent initiation of fights
Deliberate and repeated destruction of others' property
Often lies to obtain goods or favours, or to avoid obligations
Repeated stealing outside the home without confrontation (e.g. shoplifting)
Has stolen while confronting a victim (e.g. purse-snatching, mugging)
Has used a weapon that can cause serious physical harm to others (e.g. a bat, brick, broken bottle, knife or gun)
Has broken into someone else's house, building or car
Frequent truancy from school, beginning before 13 years of age
Often bullies, threatens or intimidates others
Has run away from home at least twice overnight, or once for more than a single night (unless this was to avoid physical or sexual abuse)
Often stays out after dark, despite parental prohibition, beginning before 13 years of age
Displays physical cruelty to other people (e.g. ties up, cuts or burns a victim)
Displays cruelty to animals
Has engaged in deliberate fire-setting, with a risk or intention of causing serious damage
Has forced another person to engage in sexual activity against their wishes

---

Box 6.2: Behaviours seen in oppositional defiant disorder

Unusually frequent and severe temper tantrums for the child's developmental level
Often argues with adults
Often actively refuses adults' requests or defies rules
Often deliberately annoys people
Often blames others for his or her mistakes or behaviour
Is often touchy or easily annoyed by others
Is often angry or resentful
Is often spiteful or vindictive

Should behaviour problems be regarded as a health problem, or as exclusively the province of social services and education? There is an ongoing debate about this at present, which will continue as long as funding for the three services remains separate. Ideally, all three services should work together to help these unfortunate children and their parents.

In practice, unfortunately, the different helping services work in a haphazard way that varies widely from one geographical area to another, and in some areas there is a significant contribution from the voluntary sector (e.g. Homestart,[6.2] Newpin,[6.3] Parentline[6.4] or OPUS[6.5]). This means that there are sometimes gaps in service provision, sometimes overlaps, and sometimes a lack of clarity about where might be the best place for a child or family to be referred. It also means that, although a particular child's general practitioner is supposed to be kept informed by all of the professionals involved with that child, there may be agencies involved who do not consider it necessary or appropriate to inform the general practitioner. Parents may not think to mention their involvement unless they are specifically asked. Although this may be appropriate for interventions that are entirely school-based, or for services for adolescents where confidentiality is paramount, in other cases it can lead to interprofessional misunderstandings which may impair the overall package of help that is given to the child.

Children whose problems are presented to primary care deserve whatever help is available. Even if the main causes of pure behavioural problems are arguably social, children may have other associated problems, many of which could be regarded as meriting medical attention in their own right, such as a conductive deafness due to glue ear, biologically based learning difficulties, or attention-deficit hyperactivity disorder.

Antisocial behaviour can develop from a number of different causes,[2] as shown in Box 6.3. Often many of these causes act together for an individual child.

Box 6.3:   Risk factors for the development of antisocial behaviour

Child characteristics
Difficult temperament from birth. In the developmental history, ask about how the child fed, slept and cried in the first year
Attention-deficit hyperactivity disorder
Specific learning difficulty, especially reading delay, speech delay or language disorder
Genetic predisposition (e.g. parental criminality, attention-deficit hyperactivity disorder or impulse control problems)
Attributional bias – a tendency to perceive neutral acts by others as hostile

Immediate environment
Postnatal depression. This seems to be a common finding in the developmental history. It is related to difficult temperament in a chicken-and-egg way (the child's temperament may influence and in turn be influenced by the mother's mood)
Child-rearing practices. Antisocial behaviour is clearly linked to five factors:[3]
  • lack of positive reinforcement and warmth
  • lack of parental involvement
  • poor parental supervision and monitoring of the child's behaviour
  • harsh or inconsistent discipline, or hostility directed at the child
  • defective problem-solving
Parent–child interaction patterns. Studies of the moment-to-moment patterns of interaction in families of antisocial children show that children are inadvertently trained to persist with disruptive behaviour if:
  • it gets them more attention (even if it is angry or irritable attention) than pro-social behaviour
  • it means that they can get out of having to do something they do not want to do
  • it enables them to get their own way more often

continued opposite

Child abuse. All four forms of abuse can present with behaviour problems

Neglect: some children *have* to misbehave, in order to receive any attention

Physical abuse: children who are the victims of violence are likely to become either withdrawn and helpless or violent themselves, modelling their behaviour on that of their abuser

Emotional abuse: this is the most difficult to define, but it overlaps with some of the child-rearing practices and interaction patterns described above. *Domestic violence* is one example of emotional abuse which often goes unrecognised, and whose effects on children are often underestimated. For instance, a child may be very distressed by watching his mother being beaten up by his father, but may later copy this aggressive behaviour

Sexual abuse: this may lead to the emergence of behaviour problems in girls or boys who were previously free of such problems

Any losses that may be important for the child (e.g. an important father figure leaving home, moving house, moving schools, or the death of a pet)

Wider environment

School factors affect behaviour problems independently of home background, particularly if they are unfriendly, poorly organised, with low staff morale and poor communication between staff and parents

Wider social influences (e.g. overcrowding, poor housing, a lack of social support and a crime-ridden neighbourhood) are strongly associated with childhood antisocial behaviour. It is not clear whether this is all due to the immediate environmental factors discussed above, or whether they have an independent effect

Interviewing tips

Emphasising some of the less blaming factors can be a great help for parents, as they may feel more able to cope with something which they can join with you to 'fight against'. This is called *externalising the problem*. Examples include intermittent deafness causing frustration and leading to bad behaviour, a difficult start to life for both mother and child (from which they both took some time to recover), and being born with a difficult temperament. The danger is that the child will become even more scapegoated, so it is important to describe the problem in terms that make it clear that it is no-one's fault. You could say, for instance, how many parents with a first child who does not sleep, will not feed and cries all the time are scared to have another, but that if this is the second child, they realise how lucky they have been with the first one (*see* Chapter 4 on temperament).

Presenting the problem in a new light in this way is a form of *reframing* (*see* Chapter 7 on interviewing families). To give another example, if the child was being very disruptive during the interview, you could say how helpful this was in demonstrating the type of problem the parents had to cope with at home.

Another family therapy technique that can be very useful in brief interviews about children with behaviour problems is *looking for solutions rather than problems*. Finding out what the parents have done that works can be affirming for them, and may lead to the development of more solutions. It also avoids the undesirable situation of discussing everything the parent dislikes about the child in front of him.

Behavioural management principles

Common disciplinary strategies often fail because of the lack of a positive basis to the relationship between parent and child. One example of this is the *positive reinforcement trap*, which refers to the situation in which a parent neglects opportunities to praise good behaviour, and only pays attention to naughty behaviour (*see* Figure 6.1). The reprimands or punishments that are given for unwanted behaviour become rewarding to the child, so that the behaviours are maintained. For instance, if a child is ignored while he is playing quietly, but is told to shut up whenever he whines, he is more likely to go on whining than to be quiet.

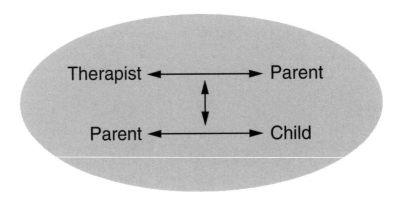

Figure 6.1:   The relationship between parent and adviser in behavioural techniques.

Another way in which unwanted behaviours are maintained is by the *negative reinforcement trap* (*see* Figure 6.2). Negative reinforcement refers to the rewarding of behaviour by omitting or ceasing a punishment or sanction. If a parent gives into a child's whining and abandons any attempt to set limits, then the child will be more likely to whine again. If a child gives in and stops attention-seeking behaviour only when their parent becomes really angry (shouting or hitting the child) then the child's reaction will negatively reinforce the parent's coercive behaviour.

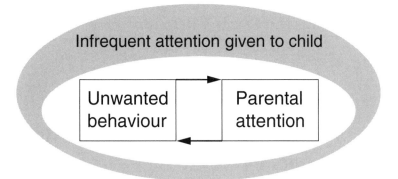

Figure 6.2: The positive reinforcement trap.

It can be quite an effort for some parents to establish a positive relationship with a difficult child. The health visitor may be ideally placed to facilitate this from an early age, by encouraging the parent(s) to make appropriate use of play, praise and other rewards. It is essential that the professional models with the parent the relationship that she hopes the parent will foster with the child (*see* Figure 6.3). If the professional points out only what the parent is doing wrong, this will mirror the parent's management of the child. Rather, the task for the professional is to emphasise all of the things that the parent is doing right, and to praise effusively any small improvement in this, or any attempts at new techniques, even if these are initially unsuccessful. This is surprisingly difficult to do – demonstrating how difficult it must be for parents who are unused to adopting this approach with their children.

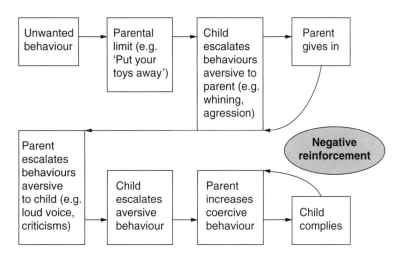

Figure 6.3: The negative reinforcement trap.

Below we shall present a practical approach to behaviour problems according to both age (pre-school, primary school and secondary school) and commonly presented problems. We have included all of the issues in one chapter, as many of the same principles can be applied to a variety of problems and across a wide age range.

Behaviour problems that are seen in pre-school and primary school children.

The commonest behaviours about which parents complain in pre-school children[4] are feeding and sleeping difficulties (which are dealt with in Chapters 18 and 19), hyperactivity (which is dealt with in Chapter 22) and tantrums and aggression, which are dealt with here. We shall also discuss sibling rivalry, which parents commonly find difficult to manage. Techniques that can be applied to non-compliance in general, and that are suitable for use by health visitors or others in the primary care team who are prepared to commit time to these problems, are described in Chapter 38.

Tantrums

Tantrums are a normal feature of development in the pre-school years. They are particularly likely to occur when the child is tired, ill, or feeling insecure or stressed in any other way. They become a problem when they are too frequent or too intense, or if the child is becoming old enough for the parents to feel concerned about their persistence.

Assessment

Assessment should be both specific (involving one or two recent examples) and general (thinking about background factors). There are several options for management, some of which are discussed again in a more general way in Chapter 38.

The most effective way of obtaining relevant details about recent examples of tantrums is to use the ABC mnemonic – **A**ntecedents, **B**ehaviour and **C**onsequences (*see* Table 6.1). This can also be used for almost any other behavioural problem.

Table 6.1:   An example of an ABC diary

Date, time and place	Antecedents	Behaviour	Consequences
Tesco's checkout, Friday, 11.00 a.m.	Being bored; seeing the sweets on the rack	Screaming, shouting, kicking	I was embarrassed – everyone was watching. I had to give in; then the screaming stopped

Start with B. What exactly constitutes a tantrum? Next establish C. Who does what, exactly, during and after a tantrum? If the parent says that she ignores the child, be sure to check on this. Exactly what does ignoring consist of? Finally, establish the nature of A. What were the immediate precipitants? These might include the parent having a tantrum or otherwise behaving unreasonably. Few parents will tell you this spontaneously or early in the consultation, so leave it until after you have established the behaviour and consequences, and then ask 'What exactly were you doing just before he started to shout?'.

The general assessment should consider the following points:

- the *general health of the child*, including pain or other discomfort, and fatigue (usually due to insufficient sleep). Has there been a head injury?
- *delayed language development* will lead the child to be frustrated by his inability to communicate his needs. Check that hearing has been adequately assessed
- *the child's mental age* – a child with developmental or intellectual delay will be slower to grow out of childish practices, and slower to learn tolerance, adequate communication or postponement of gratification
- *consistency of parental discipline* – parents who say one thing one day and do another the next, or who frequently disagree with each other, can breed muddled and irritated children
- *modelling* – a child who has witnessed older siblings or parents having a tantrum is more likely to maintain this behaviour, and less likely to learn alternative ways of resolving frustration or conflict
- *medications* – some medications can affect behaviour (e.g. anticonvulsants, nocturnal sedatives)
- *the mental state of the child* – is he distressed about bullying or domestic violence, or is he irritable or depressed for some reason?
- *does the parent have particular stresses* that are making child management more difficult?

A mnemonic for the above list is the eight Ds:

*d*iscomfort in child due to ill health
*d*elay in language
*d*evelopmental delay
*d*iscipline inconsistent or muddled
*d*isplay of tantrums by others
*d*rugs that may affect behaviour
*d*istress in child due to external pressures such as bullying or abuse
*d*istress in parent due to external pressures.

The assessment may provide some opportunities for giving advice. Management can be divided into the following three broad areas:

- avoiding provocation or dangerous antecedents (planning to minimise situations that make the child feel thwarted, or giving the child some distraction *before* this happens)

- teaching the child alternative strategies. Children need to have some way of responding to frustration and calming themselves down. One of the reasons why tantrums persist in some children is because they have not learned any other response. It could be helpful to discuss with the parents what they think this alternative response should be
- withdrawing attention which would reinforce the behaviour (ignoring or time out; *see* Chapter 38).

To take a simple example, consider a three-year-old boy who has a tantrum every time his mother takes him shopping. This is usually in the checkout queue of the supermarket, where there are enticing sweets displayed. He will not stop the tantrum until his mother gives in and buys him some sweets. This behaviour could be modified by changing the antecedents or consequences in the following ways:

- not taking him shopping
- going to a supermarket that does not have sweets at the checkout
- saying that he can have a limited number of sweets, and buying these *before* the tantrum begins
- *distracting* him from his desire for sweets by buying him something else, such as a comic, which is not so bad for his teeth
  (*these four strategies avoid provocative **A**ntecedents*)
- *praising* him profusely every time he manages to visit the supermarket without having an outburst, and possibly backing this up with tangible rewards
  (*this strategy teaches an alternative **B**ehaviour to cope with frustration*)
- *ignoring* the tantrum until it stops. This approach may be difficult if other people in the queue are watching critically (within a supermarket, withdrawing attention can be extremely difficult)
- putting the child in *time out* just outside the supermarket
  (*these two strategies are designed to limit the reinforcing **C**onsequences*).

Avoiding provocation includes manipulating the environment as much as possible in order to minimise temptations and frustrations. Examine the antecedents, and you may come up with specific ideas. For instance, some children may be particularly helped by forewarning of events that are known to produce tantrums, such as having to stop a favourite activity or go to bed.

Tuition in alternative ways of responding to frustration is very useful. If the child does not have a tantrum, what should he do instead? Discuss this with the parents in relation to the examples of tantrums elicited. If the answer is that he should comply with a parental command, then compliance must be rewarded with labelled praise (i.e. praise that specifies exactly what has been done well). A star chart or other reward system can be used for compliance with a particular type of command, such as getting ready for bed without making a fuss. Effective types of command, reward systems and other methods of improving compliance are also discussed in Chapter 38.

Many parents become discouraged when trying new techniques for managing a child's behaviour. They may find that the behaviour gets worse, and then give up the technique. It is helpful to warn parents that this is to be expected. An undesirable behaviour will usually become more frequent before it gets less frequent (the so-called '*extinction burst*'). For instance, the first time a parent tries to ignore a tantrum, it is likely to become louder or more desperate.

Withdrawing attention is the mainstay of management for many undesirable behaviours, tantrums included. The basic principle is that behaviours are maintained by the attention which they receive, so they will be extinguished when that attention is removed. This is likely to be more effective if attention is given to reward desired behaviour (something that many parents forget to do). There is nothing wrong with the traditional advice to ignore a tantrum – it is just very difficult to put into practice. Simply suggesting it is not enough.

There are three ways to withdraw attention – the parent can remove herself, she can stay in the same place but attend exclusively to something else (ignoring), or she can remove the child to an environment that is completely unstimulating (time out). It is not always possible to leave the child alone (e.g. if the parent is cooking), nor can dangerous behaviours (e.g. beating up a baby sibling) be ignored. It is also important to develop a positive relationship with the child, (e.g. by play), and to get into the habit of praising and rewarding whenever possible. Play, praise, rewards, ignoring and time out are all discussed in more detail in Chapter 38.

Parents need continuing encouragement to make behavioural techniques work. Frequent appointments and home visits may be necessary, and a diary in the form of the above ABC chart may be helpful.

Referral

When should a referral be made? Much depends on the local service. In a district with well-organised child mental health provision, health visitors should receive regular training in dealing with behavioural problems, which should also provide opportunities for consultation. There will then be very few pre-school behaviour problems that require referral. Children with tantrums may need referral if there are concerns about the underlying mental state of the child, if family issues are thought to require detailed discussion, or if appropriate behavioural management (with motivated parents) has failed to alter the behaviour. There is no age above which tantrums should be referred. In the case of older children much depends on the associated problems. The older the child, the fewer opportunities there are for behavioural change.

Box 6.4:   Practice points for managing tantrums

- As well as details of the behaviour, find out about the antecedents and consequences (ABC).
- Assess the possible background factors.
- Try either:
  avoiding provocative *antecedents*
  teaching alternative *behaviours* or
  withdrawing attention or other reinforcing *consequences*.

Aggression

The causes of aggression are multiple, and it may be worth remembering the following points.

- Aggressive responses can be *learned* by modelling (e.g. witnessing a violent parent), by being rewarded for aggressive behaviours by parents (e.g. by a father who believes that fighting is the best way to deal with any conflict with peers) or by finding that aggression works as a way of resolving conflict.
- Aggressive responses are *primitive*, and are likely to be used when the child has no alternative strategies. Therefore they are common in younger children and in those who have not been taught alternative ways of dealing with provocation. It also means that there are opportunities to teach more sociable responses.
- Aggressive behaviours are often *an expression of feelings* which may be difficult to express in other ways (e.g. anger, irritability, resentment, grief or sadness). Feeling threatened or provoked may also lead to aggression, so the latter is a common end-point to a variety of situations.
- Aggression is a remarkably *stable* characteristic of behaviour. Once established as a general way of coping, it does not usually go away. Thus reassurance that it will subside in time is likely to be misleading.

Assessment

As with many other psychological disorders, several factors may be responsible for an excessively aggressive child. A family in which the parents demonstrate aggression in personal relationships (e.g. with rows, harsh physical punishments or verbal threats) may also be a family in which problem-solving is limited, so that self-restraint or negotiation are not options. Aggression may arise out of a combination of learned unacceptable responses and a failure to learn acceptable ones.

On being given a parental complaint about a child's aggressive behaviour, it is important to review the general factors mentioned under tantrums, such as the child's medical status, mental state and intellectual abilities. There should also always be a specific enquiry about bullying, as many bullied children retaliate aggressively and get into trouble for continuing a fight initiated by someone else.

The state of the family is also important. Is a preferred sibling getting a better deal? Is the problem mainly a relationship with a step-parent? Is one of the parents stressed or unwell? Marital violence is a potent progenitor of aggressive behaviour in children, particularly in a son. Such a child may have witnessed behaviour that he then copies, he may have a genetic predisposition, and he may have a whole host of unresolved feelings about his parents' relationship.

An ABC analysis may be helpful in highlighting unreasonable or unrecognised provocation, and unwitting encouragement from others.

Management

The assessment may provide opportunities for straightforward advice. Beyond this, it may be necessary to see both parents and:

- put forward the view that aggression indicates a *deficiency state*. Alternative and more mature ways of coping have not been learned sufficiently well
- advise parents to tell their child when he is behaving aggressively (*labelling*), and what else he could be doing which is acceptable (*identifying desired alternatives*)
- suggest to them that they should demonstrate through their own actions and interactions how problems between people can be resolved without aggression
- teach them some of the techniques described in Chapter 38, such as rewarding prosocial actions with labelled praise or a points systems, or using time out.

When to refer

If a child with aggressive behaviour is going to be referred, this should be done earlier rather than later. Aggressive behaviour can easily become habitual, and at present there is little that can be done in the UK for children over eight years of age whose aggression is long-standing. Pre-school children are much more likely to change their habits, and children with behaviour problems at school should receive help when the problem is first recognised, not when they are on the verge of permanent exclusion.

Pressure on tier 2 (single specialist) and tier 3 (multidisciplinary team) services has led some of these services to refuse to see children with behaviour problems altogether. This puts the onus on social services and primary care to help parents and schools deal with their anxieties about children whose aggression is causing problems at home or at school. What can be done in primary care to help such children and their families? Some of the above principles can be applied in primary care. Parents can be encouraged to ask for help from social services, although in many areas this will not be available unless there are clear risks to the children. Alternatively, parents can simply be told that there is no help available, and advised to complain to their local councillor or member of parliament. Unfortunately, it is often the families who are most in need of help who are least able to complain effectively.

In areas where there is a child mental health service for children with behaviour problems, care should be taken with regard to the way in which a referral is made. Referral will be worthwhile if the parents either want the child to talk to someone outside the family, or want to discuss what goes on between family members with a professional. If they just want the child to receive a good telling off, then a referral is unlikely to achieve very much. As with other referrals, it is important to give the family an idea of what can be expected of the local service, and to clarify whether this is what they want. In the case of behavioural problems it is particularly important not to raise unrealistic expectations, and to emphasise that the longer the habits have been present, the less easy it will be to alter them.

Primary school children are often brought to the family's general practitioner because of a problem at school. Frequently such problems may include an element of aggressive behaviour. There is little point in referring to a child and family service unless the parents believe that there is something they could do differently at home that would improve the child's behaviour at school. If the parents acknowledge only a school problem, then it might be more constructive to support them in pressurising the school to allow the educational psychologist to see the child. (In most education authorities, the referral path to the educational psychology service is now solely via schools, and there is no longer a referral route from other services.)

Case study 6.1

Vicki, a 22-year-old single parent, brought her three-year-old son Morgan to afternoon surgery, complaining to the doctor that Morgan would not do anything that she told him, and that he screamed and kicked when he could not get his own way. She was becoming afraid to take him anywhere, so was going out of the house less and less. The doctor's ability to listen to the history was threatened by Morgan's behaviour, as he moved from one part of the surgery to another, knocking things from the desk on to the floor, and throwing out all the toys from the toy box in the corner of the room.

The general practitioner was aware that Vicki had had a difficult pregnancy and a prolonged labour, requiring forceps because of a slow fetal heart rate. Morgan had always been a difficult child to feed, and he woke frequently at night. He had had a series of upper respiratory tract infections recorded in the notes, and the doctor noted that he had failed his first hearing test, but had passed the second one.

The doctor tried her usual approach of holding out her arms to Morgan, who responded by coming and standing in front of her. The doctor was able to examine him whilst talking to him and smiling at him frequently. The examination revealed signs of glue ear on both sides, and the doctor explained to Vicki that part of Morgan's behaviour might be due to his being deaf. She explained carefully that Vicki would need to be sure that Morgan had heard her before she should assume that he was just being naughty. The doctor referred Morgan for a hearing test, and she also asked the health visitor to call in order to discuss with Vicki strategies for dealing with Morgan's difficult behaviour.

continued opposite

At follow-up four weeks later, Vicki and Morgan were attending a mother and toddler group two afternoons each week, and Morgan was going to a play group for three mornings each week. However, his behaviour at home seemed to be no better. The doctor examined his ears, which appeared to be quite normal on this occasion. Vicki was still very concerned that something should be done about Morgan's behaviour. She explained that the health visitor had advised her to ignore him, but that she found this impossible in a small flat on her own. She often ended up smacking Morgan, and subsequently feeling guilty about this.

The doctor asked Vicki what types of games Morgan liked to play, but Vicki said that he just tended to sit and watch television until bedtime. Vicki had had some discussions with the health visitor about how to play with Morgan, but she had found it very difficult to put into practice, because no one had ever played with her when she was a child as far as she could remember.

The general practitioner began to explore other ways of tackling difficult behaviour, including giving praise, or alternatively trying some form of time out. She did not get very far with this exploration before Vicki burst into tears and said that she really could not tolerate the situation any more. She was sleeping poorly, had lost her appetite and was almost suicidal at times. The doctor decided to offer her treatment for depression, and advised her that she would discuss with the health visitor a possible referral to the child psychiatry out-patient department.

Box 6.5:   Practice points for managing aggression

- Discuss examples of the aggressive behaviour.
- Do an ABC analysis.
- Consider what feelings the aggression might be expressing.
- Whose behaviour might it be copying?
- Ask the parents to deal with aggression calmly.
- Advise the parents to reward alternative behaviours.
- For out-of-control aggression, encourage the use of time out.
- For situations that give rise to aggression, encourage problem-solving.

Sibling rivalry

This should be considered from a *developmental perspective*. The birth of a younger sibling is bound to give rise to feelings of jealousy, particularly in the first child, as the older sibling(s) have to share parental attention as well as material things such as living space and toys. Grandparents may show an excessive interest in the new arrival, and the parents may be preoccupied or exhausted. There is scope for some preventive work here.

Before the birth, siblings can be involved actively in preparations, given a doll to care for themselves, and made to feel special.

After the birth, the parents must ensure that they are devoting attention to the older children as well as to the baby. If gifts are bought for the baby, the older child (or children) must be given presents as well. Older children can be involved in baby care, such as unfolding nappies, choosing clothes, brushing hair and other safe tasks that can be supervised easily. This gives each older child an active role in the newly enlarged family. When the baby starts to smile, the parents can emphasise to the older child that she is smiling at him. The father may sometimes become more distant after the birth of a second child, and it should be pointed out how important his involvement is for his children.

It is often *later on*, once the baby is crawling or walking and breaking or taking toys, that rivalry begins in earnest. Learning how to cope with disagreement is a necessary developmental task, and may be sorely lacking in only children. Positive outcomes include becoming assertive, expressing feelings and learning how to resolve conflict. Mild teasing by an older sibling may not only be a playful way of communicating affection, but it can also teach strategies for coping with more hurtful teasing at school. As conflict becomes more severe, the parents must decide at what level they will refuse to tolerate abuse of younger siblings (whether physical or emotional).

Assessment

Consider the factors that contribute to conflict between members of a sibling pair.

- Rivalry tends to be greatest between two children of the same sex.
- Do the parents have favourites? Sometimes the older child has been labelled as difficult or hyperactive, leading to dislike or rejection by the parents (which they disown), so that the younger child has to act this out.
- Is the younger child receiving more attention because they are more dependent? Older children seldom accept this as an explanation from the parents, but instead feel that they are being short-changed:

Sarah: Mummy, Daniel hit me!
Daniel: She started it. She borrowed my game without asking.
Mother: Daniel, don't be cruel to your little sister.
Daniel: You always take her side!

- An older child who is developmentally delayed, or even just academically less able, will deeply resent a younger sibling who catches up with them.
- Are the fights between the children a mimicry of fights between the parents, or an overt expression of conflicts that the parents think they have kept concealed? Such children may also fight in an attempt to divert their parents from marital problems. They may hope (not necessarily consciously) that their own misbehaviour will force their parents to be closer to one another.

Management

Research using concealed video cameras has shown that siblings who fight generally do not do so if they think there is no one watching or within earshot (Mark Dadds, behavioural family therapist, personal communication). The implication of this is that *ignoring* will work if it is applied with sufficient persistence. As discussed in Chapter 38, it can be extraordinarily difficult to ignore effectively. It may sometimes be enough for the parents simply to say 'Settle it yourselves'. More often, a parent will have to completely remove him- or herself.

It is particularly important *not to take sides*. Whatever a parent does must be seen as even-handed. For instance, time out or consequences (*see* Chapter 38) can be used for fights that parents consider are excessive, but they should be applied equally to both children. Parents should avoid expressing favouritism, and they can allow for differences in age or skills by emphasising the particular strengths of each child. They should steer clear of comparisons in which one child comes off worse than the other (e.g. 'I wish you would keep your room as tidy as your sister' or 'Please try a little harder with your reading – your brother could do this when he was your age').

Parents can use sibling fights as an opportunity to teach problem-solving. For instance, a parent could show her squabbling children two puppets who are fighting over a toy, or say that one of them wants to use a toy that the other will not let him have. She could then guide her children in generating possible solutions to the dilemma, and discuss the consequences of each solution. With school-age children, a family meeting can be a useful opportunity to explore solutions to conflicts between two family members. This could take place at a regular time each week.

When to refer

Sibling quarrels are a normal and healthy phenomenon. Most parents who present them as a problem can be helped to view them as a developmental challenge and as an opportunity for learning interpersonal skills, as suggested above. In some cases, fights between siblings may be part of a broader behavioural problem, in which case referral to a child and family service may be justified. In other cases, children may be at risk of significant abuse from their siblings, in which case Social Services should be involved. A further possibility is that difficulties in the parents' relationship are at the heart of the problem, in which case relationship guidance counselling should be suggested.

Box 6.6:   Practice points for managing sibling rivalry

- Describe how a certain amount of quarrelling helps to develop skills.
- How did the problem develop?
- Is there a favourite?
- Are there differences in ability?   *continued overleaf*

- Is there marital conflict?
- How are the parents dealing with the conflict? Does this calm the situation or fan the flames?
- Advise ignoring if no one is coming to harm.
- Advise time out or consequences if someone is getting hurt.
- Is there scope for problem-solving when the situation is calm?

Specific issues for young people at secondary school (11–18 years)

Stealing

Why do parents sometimes seek medical advice about the fact that their child is stealing? Perhaps they have been pressurised by others to go to the doctor, or perhaps they have found that nothing else they have tried works, and they are therefore desperate to obtain some help from outside the family.

Assessment

There are six patterns of theft.

- *Marauding.* A group of children or young teenagers go shoplifting together, or raid unattended premises. This is essentially a recreational activity, on a par with group truancy, trespassing or vandalism. There is seldom anything wrong with the children or their families except for the fact that they are poorly supervised.
- *Proving.* A teenager steals something that can be exhibited to friends and elicit their admiration. Such an activity is usually fuelled by low self-esteem or difficulties with peer relationships. Something has to be done to enhance prestige within the group, and to help to establish some self-worth. Low self-esteem of the type that leads to such behaviour may be due to a number of factors, including family scapegoating (*see* Chapters 2 and 4), poor academic ability, clumsiness, short stature, delayed puberty and previous head injury.
- *Comforting.* A child steals money from home as a way of compensating for a lack of parental attention, approval or love. The money may be hoarded or spent privately. This may be combined with partial recognition that the theft is a way of paying the parents back for not providing adequate nurturing. It is an indicator of a poor relationship between parents and child, and of itself does nothing to improve this. When seen professionally, the parents of such children are often on the point of rejecting the child altogether.

Solitary theft outside the home, with hoarding of the booty, is comparable. A child who steals from other children at school may be expressing a similar need for personal comfort in the face of hostility or rejection by other children. Teenage girls who steal babies or pets are commonly looking for something to look after in order to compensate for feeling uncared for themselves (some may decide to have their own child for this reason); a few of them may be compensating for a recent termination of pregnancy.

An apparent 'hybrid' between proving and comforting occurs when the child steals money from home, and then uses it to purchase sweets that can be handed round at school in order to 'buy' friendship.

- *Secondary.* Some children steal because they receive insufficient pocket money, they have been directly instructed to steal by parents, to pay off a bully, or out of necessity while running away from home.
- *Addiction.* Stealing can become necessary to finance an addiction (e.g. to street drugs, volatile substances or arcade machines).
- *Depression.* Stealing may be driven by a desire to alleviate depressive feelings, either by helping oneself to a present, or by the thrill of the act itself.

Management

Does the stealing fall into the *secondary* category described above? If it is prompted by a straightforward motive such as greed or parental instruction, then there is no need to become involved.

Is there any reason to believe that the child may be *depressed* or *addicted*? Depression will need treatment, which could be provided in primary care. Addiction is only treatable if there is some motivation to change, which is rare in teenagers, but the threat of court proceedings for the stealing can be useful. Cases of addiction to substances (*see* Chapter 37) could be referred to a drugs rehabilitation service. Cases of addiction to gambling or arcade games could be referred to a psychologist.

Otherwise, the key issue is whether the theft took place inside or outside the home. *Marauding* theft is of no medical interest, but the parents can usefully be advised to increase their supervision of the child. They should know where he is and with whom all the time.

From a management point of view, solitary theft outside the home can be divided into two categories. If the goods are hoarded, it should be treated as *comforting*. If they are shown to others or given away, a *proving* motive should be assumed in the first instance. The latter can be managed by counselling and/or social skills training. Local resources for this type of resource vary, but the primary care counsellor, youth clubs, a school counsellor or a child psychologist are all possibilities.

Stealing from home is likely to be *comforting*, but it is necessary to check first if the child is receiving enough pocket money. Comforting stealing is difficult to treat, and referral to a multidisciplinary team is probably necessary. If this is likely to involve a long wait, a sensible first move is to advise the parents to lock money and valuables away in a secure place (they are often curiously reluctant to do so, citing the need for trust). They should then find ways of building up their approval of the child (*see* the sections on *praise* and *tangible rewards* in Chapter 38).

Box 6.7:   Practice points for managing stealing – including when to refer

- Is the stealing secondary? If so, you can do nothing to help.
- Is the child using street drugs in a potentially addictive way, or obsessed by arcade games? If so, tackle this problem (*see* Chapter 37).
- Is the child depressed? If so, provide treatment for this (*see* Chapter 33).
- Is the child marauding? If so, insist that the parents provide more supervision.
- Is the child proving? If so, clarify any underlying cause of low self-esteem, and encourage the parents to bolster the child's self-image and arrange after-school activities. You may or may not need to involve other services.
- Is the child comforting? This will probably need referral, provided that the parents agree, to a multidisciplinary (tier 3) service.

Delinquency

The definition of a *juvenile delinquent* in the UK is a person between the ages of 10 and 17 years inclusive who has committed an offence that would be regarded as criminal in an adult. Thus the definition is legal and not directly related to mental health.

In simple terms, there are two categories of delinquent:

- those whose conduct disorder has started in early or middle childhood, and whose offending tends to persist beyond adolescence
- those whose offending starts and ends in adolescence.

There is little need to do anything for the second group, who could merely be regarded as experimenting and rebelling, usually with few harmful consequences. The first group constitute a major public health problem, not only because of their offending itself, but also because of the other problems this group often experiences (e.g. special educational needs, a high proportion of care away from their family, and a variety of psychiatric disorders). The public cost they incur comes mainly from budgets other than health, such as Social Services, education and the criminal justice system.

What is the role of the primary care team in delinquency? Probably the most important role is in the prevention of delinquency at an early stage by improving the parenting skills of mothers of under-fives. Once delinquency is established, there is little that the health service can do, as no effective therapeutic interventions are yet available in the UK. The most that the general practitioner can do in these circumstances is to support the parents.

However, there is a treatment package available in the USA specifically for offending teenagers and their families. Since this could well become available in the UK during the shelf-life of this book, and as general practitioners are playing an increasing role in the setting of priorities in the health service, it is worth mentioning here.

Box 6.8:   Components of multisystemic therapy

Family therapy that focuses on effective communication, systematic reward and punishment systems, and taking a problem-solving approach to day-to-day conflicts.
Encouragement to spend more time with peers who do not have problems, and to stop seeing other delinquents.
Liaison with school to improve learning and homework performance, and to restructure after-school hours.
Individual development, including assertiveness training to protect against negative peer influences.
Empowerment of young people and their parents to cope with family, school, peer and neighbourhood problems. The emphasis is on promoting the family's own problem-solving abilities, not on providing ready-made answers.
Co-ordination with other agencies, such as juvenile justice, Social Services and education.

'*Multisystemic therapy*', as its name implies, addresses the various systems or contexts in which the adolescent's behaviour occurs, including the family, school, peer group, the adolescent's own internal world, and any other agencies involved. A summary[2] of the elements of this package is shown in Box 6.8. Although it is very labour-intensive, with each therapist having only a small caseload and requiring extensive training and supervision, multisystemic therapy has been shown to be cost-effective, as it saves some of the money that would otherwise be spent in the courts, on institutional care and on fostering.

Referral

In the UK, it is currently difficult to obtain effective help for adolescents who present with behaviour as their main problem. Adolescent mental health services and Social Services have patchy provision, and in many parts of the country they provide little of substance for this group. Where there are well-developed adolescent services, adolescents may refer themselves, or be referred by other agencies, thus bypassing the general practitioner altogether.

Thus in primary care referral may not always be a very constructive option. In these circumstances, it is important to look hard for *treatable aspects* of the problem. These include mood disturbances, specific learning disabilities such as dyslexia, and the consequences of parental separation.

The most important treatable aspect in the 11–18 years age range is probably *depression*, which may be concealed beneath a range of behaviours that concern everyone. Many adolescents are difficult to interview, and may not give a sufficiently coherent account to enable a clear diagnosis of depressive disorder (*see* Chapter 33). In these circumstances, particularly if there has been a recent loss (e.g. departure of an important father figure, or death of a favourite grandmother) or a recent deterioration in functioning, it may be worth suggesting to the adolescent and their parents a therapeutic trial of antidepressants. These have been shown to improve behaviour problems as well as mood disorder when these coexist. Antidepressants may be given as well as or instead of a referral.

Box 6.9:   Practice points for cases of delinquency

- Adolescent-onset criminal activity can be regarded as experimental, and has a good prognosis.
- Delinquency leading on from pre-adolescent behaviour problems has a poor prognosis, and may lead to adult criminality or even antisocial personality disorder.
- In many cases, there may be no local services that can effectively help the adolescent or his family. It is nevertheless worth conducting a minimal assessment in primary care, to look for treatable components, before concluding that nothing can be done.
- If there is any suggestion of a depressive disorder, which is difficult to diagnose in this group, a trial of antidepressants should be offered.

Box 6.10:   Practice points for cases of conduct disorder

- The easiest time to intervene is when the child is between 3 and 8 years of age.
- The most effective intervention in primary care is an intensive input for mothers of pre-school children.
- In primary school children with disruptive behaviour, consider the following:
  attention-deficit hyperactivity disorder
  specific learning difficulties
  bullying
  abuse
  conflict within the family.
- In secondary school children with disruptive behaviour, consider all of the above factors, but also especially depression.

Notes

6.1   Both boxes are adapted from a combination of ICD-10 (World Health Organisation (1993) *The ICD-10 Classification of Mental and Behavioural Disorders: Diagnostic Criteria for Research.*

World Health Organization, Geneva) and DSM-IV (American Psychiatric Association (1994) *Diagnostic and Statistical Manual of Mental Disorders*. American Psychiatric Association, Washington, DC). The conduct disorder behaviours are sorted roughly in the order in which they most commonly present.

6.2   Homestart UK, 2 Salisbury Road, Leicester LE1 7OR. Tel 0116 233 9955.

6.3   National Newpin, Sutherland House, 35 Sutherland Square, Walworth, London SE17 3EE. Tel 0171 703 6326.

6.4   Parentline, Endway House, The Endway, Hadleigh, Benfleet SS7 2AN. Helpline 01702 559900. Tel 01702 554782. Fax 01702 554911.

6.5   Organisation for Parents Under Stress (OPUS), Rayta House, 57 Hart Road, Thundersley, Essex S57 3PD. Tel 01268 757077.

References

1   Spender Q and Scott S (1997) Management of antisocial behaviour in childhood. *Adv Psychiatr Treat.* **3**: 128–37.

2   Goodman R and Scott S (1997) *Child Psychiatry*. Blackwell Science, Oxford.

3   Patterson GR, Reid JB and Dishion TJ (1992) *Antisocial Boys*. Castalia, Eugene, Oregon.

4   Hall D, Hill P and Elliman D (1999) *The Child Surveillance Handbook* (2e). Radcliffe Medical Press, Oxford.

CHAPTER SEVEN

Family issues

This chapter, rather than focusing on a particular clinical problem and its management, examines theoretical perspectives that may be helpful for improving understanding of families. We shall try to focus as much as possible on the practical relevance of these concepts. We start with an outline of family therapy, then discuss attachment theory, and finally examine what happens when care within the family is not the best option. The consequences of parental separation are examined in Chapter 8.

Systems theory and general practice

Introduction

Families provide a powerful learning environment for children and adolescents, who in turn both influence the family with their attitudes and behaviour, and are influenced by it. Many of the ideas in family therapy are rather different to those in the rest of medicine. Key concepts include the following.

Systems theory

Family therapy is based on the idea that the family is a *system*. Just as a human being is a collection of cells held together by mutual benefit and the need for homeostasis, so a family is a collection of individuals held together by shared attitudes, beliefs and cultural practices, power differentials between different members, its own style of problem-solving, and some degree of resistance to change (homeostasis). Systems theory can equally be applied to groups of professionals, such as the primary care team.

Circular causality

Linear causality can be symbolised as follows:

$$X \qquad \rightarrow \qquad Y \qquad \rightarrow \qquad Z$$

where X might be liver cancer, Y a brain secondary and Z the sudden onset of blindness. In contrast, circular causality can be symbolised as follows:

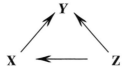

An example of circular causality might be a toddler whose mother is preoccupied with her own concerns. When the toddler behaves badly (X), the mother becomes angry and shouts (Y). Because the child does not receive any other type of attention, he finds this rewarding (Z) (*see* Figure 6.2: the positive reinforcement trap, in Chapter 6). This therefore encourages him to be naughty again at the next opportunity. The same patterns of behaviour can be described in behavioural language. The mother's shouting form of attention (Y) provides positive reinforcement (Z) for the child's bad behaviour (X), which then in turn provokes more shouting (Y).

Hypotheses

A systemic view of a symptom is that it serves a useful function for the family. For instance, a child may become ill in order to draw the parents together. Hypotheses are reviewed and redefined during the course of getting to know a family.

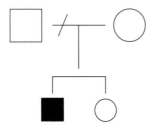

Figure 7.1:   A child of separated parents may be defined by them as having the problem.

In the example shown in Figure 7.1, the child's difficult behaviour may be seen as functioning to bring his estranged parents together. If they can be brought together more effectively to discuss how best to meet his needs, he may no longer need to behave badly.

Boundaries and hierarchy

Boundaries are the invisible lines between different subsystems, most importantly between parents on the one hand and their children on the other. A well-functioning family has clear demarcations between the roles of different members, and effective channels of communication. Problems may arise when, for example, a mother is closer to her child than to her partner, or when a parent is ill and an older child assumes responsibility for the younger children. The hierarchy in the family is the answer to the question 'Who has the power?'. Ideally, this should be shared between the parents, who act together. Problems may arise if a child has too much power (either real or perceived). An example of this would be a child whose behaviour no one will control, or whose illness or disability governs all of the family's actions.

Life cycle challenges

Different stages of life present different challenges. It helps to have a developmental view of this in order to understand what different family members may be going through at different life stages (*see* Box 7.1).

Box 7.1:   Challenges at different stages of the life cycle

Birth and infancy	Parents must make space in their relationship for new individuals, develop a new co-operative relationship to cope with child-rearing, and realign with the extended family, particularly grandparents
First school	The main caregiver and the child have to cope with separation, the child has to develop social relationships, and both child and parent have to cope with being compared with other children and parents
Adolescence	Both parents and offspring have to balance freedom and dependence, the adolescent has to develop a sense of identity (in opposition as well as in alignment to parents), the parents may have to cope with career changes and changes in their relationship, and possibly having to look after their elderly parents
Leaving home	Young people have to cope with the demands of higher education or getting a job and finding somewhere to live, and they need to develop more of an adult-to-adult relationship with their parents. Parents have to cope with being alone again, possible work-role, financial or physiological decline, and perhaps becoming grandparents themselves
Cohabiting	Young people have to form a co-operative relationship between two people, deal together with financial needs and household tasks, and realign relationships with friends and family

---

Life cycle challenges can also be illustrated diagramatically (*see* Figure 7.2).

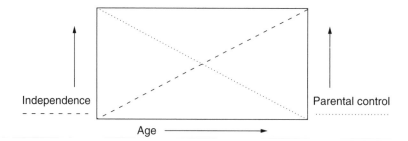

Figure 7.2: A delicate balance: parental control can gradually be relaxed as independence gradually increases.

Types of family therapy

All family therapists share certain techniques, such as drawing a genogram (family tree), joining with the family in a variety of ways (different techniques may be used for the children and the parents) and exploring the nature of differences between family members. There are three main schools of family therapy, namely *structural* (which is probably most akin to traditional medical ways of thinking), *Milan systemic* and *strategic*. However, concepts continue to evolve, and consequently new techniques are appearing all the time.

The basis of *structural* family therapy is a focus on the nature of family relationships in the here and now. How close or distant are family members in relation to each other? Are boundaries too weak or children too closely involved (enmeshed)? For example, a child who has to stay at home with his anxious and overprotective mother is at risk of developing school refusal. The therapist may reinforce a relationship or boundary that needs strengthening, (e.g. by involving a father more in supporting the mother's authority, or by setting tasks that demonstrate the authority of the parental subsystem).

In *Milan systemic* therapy, the focus is more on the beliefs held by the family and the meanings that they attribute to any symptom or behaviour. Changing these may alter the behaviour or the ways of dealing with it. For example, a child's bad behaviour may be explained as his taking after an uncle who went to prison, which may prevent anyone taking his behaviour in hand, since they believe that this is 'just the way he is'. Key techniques in this school of therapy include hypothesising (see above), circular questioning and reframing. *Circular questioning* involves asking one member of a family to give a view on another member's thoughts and feelings, such as 'What do you think everyone else in the family thinks is wrong with you?' or 'Who worries most when you are ill?'. *Reframing* involves phrasing things in a way that helps family members to see them differently. For instance, a hypochondriac is seen as someone who is good at being in touch with his bodily sensations, and a child who stays at home rather than going to school may be framed as caring a lot about his mother and not wanting to leave her alone.

Strategic therapy is now mainly solution-focused. This involves examining approaches that have been tried and that work, and looking at the exceptions to the family's story of gloom, rather than focusing exclusively on everything that is wrong. For instance, the parents of a child who never does what he is told can be asked to think of occasions when he has complied with a request, and a depressed teenager can be asked what still makes her happy. The miracle question is 'What would it be like if you woke up tomorrow morning and the problem was gone – how would things be different?'. This helps to engender a new freedom of thought, which can lead to possibilities no one had previously considered.

Relevance of family therapy

Family therapy has been shown to be effective in a number of randomised controlled trials (e.g. in poorly controlled asthma and anorexia nervosa). Can it be used in primary care? Some practices employ family therapists to conduct evening sessions with self-selected families. If this facility is unavailable in your practice, and you consider that family therapy is necessary, then you will have to make a referral to a specialist service. Most services will want to undertake their own assessment before deciding whether to commit to such an expensive resource.

More important than employing specially trained professionals to see a small number of families is to develop a systematic perspective in dealing with all of the families you see, and also in dealing with professional organisations, including your own. For instance, a useful question to ask yourself of any symptom in a child is 'What function is this symptom serving for this family?'. Another appropriate question is 'What life-cycle stage is contributing to this symptom?'. Reframing can also be useful. If a child is wrecking the surgery, try saying something like 'Well, he's being very helpful in showing me what sort of difficulties you must have with him at home.'

Box 7.2:   Practical applications of family therapy ideas in primary care

For any illness, think about its *function* for the family, as well as its *cause*.

Think about repeated patterns of interaction, rather than one person causing another's behaviour. For instance, a mother's behaviour towards her difficult child will be as much effect as cause.

Does the parental subsystem need to be strengthened? If so, seeing both parents together may be invaluable.

Try to find opportunities to reframe things positively, while still paying attention to feelings. For instance, of a teenager who is depressed after her grandmother's death you could say 'She's doing a good job of showing how sad you all are'.

Try thinking about the power imbalances, subsystems and boundaries within the primary care team. This can be particularly useful when you are caught in the trap of thinking that interprofessional problems are due to personalities.

Attachment theory

John Bowlby (1907–1990), child psychiatrist and psychoanalyst, was the first to describe the importance of attachment in human development. His interest in ethology (the study of animal behaviour) led to his theory that human children, like young animals, have a need for a figure who provides a source of safety, comfort and protection.

Bowlby's early research focused on the effect of separation on young children in residential care and hospital. In the 1940s and 1950s, parental visiting was extremely restricted and sometimes forbidden in hospitals, because of the belief that contact with the parents would upset the child. Bowlby and two other researchers, James and Joyce Robertson, filmed young children over periods of separation lasting a week or more, and demonstrated that the children were highly distressed by the experience. (Such research could not be conducted now, for ethical reasons.) The results may seem obvious today, but they were revolutionary at the time. These researchers observed that during lengthy separations the child went through three stages of response. First, he *protested* at the mother's absence, usually by crying. After a few days he became withdrawn, often refusing to eat or play, and seemed to *despair.* After several more days, *detachment* set in, so that the child began to eat and play again and appeared not to react if the mother returned. Before this stage, the child might react by clinging and being upset if the mother returned. Bowlby's legacy is summarised in Box 7.3.

Box 7.3:   The main points of Bowlby's theory of attachment

Human beings have a need for attachment to specific others throughout the life cycle.

During the second half of the first year of life, specific attachment behaviours develop, namely clinging to and following of the attachment figure.

Unwilling separation from an attachment figure leads to emotional distress.

In young children this distress is manifested as protest, despair and detachment.

Loss of an attachment figure in adults leads to a grief reaction, with shock and anger followed by numbness and finally acceptance and reorganisation.

The clinical relevance of attachment

A more ethical experiment can be performed with one-year-old children and their caregivers. The child is left alone with a stranger for three minutes, and then the nature of their behaviour on reunion with the caregiver can be categorised as either secure (about 60% of cases) or insecure (about 40% of cases). Secure children are likely to be pleased to see their caregiver again, and will seek comfort in a smile or touch, and then return to play. Insecure children will either become clingy and angry, or completely avoid the caregiver after her return, or alternate between the two behaviours. Insecure attachment should be regarded as part of the range of normality.

Securely attached children are better (in general) at forging relationships with children and adults than are insecurely attached children. For instance, they are more likely to be able to ask a teacher for help when there is something which they cannot deal with in the classroom. They are also more able to cope with separations from parents, such as staying overnight with friends and the first day at school, presumably because they are confident that their parents will still be there for them (both physically and emotionally).

Insecurely attached children are more clingy, which can provoke more rejection from their caregiver. They are also less empathic, more non-compliant, more likely to fight with siblings, and more likely to be either the victim or the perpetrator of bullying. Insecure attachment in infancy has been linked to school refusal, low self-esteem and anxiety disorders in later life.

Attachment behaviours, such as clinging to or following the caregiver, are biologically important because the infant's survival may depend on staying close to the caregiver. They are also psychologically important, as they provide the foundation for emotional and social relating. They are apparent from about six months of age, usually reaching a peak between two and three years, and then gradually subsiding with increasing maturity. Older children may display such behaviours when under stress (regression). They are more likely to occur, at any age, in the presence of illness, tiredness or anxiety. They can be regarded as signs of *separation anxiety*, but it is important to remember that this is a normal phenomenon. One way in which children manage their anxiety is by having a *transitional object*. This is a favourite blanket, cuddly toy or some other object which can be used as a substitute for the mother, and which becomes emotionally invested with the same comforting qualities. Another normal behaviour that may be observed during a consultation is *stranger anxiety*, which refers to shyness and wariness towards strange people, and is often associated with an increase in the other attachment behaviours.

Some children with autistic disorders (*see* Chapter 5) do not display ordinary attachment behaviours. Lack of attachment to people is a feature of these disorders, sometimes associated with an attachment to an inanimate object (e.g. Thomas the Tank Engine).

An *attachment disorder* is defined as a failure to make specific attachments, associated *either* with a complete lack of interest in initiating or responding to other children and adults, *or* with indiscriminate but superficial attachment to any adults who are encountered. There may be many features identical to attention-deficit hyperactivity disorder. There may also be aggressive behaviour, defiance and ambivalent feelings towards adults (i.e. needing love but showing hate).

Internal working models are the legacy of early attachment relationships (or a lack of them). An adult's parenting style is likely to be based largely on her own experience of being parented when she was a child. She will tend to treat any offspring in the same way as she has experienced her internal parent as having treated her. She will also tend to have a similar relationship to authority figures, including doctors, nurses and social workers, as she had to parental authority. This may result, for instance, in lack of co-operation, or in idealisation.

Box 7.4:   Practical applications of attachment theory

Use your knowledge of families gleaned over time, and your observations of relating within the consulting-room, to hazard a guess as to whether a child is securely or insecurely attached. The history of response to separations may also provide you with a clue. Insecure attachment can be one risk factor among many for a variety of child mental health problems.

Be aware of the attachments that your patients make to you. This is likely to be influenced by their internal models of childhood attachment figures.

Be on the lookout for multiple pathology in 'looked-after children'. These are children who are likely to move from one carer to another, and may not be registered with one general practice for long. They are likely to have had disrupted attachments, and they may have an attachment disorder.

Case study 7.1

William, by the age of ten years, had been in seven foster placements and had had one failed adoption. He was brought to the general practitioner by the key worker at his children's home. His behaviour was proving challenging, and his social worker wanted him to have individual therapy. The general practitioner referred him to the local child and adolescent mental health service.

After a long wait for an appointment, William and his key worker and social worker were seen jointly by a psychologist and clinical nurse specialist. By this time, his class teacher was finding him a disruptive influence in the classroom. The psychologist who saw him discovered the early care history from the social worker. William's father had left when he was born, his mother had neglected him, he and his siblings had been adopted separately (he still had yearly contact with them), and his placements had broken down partly because his behaviour was so challenging.

The psychologist and nurse made a diagnosis of attachment disorder and oppositional defiant disorder. There were features of attention-deficit hyperactivity disorder at school, and the nurse arranged for the clinic psychiatrist to prescribe a trial of stimulant medication, which was unsuccessful. The psychologist said that she thought individual therapy would be inappropriate, as William would need to be in a stable placement for this to work. The social worker was planning to find a long-term foster placement.

William's school problems continued into secondary school. The psychologist identified specific learning difficulties, and with the aid of extra special needs help in school, William was just able to avoid exclusion. After a couple of introductions to potential foster carers, William stated that he would prefer to stay in the children's home, but with respite foster care for one weekend per month. This was eventually arranged.

continued opposite

The psychologist then agreed to involve the clinic's child psychotherapist. After four assessment sessions, she agreed to see William for weekly individual therapy. He found it difficult to express his feelings in these sessions, and felt ashamed that he was having therapy while the other inmates of the children's home, mostly short-term residents, were not. After a few months it became clear that he was becoming angry after holiday breaks, and must be developing an attachment to the therapist. After an 18-month period, he and the psychotherapist agreed to end the sessions.

William remained in the same children's home. By 14 years of age, he was finding the school environment too challenging, and his social worker found him a place at a sixth-form college that had a small unit for under-sixteens. His social worker was changed, but he and his psychologist subsequently complained, and he was allowed to have the same social worker back. He had developed good relationships with the staff at the children's home, and kept in touch with some of the resident children who had moved on. He was settled ...

Fostering, adoption and the care system

Most of the children who show abnormal attachment behaviours will come from significantly dysfunctional families, and will have a history of abuse and neglect. A proportion of them will be removed to the care of the local authority, and some of these may experience a succession of placements in foster care or children's homes. In this case, they will already be known to Social Services, and may also be known to local child mental health services.

The care system

When parental care of a child breaks down, or is not considered to be in the child's best interests, Social Services have a duty to make alternative arrangements. If the parents agree to these, the child will be *accommodated*; if not, the child will be placed on an *interim care order*. This gives *parental responsibility* temporarily to the social worker. *Parental responsibility* means having the rights and duties of a parent to determine what is in the best interests of a particular child.

Initially, a child whose parents cannot manage him at home, or who is removed from his home by social workers, will normally be placed in a foster home. Only if foster care is demonstrated not to work will a children's home placement be considered.

If there is an interim care order, then the court is involved in deciding what is best for the child. A *guardian ad litem* is appointed (more recently entitled a '*litigation friend*'). This is a professional, often with a background in social work or probation work, who focuses on the child's interests and represents these in a world of adults.

The court has to decide whether or not the child should be returned to his parents, or whether he should be returned to some other family member, or whether alternative arrangements should be made permanent. This may involve making a *care order*, which gives Social Services parental responsibility until the child is 18 years of age, or freeing him for adoption. Experts are often involved in advising the court on parenting capacity and the nature of the child's difficulties – these are usually child psychologists or child psychiatrists. There may be a phase of attempted rehabilitation, depending partly on what the experts advise.

The relevance of all this to primary care

Children in the care system are likely to move from one placement to another, which means changing general practitioners frequently. This makes it difficult for the general practitioner or health visitor to get to know the child's situation. Moreover, they are very dependent on the foster carer, who may know even less than they will when they get the records. If the child is on a care order or interim care order, it is necessary to talk to the social worker if possible, if only to agree that the foster carer can make day-to-day decisions. If the child is accommodated, then it is necessary to talk to a parent, unless you are shown written authority from the parent delegating day-to-day management to the foster carer.

If you refer a child anywhere, consent is needed from someone with parental responsibility (only one individual is necessary). A foster parent is not usually in a position to give consent.

Box 7.5:   Practice points with regard to the care system

- If a child attends with a foster carer or children's-home key worker:

    try to find out who has parental responsibility. At least one such person needs to be informed of any health service involvement

    make sure that the social worker is aware of what is happening, even if they do not have parental responsibility. They tend to resent not being informed (e.g. about a hospital referral or an unusual choice of medication).

- It is worth trying to find out why the child is in care, although this may prove more difficult than it sounds.

Acknowledgements

We are indebted to Dr Pat Hughes, Senior Lecturer in Psychotherapy at St George's Hospital Medical School, for writing a student chapter on which the section on attachment theory is based.

CHAPTER EIGHT

Separation, divorce and reconstituted families

Introduction

The effects of separation and divorce on children can be summarised as follows.[1]

- Parental separation is part of a process that begins before divorce itself and continues long afterwards. Detrimental effects on children may occur at any stage if the parents are not able to make their children's needs a priority.
- Although short-term distress at the time of the separation is common, this usually fades with time, and long-term adverse outcomes typically only apply to a minority of children who experience the separation of their parents. However, these children are twice as likely to experience specific poor outcomes in the long term compared to those in intact families (*see* Box 8.1).

Box 8.1:   Specific poor long-term outcomes reported in children of separated families

Children of separated families are twice as likely to:

- grow up in households with lower incomes, poorer housing and greater financial hardship (especially those headed by lone mothers)
- have behavioural and emotional problems, including bed-wetting, being withdrawn, aggression, delinquency and other antisocial behaviour
- perform less well in school and gain fewer educational qualifications
- visit their general practitioner more often, report more health problems and be admitted to hospital following an accident
- leave school or home when young
- become sexually active, pregnant or a parent at an early age
- display depressive symptoms during adolescence and adulthood
- have high levels of smoking, drinking and drug use during adolescence and adulthood
- experience financial hardship when they are adults.

- Research into the long-term consequences of separation and divorce has shown that the age and gender of the children make no difference, and parental absence may be less important than the factors listed in Box 8.2.

Box 8.2:   Factors that affect the long-term outcome for children who experience parental separation or divorce

- Financial hardship can limit educational achievement.
- Family conflict before, during and after the parental separation can contribute to behavioural as well as emotional problems.
- The more difficult a parent finds it to come to terms with the separation, the more difficult the children will find it, too. Parental adjustment is affected by financial and social factors, so that many of the factors are interrelated.
- Multiple changes in family structure increase the probability of poor outcomes. Experiencing the breakdown of two or more parental relationships appears to have an extremely detrimental effect on children.
- Quality contact with the non-resident parent can improve outcomes.

Although the differences in outcome are clear, they only affect a minority of cases, and it is not necessarily the separation itself that causes all of the problems. The atmosphere in the home before separation, and the relationship between the parents following separation, are also important factors.

Reconstituted families pose a whole set of new challenges for the children and adults involved. Children may have to get used to a strange adult, stepsiblings and possibly a house move. Younger children seem better able to cope with these changes than older children, who may be better off staying in lone-parent families. There are increased risks for young people in stepfamilies compared to lone-parent families in the areas of educational achievement, family relationships, sexual activity, partnership formation and parenthood at a relatively young age.

Assessment

What is the parent concerned about and why? What is going on between the parents and what are the arrangements for the children? If you can identify a problem, whose is it?

The parent who is looking after a child may well present him as the problem, when in fact he may simply be responding normally to an upsetting situation. Parents may be so preoccupied with their own feelings that they have difficulty imagining their children's points of view. Often what is lacking is any form of working co-operation between the biological parents.

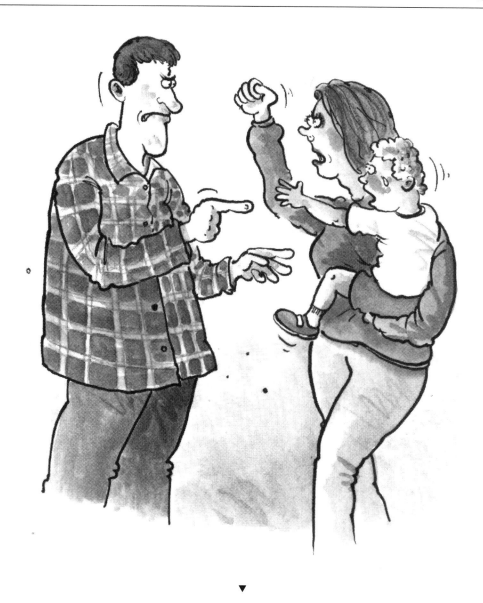

▼

Management

Members of the primary care team are in a good position to provide practical and common-sense advice. Important points include the following:

- It is important to ensure that children have received an *explanation* of the separation that they can understand, preferably from both parents – for instance, for younger children, 'Mummy and daddy aren't friends any more, just like you and your friends sometimes stop being friends'. Adolescents may need a fuller account, and honesty is essential, for instance in admitting that a new relationship played a part in the breakup of the marriage. Children invariably – and usually irrationally – feel that the separation is their own fault. It is therefore essential for both parents and professionals to reassure them that this is not the case, and that they are still loved by both parents.

- *Information* may be very helpful for parents, and can allay fears that separation *itself* can have a damaging and permanent effect on the children. It is equally important to convey the message that present and future factors such as family conflict could have detrimental effects.
- Parents should try to *agree* on what is best for the children. This may involve going to mediation. If available, this is now recommended by solicitors, in accordance with changes in divorce legislation. Alternatively, couples may obtain valuable assistance before, during and after separation from the organisation Relate. The last resort is for the courts to decide what is best for the children. As a professional, it is important not to be drawn into taking sides. In particular, if you see only one parent (as is often the case if the other parent moves away), do remember that you are hearing only one side of the story.
- If there must be arguments, advise the parents to keep these out of sight and hearing of the children. Children should not be involved in conveying messages between parents, or expected to take sides. Parents must see their role as *protecting* their children from adult matters and adult responsibilities.
- Try to ensure stability and *predictability* in the children's lives (e.g. being able to go to the same school and keep up the same friendships and activities, and having regular contact arrangements with the absent parent, which are adhered to).
- Children invariably want both parents to be *together*. If parents can meet as friends, this will help. Even if they cannot do so, each child needs an opportunity to show that they love each parent.
- Parents should obtain their own sources of adult *support*, rather than relying on their older children for emotional succour.
- Children benefit from any opportunity to *talk about* their experiences or feelings. The custodial parent may find this difficult to provide, so a family friend or relative who can remain neutral could be asked to take on this role for the child. Referral to a professional should not be necessary just for this purpose.
- Bringing *new partners* into the child's life will be difficult both for the child and for the new adult. It is important to anticipate this, to expect a variety of emotional and behavioural responses from the child, and to sympathise with the difficulties for the adult in this new role.

Referral

If there are major difficulties in helping the children to cope, it is the parents who need to address these and, if necessary, to seek outside help. This is preferable to focusing on the child as the problem or as the person who needs help, when the child's behaviour or emotional distress is in fact merely an index of what is going on between their parents. Usually the most helpful approach for the child is for the parents to sort out their differences.

Referral of the child as an identified problem to a child and family service may therefore be counter-productive. Encourage the parents to find some way of working together, such as going to mediation or Relate. Even if they are unwilling to discuss matters, silent co-operation is possible (e.g. in relation to contact visits). The custodial parent should also be able to find someone within her social network to serve as a confidant for the children.

Case study 8.1

Patricia visited the general practitioner to complain that her son Daniel, aged 10 years, was misbehaving at home and at school. She was worried that he was becoming verbally abusive towards her, just as his father had been. The general practitioner had treated Patricia with antidepressants in the aftermath of her marital separation one year earlier. He enquired about the nature of the boy's behaviour and the concerns of the school. Patricia confided that she had prevented Daniel from contacting his father recently, as she had found that he was more abusive towards her when he returned from his visits. Patricia started to describe again how awful her husband used to be, but the general practitioner gently interrupted and explained that this information would not help him to understand Daniel's problem. He arranged to see Daniel on his own on another occasion, after which he would see Patricia again on her own.

The general practitioner saw Daniel the following week, who was quite happy to talk to the doctor on his own. He reported that he missed his father very much and was angry with his mother for preventing him from going to see him. He was finding school difficult, as he was being teased and called names. He tended to react to this and was occasionally getting into trouble. He said he got on with his mother most of the time, but not with her new boyfriend. He was not sure why his parents had split up, but he thought it might be because of his own naughty behaviour. The general practitioner discussed with Daniel what he was allowed to tell Daniel's mother, and he then arranged to see Patricia the following week.

The general practitioner explained to Patricia how upset Daniel still was about the separation, and he gave her an information leaflet about the effects of separation on families and children. He urged her to discuss the bullying with Daniel's teachers, and he explained that he thought it was very important for the children of separated parents to see the absent parent regularly. He advised Patricia that Daniel needed to know that his parents were able to agree about him, and that they needed to explain to him together that the reasons why they separated were nothing to do with his behaviour. The doctor then gave Patricia the details of a local mediation service.

Three months later Patricia came in for a renewal prescription for her contraceptive pill and mentioned that Daniel had settled in well at his new secondary school, although there were occasional problems. He was seeing his father every two to three weeks and was getting on better with her boyfriend. She was trying hard to avoid saying negative things about his father in Daniel's presence.

Box 8.3:   Practice points for providing advice on the effects of parental separation

- In general, the situation improves with time.
- Remember the child's point of view. They may be right to be distressed, and they may need to be allowed to express grief and other emotions.
- Encourage the parents to work together to resolve matters for their children.
- Simple advice and support may be sufficient.

Reference

1   Rodgers B and Pryor J (1998) *Divorce and Separation: The Outcome for Children.* Joseph Rowntree Foundation, York.

Further reading

For professionals

Rodgers B and Pryor J (1998) *Divorce and Separation: The Outcome for Children.* Joseph Rowntree Foundation, York. Available from York Publishing Services, 64 Hallfield Road, Layerthorpe, York YO31 7ZQ (tel 01904 430033).

For parents and teachers

Burrett J (1993) *To and Fro Children: A Guide to Successful Parenting after Divorce.* Thorson's, London.

The Children's Society (1988) *Focus on Families. Divorce and its Effects on Children.* The Children's Society, London.

Royal College of Psychiatrists (1999) *Divorce or Separation of Parents: The Impact on Children and Adolescents.* Factsheet on Mental Health and Growing Up, No. 15. Royal College of Psychiatrists, London. Available from 17 Belgrave Square, London SW1X 8PG (tel 020 7235 2351 ext 146); e-mail booksales@rcpsych.ac.uk; website http://www.rcpsych.ac.uk/pub/pubsfs.htm.

Wells R (1989) *Helping Children To Cope with Divorce.* Sheldon Press, London.

Keeping in Touch: How to Help your Child after Separation and Divorce. Available from Young Minds, 102–108 Clerkenwell Rd, London EC1M 5SA (tel 0800 018 2138).

For children

There are many books for children of different ages and backgrounds, which are available in local libraries or bookshops. One example is given here.

Osman T and Carey J (1990) *Where Has Daddy Gone?* Heinemann, London.

Further information

The **Citizens' Advice Bureau** can be invaluable as a source of information about local mediation or for free legal advice. Local branches are listed in the telephone directory.

National Family Mediation is an organisation set up specifically to help families who are separating. It has a useful booklist that includes books for children of different ages. It is based at 9 Tavistock Place, London WC1H 9SN (tel 020 7383 5993).

Parentline offers help and advice to parents on bringing up children and teenagers. The contact address is Endway House, The Endway, Hadleigh, Essex SS7 2AN (telephone helpline 01702 559900).

Relate can help couples or one member of a couple. The central office is at Herbert Gray College, Littlechurch Street, Rugby, Warwickshire CV21 3AP (tel 01788 573241); details of local branches are available on the website, www.relate.org.uk. Some branches have a service for 11- to 18-year-olds called **Relateen**.

A longer factsheet than that published by the Royal College of Psychiatrists is printed on the next three pages, so that it can be conveniently given to parents.

How children experience parental separation and divorce

An information handout for parents

Introduction

Parents often underestimate the effect on children of the parents deciding to live apart. The three aspects of parental separation that cause children most distress are:

- rows between their mother and father
- losing an important relationship
- feeling that it is their fault.

Rows between parents

Negative feelings between parents are unavoidable, even in the happiest families. When parents part, such feelings, or the rows that result from them, may have contributed to the separation, may result from it, or both. Children often report feeling a great sense of relief that the rows in the home have stopped.

Each parent may experience powerful emotions, such as anger, guilt or sadness. It is likely to take several years (at least) to work through these feelings. Children can be caught up in these emotions by:

- witnessing continued rows between their parents
- being used as a messenger for complaints from one parent about the other
- being blamed for behaving like the absent parent. This often happens to the child who is most like the absent parent in personality, temperament or appearance.

How can parents help their children in this situation?

- Try to find another adult you can talk to about how the separation has affected you and what you feel about your ex-partner. This is preferable to confiding in one of your children about these feelings.
- If you must continue to have rows with your ex-partner, try to do this away from the children if at all possible. Sometimes it may be helpful for you both to meet with another adult who is impartial. This could be a mutual friend, or someone from a Conciliation Service. Your local Citizens' Advice Bureau will be able to tell you the location of your nearest Conciliation Service.
- Try to find a way of negotiating the practical details of sharing the care of the children (such as contact times) without letting the negative feelings interfere with this.

continued opposite

The loss of a parent

Losing a parent through separation can be just as painful as losing a parent through death, and may take much longer to get over, as there is still the possibility of seeing the absent parent. Children may have difficulty in expressing this pain, either because it is difficult to put into words, or because they feel that it is disloyal to the parent with whom they are living.

The grief may be expressed indirectly, often through various changes in behaviour. This may include difficulty in concentrating on school work, withdrawal from friendships, aggressive outbursts, or defiance of authority. Children may return to behaviours they had formerly grown out of, such as bed-wetting, whining or tantrums. Alternatively, they may set their feelings on one side and behave much older than their years, in order to take on some of the family responsibilities.

Ways to help children to cope with the difficulty of losing a parent through separation include the following.

- *Explain* to each child what has led to the separation and what will happen to him or her. For instance, children may fear that if one parent has left, the other may do so, too. Ideally, these explanations should be given by both parents together. If this is not possible, each parent should give their own explanation, preferably with some advance agreement between them, so that each gives roughly the same version of events. The explanations that are provided should be direct, honest and appropriate to the age of each child.
- Ensure that each child has as much *contact* as possible with the absent parent. This is often very difficult both emotionally and practically, but it is almost always in the children's best interests to maintain contact with both parents. Arrangements for contact should be clear and predictable from each child's point of view. Even if this is the case, it is likely that children will find the hand-over from one parent to another quite distressing, both because it reminds them of what they have lost, and because they have to adjust to two different systems of household rules. Very often the parent who is looking after the children for most of the time will bear the brunt of this distress. If contact between children and their absent parent is impossible, telephone calls, letters or cards may help. Even very young children appreciate the fact that a parent is thinking of them and that they are valued.
- It may be helpful for each child to have *someone to talk to* about their reactions to the separation. This could be either parent, but it may be easier if it is someone outside the immediate family, such as a friend of a similar age, a grandparent, aunt, uncle or family friend.

Blame

It is not only parents who feel guilty about separating. Children may also feel responsible for the separation, however irrational this may seem. A child's guilt may start long before the actual separation, when the parents' relationship is becoming difficult. Even if the parental rows are nothing to do with a child, that child may feel that he or she ought to do something to stop them. This guilt may be expressed in very indirect ways, just like the grief.

continued overleaf

Explanations that are given to children need to emphasise that the separation is the responsibility of the parents. Children also need to be reassured that their parents still love them. They also need to feel able to love both of their parents. This is made more difficult if one parent makes negative comments about the other, or interrogates the child about the time spent with the other parent.

Step-parents

Many children find that getting used to a new adult in the home is very difficult. They may blame this person for their parent's separation, even if there is no basis for this belief. They may resist the new adult's attempts at discipline, even if these are quite fair and reasonable. All of this makes it very difficult for anyone taking on the role of stepmother or stepfather. It requires a great deal of patience, tolerance and understanding of how the child is likely to feel (this is not the same as lax discipline).

Conclusions

The above comments must be treated as generalisations. For an individual child, only some of them may apply, and some of them will not. Nevertheless, a few of the comments may be helpful in understanding how a child of yours is feeling.

CHAPTER NINE

Chronic paediatric illness

Introduction

The effects of chronic illness

Acute illness may be a shock but, provided that recovery is complete, children and their families are likely to return to normal functioning and their usual routine very quickly. In contrast, the consequences of a continuing (i.e. chronic) illness permeate every aspect of the child's life, and are likely to affect every member of the family to some extent. It is normal for chronic illness to have significant psychological and social consequences, but that does not make these effects any easier to deal with. These consequences will depend on a number of factors, including the following:

- *the age of onset* – a child who develops a chronic illness after being completely well will follow a different path from a child who is born with persisting problems
- *the outcome of the condition* – parents may react completely differently if they feel that their child is unlikely to survive (e.g. muscular dystrophy or cystic fibrosis will have different implications from asthma or diabetes).
- *the nature of the handicap* (e.g. multiple congenital anomalies, or exercise-induced wheezing)
- *the extent of the disability* (e.g. overall developmental delay, or having to miss sports at school).

Assessment

It may be useful to think about the effects on different family members and on the family as a whole. One way of approaching this is to consider first the effects on the child, then the effects on the parents, then the impact on other family members living at home, and finally the effect on family members elsewhere.

The effects on the child may include the following:

- *a disturbance of self-image* – the young person may feel different in a variety of ways. Self-esteem may be affected, sometimes to the extent of causing depression. Some children express their negative feelings about themselves by behavioural disturbances. Bodily deformations are particularly difficult to tolerate in adolescence, when a sense of identity is developing. Illnesses that do not show on the outside may still lead to feelings such as 'Why me?'. This in turn may affect
- *relationships with peers* – opportunities for social activities may be reduced. For instance, a young person with diabetes may be unable to go to a sleepover because a friend's parents may be scared of the illness, or they may not be allowed to go for a long walk with friends for fear of a hypoglycaemic attack
- *disruption of school* – school attendance may be reduced because of recurrent hospital admissions (e.g. in cases of leukaemia or severe asthma) or exhaustion (e.g. in chronic fatigue syndrome). School performance may be affected by cognitive impairment (e.g. in leukaemia), physical limitations (e.g. in asthma) or the emotional distractions of being ill
- *dislike of treatment* – children with cystic fibrosis may get fed up with repeated physiotherapy, or having to take large quantities of pancreatic enzymes at every meal. Children with leukaemia may dread their visits to hospital, where injections cause vomiting, and some treatments may require prolonged social isolation. Some children learn to vomit at the thought of an injection, while others may develop a needle phobia, which can affect their access to health care.

Effects on parents include the following:

- *bereavement* for the loss of the perfect child. Parents may go through the well-described stages of reaction to being told that their child has a chronic illness (denial, anger, guilt, bargaining and finally acceptance)
- *chronic sorrow* because the child continues to be less than perfect. This could be regarded as a long drawn-out bereavement reaction. Particularly in children with significant handicap, there may be new effects emerging at different ages, and as the child becomes older the differences compared to other children become more glaringly apparent
- *over-protectiveness.* It is easy to be critical of over-protective mothers, but in general it is difficult to tell whether this is due to a mother who tends to be anxious about her child, or to the nature of the illness. It is particularly common in chronic fatigue syndrome, but may occur with any illness
- *social effects.* A chronic illness or lifelong handicap in a child may strain parents socially and financially as well as emotionally. One parent may have to give up work, and the other may have to forgo promotion, in order to be available for the child. Financial difficulties may then result. There may be little time for a social life, and other parents may show little understanding. Some marriages are strengthened by such stresses, while others collapse under the strain.

Case study 9.1

A 10-year-old boy with asthma was noted to have much poorer school attendance than could be justified by the severity of his asthma. Careful history-taking elicited first that his mother tested his peak flow rate every morning, when it was often lower than during the rest of the day, and secondly that she had *two* relatives who had died from status asthmaticus on the way to hospital. She could not be persuaded that her son's asthma was not this severe.

Effects on siblings include the following:

- *feeling left out*. It is difficult for parents not to give the sick child more attention. Unaffected siblings may feel that the ill child is more important than them, or that they have to be ill in order to obtain the same level of love and attention

---

Case study 9.2

The sister of a boy with acute myeloid leukaemia who had survived two bone-marrow transplants – involving much travelling for their parents – developed severe abdominal pain, requiring admission to hospital. No organic cause was found.

- *becoming parental* towards the ill or handicapped child. This seems to affect older siblings, particularly girls. It may have a beneficial effect on the sibling's development, provided that she also has the opportunity to be an age-appropriate child.

Grandparents or other members of the extended family:

- *can be very helpful* as temporary childminders for the siblings and a source of support for the parents
- *may at times be unhelpful* if they are critical of the parents' handling, or exacerbate their anxiety.

Management

The primary care team may need to complement a specialist team if the latter is involved. Specialist teams may focus very much on the child's needs, and not always on those of other family members.

The support that is needed by a child will depend on what has already been done by the specialist team. The general practitioner may have a co-ordinating role. Particular points to consider with regard to the child include support groups, the opportunity to meet other young people with similar conditions and charitable foundations for holidays.

Depression is more likely to occur, and ordinary intercurrent illnesses will need treatment, and may generate more anxiety. Support for the family needs to include practical considerations such as disability living allowance and other benefits, arranging respite care if appropriate, and attending to the physical and emotional needs of all family members, especially siblings.

Case study 9.3

Sophie was known to the general practitioner as an 11-year-old child with achondroplasia. Her mother brought her along to see the doctor, reporting that she had become very distressed during the last month since starting secondary school. Previously she had been coping very well in a small supportive local primary school, but now she had to take the bus into town and things had become much more difficult for her. She had started to call herself a freak, and the school had reported that she was socially isolated. Despite being of above average intelligence, with a good academic record, her standard of schoolwork in the new school was poor.

The general practitioner telephoned the school and spoke to Sophie's teacher, who agreed that she could see the school counsellor. The doctor also wrote to a local orthopaedic surgeon to ask whether Sophie could be put in contact with other children in the area with achondroplasia.

The specialist agreed to see Sophie and put her in touch with other children with achondroplasia, after obtaining the necessary consent from all concerned. The specialist also promised Sophie that when she was older he would consider performing a leg-lengthening operation.

Box 9.1:   Practice points for chronic illness

- Psychological and social problems are more common in children with chronic physical illness.
- Specific difficulties that are not always addressed include social isolation of the child and their parents, practical issues with regard to child care and respite, financial hardship and the feelings of siblings.

CHAPTER TEN

Effects of parental mental illness on children and families

Introduction

Any form of mental health problem affects not only the patient, but also all of the other family members. Clinical experience suggests that there is an emphasis within adult mental health teams on the patient alone, so that the needs of parents and children may be overlooked. Over 50% of women with serious mental illness have children under the age of 16 years, although not necessarily living with them. About 25% have children living with them, often pre-schoolers.[1] Milder degrees of anxiety and depression are more common, and have smaller but still significant effects on the children. Similarly, children may be affected by parental substance abuse (including alcohol), especially if this leads to unavailability and neglect, or domestic violence.

Children often cope well when a parent is ill for a limited period of time, especially if they can be helped to accept that their parent is unwell (implying that recovery will occur). The outcome for the children seems to depend on how well-developed attachments have been before the onset of illness, and the quality of attachments with other adults. A temporary period of foster care may be necessary in severe cases, if other members of the family cannot look after the children. Multiple episodes of illness may be more difficult for children to tolerate.

Children may experience a parent's mental illness in a variety of ways (*see* Box 10.1).

Box 10.1:   Possible elements of a child's experience of a parent's mental illness

1 Direct effects:
•   finding their parent unrousable and not knowing what to do, or having to summon help
     themselves
•   seeing their parents using drugs and not knowing what to make of this*
•   not being given any explanation of what is happening (e.g. doctors, ambulances or other
     professionals coming to the house)
•   finding their parent in a strange unfriendly place that does not look like a hospital
•   being distracted and unable to concentrate at school.
2 Indirect effects of parenting relationship:
•   being left to their own devices to an excessive degree
•   feeling frightened or insecure
•   having to look after themselves, their siblings or their parent (i.e. becoming a parentified
     child)
•   not being taken to school regularly
•   being embarrassed or frightened by their parent's behaviour and other people's reactions.
3 Effects of shared environment or genes:
•   having contact with many strange people (involved in drug use), some of whom may be
     abusive
•   being exposed to domestic violence
•   worrying about developing mental illness when they grow up.

*Case vignette: Mother says to doctor 'They don't know anything about my drug use', while
her child plays with a teddy and toy syringe, injecting the teddy ...

Aetiology

Conceptually, it may be helpful to consider three ways in which parental mental illness
and child disturbance may be connected.[2]

1   There may be a direct impact of the parental disorder on the child.
2   There may be an indirect impact on the child mediated by interaction or relation-
     ships, and especially the type of parenting.
3   The association may be due to common factors affecting both parent and child, such
     as social adversity or genetic factors.

Assessment

The main message here is to *think about the children.*

The parent's own disorder must of course be assessed, but it is important to consider the adequacy of parenting. What (if any) risk does this parent pose to her children because of her mental illness and associated difficulties? It is important to remember that children can be harmed by *acts of omission* (e.g. neglect and poor supervision) as well as *acts of commission* (e.g. involvement in delusions or excessive violence). Primary care workers are well placed to begin such an assessment, as they may be in the unique position of knowing both the parent and the child well.

The children of non-psychotic parents (i.e. those with less severe mental illness, drug use or alcoholism) often fare worse than those with psychotic parents, especially when their parents' state is combined with personality dysfunction and social and marital adversity.

Although a full *assessment of parenting* should be left to Social Services, it is important that someone (this may well be the primary care worker) begins to consider the questions listed in Box 10.2.

Box 10.2:   Aspects of parenting to consider during assessment

- What happens to the children when the parent is ill or in hospital?
- Who else is involved with the family (e.g. Social Services, education welfare officer, police, probation officer, child or adult mental health services)?
- Who is the main carer's partner? Women with mental health problems may be vulnerable and form relationships with violent or abusive men. Such women, especially those who have themselves been sexually abused in childhood, may be targeted by sex offenders with a view to gaining access to their children.
- What are the usual patterns of child care? For example, who gets the children up, feeds and clothes them, takes them to school, is at home when they get back from school, cooks their evening meal and puts them to bed?
- What does the parent feel towards her children, and how does she handle them? What is her style of discipline? Does she ever feel out of control, angry or violent towards them? Who (if anyone) would she go to for help?
- If the parent is seriously depressed or deluded, do thoughts of potential harm involve any of her children? For instance, has she thought of killing the children as well as herself?
- Are the parent–child interactions generally warm and affirming or disinterested and coercive?

Management

The safety and well-being of the children must be a priority. Confidentiality and loyalty to the adult may therefore need to take second place.

Encourage the parent to think about the child and his needs. Sometimes intervening to support the child can have a positive effect on the parent's disorder. Does the parent need more practical and social assistance in the home? Would the provision of day nursery or respite care be helpful? Would a support network, such as Homestart,[10.1] Newpin,[10.2] drop-in centres, mother and toddler groups, sympathetic nurseries or other voluntary agencies, be helpful?

Should Social Services be involved? It may be useful to have an initial discussion with a senior social worker or a consultant community paediatrician.

The child, if old enough, may benefit from age-appropriate information or attendance at a self-help or support group such as Al-a-Teen.[10.3]

Referral

* Consider whether the parent might benefit from referral (or re-referral) to the local adult mental health team.
* Consider referral to Social Services if you suspect that any form of child abuse has occurred, or may occur, or if you feel that a detailed parenting assessment is indicated (e.g. because of inadequate supervision, or because the child is becoming parentified).
* Consider referral to a community paediatrician if the child is failing to thrive.

Case study 10.1

The health visitor attached to the practice asked to be fitted in between patients during the general practitioner's morning surgery. She told the doctor that she had come back from a routine follow-up visit to Elaine, a 29-year-old single mother with one child in school and one at nursery. The health visitor was concerned that the house had become less tidy since she had last visited. Elaine seemed rather distracted, and she told the health visitor that she had been raped by an acquaintance three months previously, and that she was sure the neighbours were trying to take control of her thoughts about this incident. The health visitor had asked her whether she would agree to see a psychiatrist or a community psychiatric nurse, but the woman had refused.

The doctor visited urgently after surgery and found Elaine to be suffering from delusions of control by the neighbours and hearing voices through the walls of her flat. The doctor arranged for a joint domiciliary together with the duty consultant psychiatrist and approved social worker. Elaine agreed to be admitted voluntarily to the psychiatric ward, and the social worker arranged for placement of the two children with a foster carer.

continued opposite

The children were brought to the general practitioner one week later by the foster mother. She said that she needed to have them checked over physically, but the doctor could find no physical abnormality. The foster mother was continuing to take the children to the same school and nursery locally. The school had confirmed that the children had been arriving late, looking unkempt, and had been more socially withdrawn. However, neither the school nor the nursery had had any idea that the mother was so ill.

Two weeks later the general practitioner received a discharge letter outlining Elaine's care programme, which included regular visits from a community psychiatric nurse and a social worker, and monthly out-patient visits to the consultant psychiatrist. The general practitioner discussed this with the health visitor, who agreed to continue to visit and monitor the health of the children.

Box 10.3:   Practice points for dealing with parental mental illness

- Think about both the parent *and* the children.
- The involvement of both adult psychiatry services and Social Services may be necessary, and the primary care team may play an important role in liaising between the two services.
- Health visitors should be aware of local support services and voluntary agencies, which can be invaluable.
- The primary care team provides important continuity of care, and may be in the best position to highlight the children's needs.

Notes

10.1   Homestart UK, 2 Salisbury Road, Leicester LE1 7OR (tel 0116 233 9955).

10.2   National NEWPIN, Sutherland House, 35 Sutherland Square, Walworth, London SE17 3EE (tel 020 7703 6326).

10.3   Al-anon and Al-a-teen, 61 Great Dover Street, London SE1 4YF (tel 020 7403 0888). Al-a-teen is an organisation for young people aged 12–20 years who have been affected by someone else's drinking.

References

1   Oates M (1997) Patients as parents: the risk to children. *Br J Psychiatry.* **170 (Supplement 32):** 22–27.

2   Murray L and Cooper PJ (1997) Effects of postnatal depression on infant development. *Arch Dis Child.* **77:** 99–101.

CHAPTER ELEVEN

Child abuse

Introduction

Definitions

Child abuse is the difference between a hand on the bottom and a fist in the face

(Henry Kempe)

A child is considered to be abused when he or she is *treated detrimentally in a way that is unacceptable in a given culture at a given time.*

Prevalence

Child abuse is common, and it occurs in all types of family. One in 1000 children aged under four years suffers from *severe* physical abuse, and one in 10 000 die as a result of such abuse. The prevalence rates for child sexual abuse vary according to the definition used. On the basis of surveys of adults, it is thought that about 10% of children are sexually abused before their sixteenth birthday. Figures for emotional abuse and neglect vary from one local authority to another, because of the difficulty in agreeing on thresholds and the overlap with other forms of abuse.

Types

There are four main types of abuse:

- physical abuse or non-accidental injury
- child sexual abuse
- neglect
- emotional abuse.

Bullying can also be considered to be a form of abuse – peer abuse physical, emotional, or both.

Münchausen's syndrome by proxy is severe but less common, and is categorised as either emotional or physical abuse.

Different types of abuse often occur together in the same child. Children may be harmed both actively and passively – by acts of omission as well as those of commission. Abuse may have long-term consequences for the child's social, emotional and cognitive development.

Box 11.1:   Risk factors for abuse

Child
- Young children are most at risk. Most deaths occur in children aged under one year, and most severe non-accidental injury occurs in children aged under two years.
- First-born children are especially at risk.
- Reported sexual abuse is more common in girls than in boys. Other forms of abuse occur equally frequently in boys and girls.
- Abuse may happen to just one child in a family, or to several.

Abuser
- The abuser is usually the child's parent(s) or the parent's partner. In other words, they are likely to be previously known to the child (i.e. not a stranger).
- Young parents more commonly are involved.
- Both parents may be involved, especially in cases of physical abuse and neglect.
- There are marked sex differences among perpetrators: 90% of sexual abuse perpetrators are men, and only 10% are women; women are more likely to poison, suffocate or be involved in Münchausen's syndrome by proxy.
- There is usually *no* major mental illness.
- The abuser is often someone who was abused as a child.

Social/family factors
- Social deprivation.
- Unemployment.
- Abuse occurs in *all* social classes and *all* cultures.

Assessment

History

The general principles of assessment are to find out what has been happening to the child from the parents, the child, and other informants such as the health visitor or teacher. The accounts given should be carefully documented, as there are often discrepancies that may be highly significant. Altered stories are characteristic of child abuse, as is delay presentation.

Examination

This should be both general and specific, and the child must be completely undressed. Unsuspected signs (e.g. bruises, cigarette burns) may be detected by a general examination, which should also include height and weight (to be plotted on a growth chart, since this can provide evidence of neglect). Inspection should be made for specific injuries indicated in the history. All findings, both positive and negative, should be carefully recorded (a blank picture of a child's body may be useful for noting the location of injuries). Only a designated doctor, usually a consultant community paediatrician, should conduct a full examination for signs of sexual abuse.

Interviewing the child

Investigative interviewing is best left to social workers. The situation that is most likely to arise in general practice is with adolescents who may be on the verge of disclosing that they have been sexually or physically abused. The symptoms may suggest this, and it is important to consider it as part of the differential diagnosis in all behavioural and emotional problems.

Young people do not seem to mind being asked a routine systematic enquiry question about sexual or physical abuse. The wording should be adjusted to be appropriate for the child's age. For a teenager aged 15 years or over, an enquiry such as 'Have you ever been sexually abused?' may be appropriate. For a younger child, something like 'Has anyone ever touched you in a way that made you feel uncomfortable?' may be more suitable, but remember that sometimes the experience may be enjoyable, although it feels wrong. Such questions are unlikely to do any harm, although they do not necessarily yield any useful information. However, because of concern about the implantation of false memories in impressionable people by professionals, care must be taken not to go beyond the content of what the child says. Open questions are preferable to leading questions, and comments such as 'It sounds to me as if you were raped by your stepfather' are unwise.

If a child discloses abuse to you, you then have a duty to involve other agencies (usually Social Services or the local branch of the National Society for the Prevention of Cruelty to Children). However, there are two situations in which this may not be necessary, at least immediately. One is when the young person is at least 16 years of age and is quite clear that she does not wish to involve other agencies. Provided that neither she nor any other child is at risk, there is no justification for overriding her veto. The second situation is if you consider that the amount or quality of information that you have obtained is insufficient to trigger an investigation, and you think that you might obtain more information by seeing the young person again. This is a very difficult judgement to make, and it would be advisable to seek advice at an early stage from a senior partner, consultant community paediatrician or Social Services child protection adviser (without necessarily giving the child's name).

If you do inform other agencies, it is important to tell the young person before you do this, and to explain why you have to do so. Otherwise they may lose trust in professionals and be unable to repeat the allegations to anyone else.

Child physical abuse

Box 11.2:   Indicators of physical abuse

Delay in seeking medical help

The story of the 'accident' is vague, lacking in detail and varies with each telling and from person to person

The account of the accident is not compatible with the injury observed

Abusing parents are often more preoccupied with their own problems than concerned about their child

The parents' behaviour gives cause for concern – they may be hostile, argumentative or leave before the appointment is due

The child's appearance and their interaction with their parents are abnormal – they may look sad, withdrawn or frightened, they may show 'frozen watchfulness', or they may be failing to thrive

The child may say something, such as 'mummy did it'.

Certain patterns of injury are very suggestive of physical abuse. These include, for instance:

- finger-tip bruising
- adult human bite marks
- cigarette burns
- lash marks
- torn tongue frenulum
- unexplained subdural haematoma
- unexplained retinal haemorrhages
- bruises of different ages
- multiple fractures of different ages
- certain unusual fractures (a fracture in the first year of life should always be regarded as suspicious).

Details and numerous graphic examples of these injuries are given in the BMA's publication, *The ABC of Child Abuse*.[1]

Child sexual abuse

This can be defined as 'a child or adolescent being made to participate in sexual activities that they do not fully understand and to which they cannot consent'. These activities violate social taboos and family roles. There is usually a power differential in that the abuser coerces the abused. Child sexual abuse may occur within or outside the family, and the perpetrator may be an adult, an adolescent or (rarely) a child.

The forms of sexual abuse range from inappropriate fondling or masturbation to full sexual intercourse and buggery. Some children are involved in the production of pornographic photos or videos, and some are victims of sex rings (i.e. groups of adults who abuse children).

It can be difficult to distinguish abusive sexual behaviour, or the sexualised behaviour that results from abuse, from normal experimentation. There has been very little scientific research into normal sexual behaviour in young children. It is generally accepted that questions and curiosity about one's body, and playing with one's own genitals, are a normal part of growing up, and may occur more frequently at around the age of five years as well as in adolescence. These phases are usually transitory and private. Concern is justified if such behaviours are frequent, persistent and occur in public (e.g. at school) despite the issuing of clear adult boundaries.

Sexually abused children are usually threatened or bullied not to tell anyone about the abuse. If and when they do disclose it, they may later retract their statement. There may be many children who are abused who do not disclose the abuse. A sexually abused child may also show features of emotional abuse and neglect.

Box 11.3:   Indicators of sexual abuse

There is a history of previous sexual abuse in the nuclear or extended family

There is a new male member of the household with a record of sexual offences (referred to as a schedule 1 offender). Males with a paedophilic orientation may target vulnerable women with children

Medical presentations include symptoms due to local trauma, sexually transmitted diseases, recurrent urinary tract infection and pregnancy

Behavioural presentations include almost any emotional or behavioural problem. The only specific pointer is sexualised behaviour enacted in play or shown towards others. Inappropriate sexual knowledge is also cause for concern, as is frank sexual abuse of other children. Here it is the power differential that is important, rather than any particular age difference.

Some adolescents may present by running away from home, overdosing, cutting, bingeing, promiscuity, or misuse of alcohol and street drugs

---

Emotional abuse and neglect

Emotional abuse is extremely difficult to define, as it concerns the nature of the parent–child relationship. Difficulties include the need to examine the process instead of just merely isolated events, and the question of where to set the threshold for definition or intervention. Recent definitions have attempted to describe the characteristic patterns of parental behaviours and attitudes. These patterns of behaviour occur to a greater or lesser extent in all families, but in emotional abuse they are pervasive, long-lasting and damaging to the child.[2]

Box 11.4:   Indicators of emotional abuse

The relationship of a parent to a child can be defined as emotionally abusive if one or more of the following dimensions is sufficiently pervasive to be considered characteristic of the interaction (there also needs to be cause for serious concern about the child's functioning and emotional state):

- persistent negative attributions or misattributions to the child, which the child believes and which therefore make him feel bad about himself (e.g. 'You are a *bad* boy' or 'I'll have you put in care'). These lead to the child being given 'deserved' harsh discipline, punishment and rejection
- emotional unavailability, unresponsiveness and neglect (e.g. repeatedly failing to comfort a child when he is hurt)
- inappropriate or inconsistent developmental expectations and considerations (e.g. expecting a six-year-old girl to do everything for her two-year-old brother)
- missocialisation (e.g. involving a child in stealing, or keeping a child completely isolated from his peers)
- failure to recognise or respect the child's individuality and psychological boundaries. This may result in the child being used to gratify the parents' own emotional needs (e.g. an agoraphobic mother relying on a child to do all the chores, such as shopping, to the exclusion of schooling).

For the definition to be complete there also need to be effects on the child. As with sexual abuse, there may be a wide variety of emotional and behavioural difficulties, which may be non-specific. A younger child may show developmental delay. The child may behave badly, perhaps in an attempt to attract some attention. The child may blame himself, feel sad or worthless, or fear being abandoned. He may have difficulties in peer relationships and accepting discipline from teachers, and may be anxious (e.g. about becoming independent).

Domestic violence is a type of emotional abuse that is invariably anxiety-provoking for both parents and children, and it is often kept secret. Parents sometimes say that their children are unaware of the violence that occurs after pub closing-time, because they are asleep, but most children do know what is going on, even if they have gone to bed before the violence occurs. Children may be very upset by it and far too frightened to talk to anyone. There is also a risk that they may subsequently display violent and aggressive behaviour (presumably because of a mix of modelling and genetics).

If a member of the primary care team becomes aware of the existence of a violent relationship, it is important to consider carefully the well-being of the children. There are now guidelines for a multi-agency response to domestic violence, and the police and casualty departments are much more pro-active than has been the case in the past. It is important for all members of the primary health care team to contribute to this in a constructive manner.

Neglect

This overlaps with emotional abuse, and the two often coexist with other forms of abuse. Neglect is often ignored or overlooked.

Box 11.5:   Indicators of neglect

Lack of care for the child's *physical needs* may lead to nappy rash, failure to thrive and frequent accidents, which may lead to repeated attendance at Accident and Emergency departments

Babies need encouragement and *social stimulation* in order for them to acquire motor and social skills. If such encouragement and stimulation are significantly lacking, delayed development may occur, particularly with regard to language. Under-stimulation may lead to compensatory self-stimulatory behaviours (e.g. head-banging or rocking)

Neglected and abused children may show *avoidant* or *anxious attachment*. The former show little apparent attachment behaviour. They either roam around the room in a non-directed way, or observe what is happening warily ('frozen watchfulness'). The latter do not feel safe and secure with their primary caregiver, they lack the confidence to explore their surroundings, and they are whiny, unhappy and cling to their caregiver, who (usually) responds with irritation

---

Münchausen's syndrome by proxy (factitious disorder by proxy)

This term was first used in 1977 to describe children whose mothers invented stories of illness about their child and substantiated them by fabricating false physical signs. It is a rare but serious form of child abuse and is potentially fatal. In UK use, the term describes a relationship and a behaviour pattern between a parent and child, rather than a psychological disorder in either of these individuals, although the mother may have diagnosable psychopathology (most commonly personality disorder).

Box 11.6:   Indicators of factitious disorder by proxy (Münchausen's syndrome by proxy)

The illness is fabricated by one of the parents, usually the mother

It may take many different forms, including poisoning, apnoeic episodes (actually due to suffocation), tampering with urine samples, stating that the child has had fits, or claiming that the child cannot walk

The situation can be life-threatening

Fabricated symptoms may be primarily psychological (e.g. a mother may give a very convincing history of developmental problems such as Asperger's disorder, or attention-deficit hyperactivity disorder)

The child is presented to doctors, often repeatedly

The perpetrator (initially) denies causing the child's illness

The illness clears up when the child is separated from the perpetrator

The parent may have a partial training in nursing or other paramedical specialty.

The father is often separated, peripheral or uninvolved

There may be a history of previous child deaths, multiple illnesses or allergies. The motivation is seldom clear, but often the involved parent is a 'hospital addict' who derives satisfaction from receiving professional attention. At times there may be an element of financial gain from a disability living allowance

---

Management of child abuse

All doctors should be aware of the procedures to be followed in cases of suspected child abuse. These are contained in local guidelines and in national documents such as *Working Together*.[3]

General principles

- *Medical confidentiality.* Doctors have a legal and ethical duty to maintain their patient's confidentiality. Knowledge of or suspicion of abuse and neglect is one of the exceptional circumstances that will justify a doctor disclosing information to an appropriate, responsible member of a statutory agency. The General Medical Council Guidelines state that *'where a doctor believes that a patient may be the victim of abuse or neglect, the patient's interests are paramount and will usually require a doctor to disclose information to an appropriate, responsible person or officer of a statutory agency'*. The statutory agencies are Social Services, the National Society for the Prevention of

Cruelty to Children and the police child protection team. They have a statutory duty to investigate suspected cases of abuse and to decide what action, if any, is necessary to protect the child.

- *The child's interests are paramount at all times.* The child's welfare trumps that of the parents. The professional often needs to make a balanced judgement between the justification for breaching confidence and the need to maintain confidentiality. Sometimes this is a matter of choosing between the interests or feelings of an adult and the need of a child to be protected from abuse. However, the choice is often less clear-cut than this, due to uncertainty as to whether abuse has occurred. One of the particular difficulties that arises in the primary care setting is that the professional needs to have an ongoing relationship with each family member, including those who are (or may be) abusers. This means that the situation has to be handled sensitively.

- *Communication with the child, parent(s) and other professionals.* One of the issues that has to be decided is whether to inform a parent before telling Social Services. This is more likely to preserve your relationship with the parent, but in some circumstances it may put the child at greater risk. Rather than being accusatory or confrontational with the parents, try to engage their natural concern for the child. For instance, you could say that you are sure they would want to investigate a situation in which their child might have been abused, and you could perhaps imply that it could be someone else. If a child is old enough to be informed of your intentions, then it is best to do so if possible – in an age-appropriate way – before telling statutory professionals. Otherwise the resulting sequence of events is likely to be very bewildering for the child. Having decided to breach confidentiality, it is then important to work together with all the other professionals involved, if possible in partnership with the parents, towards the best interests of the child (Children Act 1989).[4]

Stages in the management of individual cases

1   *Preliminary consultation.* Careful thought may be needed before you refer to Social Services. This may include discussion with a senior colleague, a consultant community paediatrician, or even a senior social worker on condition that identifying details are not revealed.

2   *Referral.* When it is felt that the child is suffering significant harm or is at risk of significant harm, *you have a duty to refer the child.* Doctors, health visitors or other members of the primary care team must share their concerns with the statutory agencies for further evaluation and discussion within a time frame that is not detrimental to the child's interests. In other words, you can take longer over a case of emotional abuse or even a case of sexual abuse than over a case of physical abuse where the child's life may be at risk.

3   Sometimes a *strategy discussion* is held in order to decide what steps are appropriate, whether an investigation should take place, and whether a child protection case

conference is necessary. This is usually a professionals' meeting that includes the child protection police, but not the parents.

4   The *Child Protection Case Conference* follows on from the stages of recognition and referral, strategy discussion and investigation. It is an opportunity for all of the professionals involved to pool any information of which the others may not be aware. It is also an opportunity for joint planning of how to ensure the child's safety – that is, deciding the *child protection plan*. Attendance by members of the primary care team is always requested. In practice, this may be difficult due to competing commitments, but the presence of a professional who knows the family well is invaluable. In many cases, the health visitor may be able to represent the primary care team's views, following appropriate discussion.

5   The *Child Protection Register*. Each Social Services area has a central register listing all of the children in the area who have been abused or who are considered to be at risk of abuse. There are usually four categories of registration, equivalent to the four main types of abuse. This register is available to all Accident and Emergency departments and health centres.

6   Each child on the Child Protection Register should have a *child protection plan*. This aims to involve professionals and the parents working together to prevent further abuse. It may specify particular roles for members of the primary care team. For instance, in the case of under-fives, the health visitor may be a member of the *core group* that reviews progress with the child protection plan.

7   A child's name is only *removed from the register* when it has been agreed at a case conference that formal inter-agency working is no longer necessary to protect the child.

The flow diagram in Figure 11.1 (opposite) shows the management pathways.

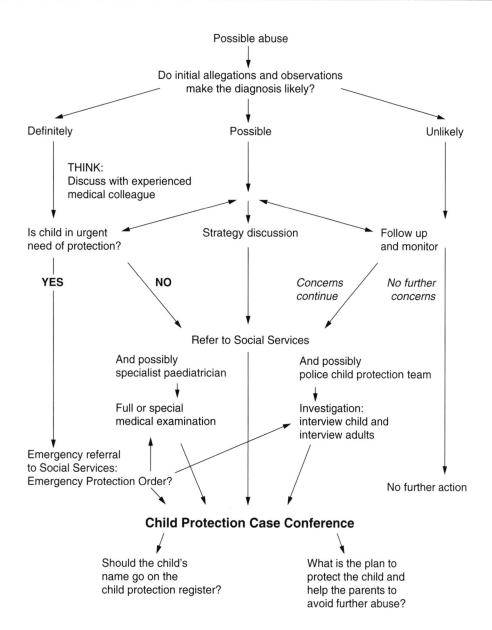

Figure 11.1: Management of suspected cases of child abuse.

Case study 11.1

At the weekly practice team meeting, the health visitor highlighted her concern about a child aged 18 months called Hayley. The health visitor had received notification of three visits to different casualty departments with minor injuries during the last month. The general practitioner had previously visited the home on more than one occasion and was aware that the family, which included two other pre-school aged children, was living in very cramped conditions. The father had a low-paid job and there was a lack of family support for the young mother. It was decided that the health visitor would visit the family and encourage them to bring Hayley for her routine immunisation, which was overdue.

Ten days later Hayley was brought to the immunisation clinic by her mother. On undressing her, the health visitor noted bruising on the upper arms and around the rib-cage, and asked the general practitioner to see her urgently, which he did immediately. Hayley's mother told him that she had fallen down some steps a few days before. The general practitioner considered calling Social Services immediately, but instead decided to arrange for the duty community paediatrician to see the child later the same day. He explained to Hayley's mother that he was concerned about Hayley's repeated bruising, and told her that he was concerned that she might have a blood disorder that made her bruise easily or that, alternatively, someone might be hurting her. He asked who, apart from the mother, had looked after Hayley recently, but the mother confirmed that the child had not been left with a child-minder.

Later that evening the general practitioner received a telephone call from the community paediatrician, who had found more bruising inside the thigh and had arranged for a skeletal survey. The X-rays had shown multiple fractures of different ages, and Hayley had been taken to the local paediatric hospital ward. The community paediatrician asked the general practitioner about his availability for a case conference over the next few days.

Box 11.7:   Practice points for child abuse

- Is the child suffering significant harm (one of the four forms of abuse), or is he likely to do so?
- Consider the child's interests and the parents' interests separately. Is there a conflict? If so, seek advice.
- If you report actual or potential abuse to a statutory agency, this will set in train a sequence of events that is dictated by local guidelines.
- If you fail to report abuse that may harm a child, you are failing in your duty to that child.

References

1   Meadow R (ed.) (1997) *The ABC of Child Abuse* (3e). BMJ Publishing Group, London.

2   Glaser D (1995) Emotionally abusive experiences. In: P Reder and C Lucey (eds) *Assessment of Parenting: Psychiatric and Psychological Contributions*. Routledge, London.

3   Home Office, Department of Health, Department of Education and Science and Welsh Office (1991) *Working Together Under the Children Act 1989. A Guide to Arrangements for Inter-Agency Co-Operation for the Protection of Children From Abuse*. HMSO, London.

4   (1991) *The Children Act 1989: Putting it Into Practice. Reference Pack*. Open University, Milton Keynes.

Further information

Always consult your local child protection guidelines.

Meadow R (ed.) (1997) *The ABC of Child Abuse* (3e). BMJ Publishing Group, London.

Royal College of Psychiatrists (1999) *Child Abuse and Neglect – the Emotional Effects*. Factsheet on Mental Health and Growing Up. No. 20. Royal College of Psychiatrists, London (tel 020 7235 2351, ext 146); e-mail booksales@rcpsych.ac.uk; website http://www.rcpsych.ac.uk/pub/pubsfs.htm.

Childline provides a free and confidential service for children. Posters stating the free number (tel 0800 1111) should be displayed in the health-centre waiting area where children can see them. The address is Freepost 111, London N1 0BR; website http://www.childline.org.uk/. Childline is also a useful source of factsheets.

Kidscape is a useful source of information about all types of abuse (not just bullying) for children, parents and teachers, including advice on keeping safe. The postal address is 2 Grosvenor Gardens, London SW1W 0DH (tel 020 7730 3300; fax 020 7730 7081); e-mail contact@kidscape.org.uk; website http://www.kidscape.org.uk/.

CHAPTER TWELVE

Sexualised behaviour

Introduction

What should you do if a parent asks you whether or not she should be worried by the sexualised behaviour her child is showing? How can you tell which behaviour is normal, whether it is just exploratory play, whether it is based on observing adult sexual activity or videos, or whether it is a result of participative sexual abuse? Should you reassure her and ignore it, or should you take it seriously enough to ask Social Services or a community paediatrician for a further opinion?

We are not aware of any definitive studies of what constitutes normal and abnormal sexualised behaviour in childhood. A moment's thought will reveal the difficulty inherent in conducting community studies. For example, whom do you ask, and how can you be sure that the reports represent a true account? Many parents ignore their children's masturbation, or do not regard it as sexual in any sense.[1] Retrospective accounts provided by adults are likely to be inaccurate.

Assessment, management and referral

Pre-school children

Self-stimulation of the genitals is common in both sexes in pre-school children. For parents who wish to limit this (although there is no need to do so), it usually responds to common-sense techniques such as ignoring or distraction. Alternatively, encouragement to do it in private may be sufficient to satisfy social propriety. Persistent or compulsive masturbation may be due to developmental delay or an overall lack of affection. In the absence of such a simple explanation, further investigation (by a social worker or community paediatrician) is advisable.

Primary-school-aged (latency) children

Freud believed that sexual impulses were present during the first five years of life, and then subsided until they were reawakened in adolescence (hence the term 'latency').

Sexualised behaviour is less likely to be a problem in this age group, but when it is, it may be of more concern.

Individual genital play may progress to exploratory play involving others' bodies in situations where children are allowed to play with inadequate supervision. When does play become abuse?[2]

- The greater the age difference between children, the more likely the activity is to be abusive. This is more to do with coercion and freely given consent than age itself, and it applies to the definition of sexual abuse at any age.
- Another dimension is the degree of sexual arousal. Evidence that a child is being sexually aroused and obtaining more than just tactile satisfaction should raise questions about how this arousal has developed before adolescence.
- Sexualised behaviour involving other children may have been copied either from actions observed or from actions experienced.

It is worth asking the child whether anyone has touched them on a part of the body where they should not be touched, and whether they have seen anyone doing the things they have been doing. In general, if sexualised behaviour in pre-adolescents involves other children, it is wisest to refer the case, probably to Social Services, in order to let them make the decision as to whether or not it is abuse. They may have information about the family of which you are unaware.

Adolescence

Masturbation is virtually universal among adolescent boys, but probably occurs in a smaller percentage of girls. Some learning-disabled or autistic young people lack a sense of public propriety, and need to be taught where they can and cannot masturbate. Occasionally it represents a crude sexual overture by a socially naïve or mentally handicapped boy to one or more girls, who then complain, so that the boy is subsequently accused of indecent exposure. Recognition of his lack of social skills will lead to a more sympathetic response than regarding him as perverted.

Experimental sexual behaviour among adolescents should be consensual, and problems arise when it is not. An arbitrary age gap of five years is used in some definitions of sexual abuse, but it is really the degree of mutual willingness that is important. There is increasing awareness of the extent to which girls may be involved against their will in sexual acts with boys, but other combinations can occur. For instance, a promiscuous girl may involve a naïve boy (who may be too ashamed to say no) in some form of sexual activity. He may feel just as ashamed about this as a girl who has been raped or a boy who has been buggered, and will have just as much difficulty telling anyone about the experience.

An abusive incident such as a rape may be disclosed to the general practitioner several years after the event. The victim's account should make it clear whether the episode was consensual or not. She should be encouraged to report the incident to the police or Social

Services, even if it happened a long time ago. This will enable the involvement of victim support services. However, the Children Act rules of consent apply (*see* Chapter 2 on consent), and the victim may be of sufficient age and understanding to veto the involvement of other agencies. If she requests someone to talk to (make sure that this request is made by the young person and not just the parent), she will need to be referred to a practice counsellor, adolescent counselling service or child and adolescent mental health service.

Case example 12.1

Sandra called her health visitor in great distress about her three-year-old daughter Amy. The nursery had asked her to take Amy home after she had tried to stick a pencil in another child's bottom. The health visitor went round later the same day. She knew Amy well, and asked her what she was trying to do. Amy said she had been trying to stick the pencil in the other girl's bum. Undaunted, the health visitor explored this further. Eventually it emerged that Amy's baby sister had been in hospital out-patients that week, and Amy had seen her having a rectal temperature taken.

   With Sandra's permission, the health visitor called Social Services to confirm that she did not need to refer this case. As she suspected, the nursery had already made a referral, stating their concern about the sexualised behaviour and its possible significance. The planned investigation was quickly halted, and the nursery staff were reassured. Sandra apologised on Amy's behalf to the other girl's mother, who was able to laugh about it.

Box 12.1:   Practice points on sexualised behaviour

*   Masturbation is usually normal behaviour. The issue of its social acceptability is generally the problem.
*   Sexualised play between pre-adolescent children may be normal, although it suggests a worrying lack of supervision. Any sexual activity involving other children has the potential to be abusive, and should normally be referred.
*   Sexualised activity between adolescents should be regarded as a form of abuse if one party has experienced it as coercive.

References

1   Deehan A and Fitzpatrick C (1993) Sexual behaviour and knowledge of normal children as perceived by their parents. *Irish Med J.* **86**: 130–2.

2   Lamb S and Coakley M (1993) 'Normal' childhood sexual play and games: differentiating play from abuse. *Child Abuse Neglect.* **17**: 515–26.

CHAPTER THIRTEEN

Post-traumatic stress disorder and adjustment disorder

Introduction and definitions

Children, like adults, can react adversely to catastrophes such as a car crash or an episode of extreme violence. Symptoms may include nightmares or flashbacks, avoidance of similar situations, and increased arousal. Children may have similar symptoms after any form of abuse (e.g. sexual abuse or bullying). The following is a useful definition of *post-traumatic stress disorder* in childhood,[1] which allows for the different ways in which symptoms may present at different ages:

1 *exposure* to a traumatic event
2 *re-experiencing* the event in nightmares, flashbacks, memories, response to reminders or in play – which may be uni-themed
3 *non-specific effects* such as social withdrawal or regression (in language skills, toilet training or a return of earlier behaviours)
4 *increased arousal* (e.g. night terrors, decreased concentration, hyper-vigilance or an exaggerated startle response)
5 *new fears* (e.g. of the dark, of separation or of toilets), or *new aggression*
6 symptoms must last for *at least one month*.

Minor variants of this picture can occur. For instance, a child's tantrums may become more frequent again after the death of a pet, or bed-wetting may recur when their parents separate. Such milder variants are common and are often labelled as an *adjustment disorder*. There is some debate as to whether this is a part of normal experience or a psychiatric condition. The symptoms are usually self-limiting unless they are maintained by factors such as parental anxiety or continuing parental conflict.

Alternatively, other conditions can be triggered, such as a generalised anxiety disorder, panic attacks or depression. The whole family is likely to be affected, even if only one member experienced the trauma. How the family copes will depend partly on communication style – families who tend not to share their feelings and experiences are more likely to develop difficulties.

Assessment

- Take a brief history of the trauma. This should only go into as much detail as is comfortable. It is sufficient to obtain an idea of the type of emotional upset that has been experienced.
- Be clear whether there are legal proceedings pending. If there are, it is more likely to be the parent than the child who is eager to emphasise the severity of the symptoms.
- Go through the above list of symptoms. Probably the easiest way to remember these is to ask first about new behaviours that are linked to the traumatic experience, and then about any other new behaviours, prompting for *increases* (e.g. in fearful behaviours or separation anxiety) and *decreases* (e.g. in friendliness or maturity).

Given that you have previous knowledge of the family, this should provide enough information for a provisional diagnosis.

Management

In cases of *post-traumatic stress disorder*, it may be helpful to tell the parents that talking about the trauma will help them to deal with the memories and associated emotions. Symptoms often seem to be prolonged when something is holding up emotional processing, and the feelings and thoughts may recur unchanged until they can be understood and tolerated.

On the other hand, insistence on a child's talking may be counter-productive if she is quite clear that she would prefer to deal with the situation by *not* talking about it. Younger children may indicate whether the trauma is preoccupying them by the themes in their play, which other family members may be able to use as a cue for discussion. Some families may be unwilling to communicate due to fear of opening things up. It is important to respect this attitude, while not necessarily agreeing with it.

Evidence obtained in adults suggests that pressurising trauma sufferers to talk immediately after the event may make the long-term outcome *worse*.[2]

The prognosis is usually good once communication within the family about the events has been established. Teenagers who bottle things up for years can be an exception to this, an extreme example being rape, which often seems to dictate secrecy. Such a teenager may need someone outside the family to talk to when she is ready, but there is little point in trying to force this to happen before she is prepared to speak about it.

In cases of *adjustment disorder*, it should be sufficient to explain to the parents that symptoms such as regression or worsening behaviour are common at times of emotional upset, and will improve provided that the distressing events do not continue. This does not mean that they should be dealt with any more leniently than usual, although the child may need to be shown more affection until the emotional disturbance has subsided. Parents may underestimate the effects on children of changes and losses such as a house move or the death of a grandparent (which also has indirect effects via parental grief). Parents should be encouraged to deal energetically with any continuing source of distress (e.g. bullying or the aftermath of divorce).

Referral

If litigation is pending, then any referral for an expert opinion should be made by the solicitor who is representing the child.

In *post-traumatic stress disorder*, referral for therapeutic input should only be made if the child appears to be willing to talk to someone outside the family, and there is reason to believe that family members cannot provide enough of a sounding-board. Sometimes it is more useful for the whole family – or a sibling group – to have outside help in sharing their experiences and feelings, rather than an individual child.

In *adjustment disorder*, referral may be necessary if there is real doubt about the diagnosis, or if parental concern requires a specialist opinion.

Case study 13.1

Joanna Harvey brought her two daughters, Kate (aged 13 years) and Alice (aged 15 years) to see the general practitioner. The two girls had been involved in a car crash in their grand-parents' car two years previously. Since that time Alice had suffered nightmares, usually only two or three times a month, but recently she had had a series of nightly bad dreams. Mrs Harvey told the doctor that the girls had both been assessed by an independent expert a year after the accident (this had been arranged through the insurance company) and had subsequently received financial compensation. Kate had not been significantly injured, and was checked briefly in casualty and allowed home. Alice had been admitted to hospital for several days with a head injury and an injured arm that had left her with a long scar. Mrs Harvey said that the girls had both found talking about the accident with the independent expert helpful, but there had only been a single appointment. Although the family had talked together about the accident before this interview, the expert's presence had helped them to think of things they had not remembered previously. Alice did not want medication, and Mrs Harvey explained that both girls would like another opportunity to go over the events of the accident together. The general practitioner agreed to see them together without their mother in a special half-hour appointment.

The doctor saw the two girls together for three half-hour sessions over the next three weeks. They talked through their respective memories of the accident and its aftermath, and Alice in particular, was encouraged to talk through and consider the effects on her of the head and arm injuries. Alice's nightmares again became much less frequent, and both girls agreed at the end of three sessions that they felt better.

continued overleaf

A few months later Mrs Harvey came to see the general practitioner with the flu. She reported that Alice was still having occasional nightmares, and still became frightened sometimes when riding as a passenger in a car, but that she was coping with these persisting symptoms.

References

1   Scheeringa MS, Zeanah CH, Drell MJ and Larrieu JA (1995) Two approaches to the diagnosis of post-traumatic stress disorder in infancy and early childhood. *J Am Acad Child Adolesc Psychiatry.* **34**: 191–200.

2   Mayou RA, Ehlers A and Hobbs M (2000) Psychological debriefing for road traffic accident victims: three-year follow-up of a randomized controlled trial. *Br J Psychiatry.* **176**: 589–93.

CHAPTER FOURTEEN

Death, dying and bereavement

Introduction

Members of the primary healthcare team can have an important role in helping children and their families to come to terms with dying and bereavement. Since the death of a child is a comparatively rare occurrence in the community, professionals may feel ill equipped to deal with this situation. An important first step is to gain an understanding of a child's concept of death that is helpful for both dying and bereaved children.

A child's concept of death

The way in which a child understands death depends very much on his age and developmental level. The development of this understanding has been studied in detail by child psychologist Richard Lansdown.[1] Most three-year-olds will have some realisation of the nature of death, but an understanding of the universality of death and ideas of causality do not develop until six or seven years of age. In general, a full understanding of death is not acquired until eight years, but many younger children do have a good although more limited understanding. Interestingly, most children up to the age of about eight years seem to have some concept of heaven, regardless of their religious background. Dying is often viewed as a journey, and children may ask very practical questions about the mechanics of getting into heaven. It is important to gain an idea of how much a child understands about death, and to be led by him in the way that you approach the subject.

Bereaved children

It is widely believed that children are bereaved and suffer grief reactions in much the same way as adults, with milder and shorter reactions in younger children. However, the available evidence does not appear to support this view.[2] Children vary tremendously in how they express grief, and they may not show the conventional stages. They are more resilient than adults in the face of bereavement, and in general they appear to be less affected in the long term by death than by parental separation. Children's resilience to adversity such as bereavement depends on a number of factors, including temperament, high self-esteem and the ability to form new relationships, as well as having a confiding relationship with a surviving adult.

It remains an open question how much children should be protected from death. Current ideas about how feelings are processed suggest that children may cope better with the death of a parent if they are allowed to participate in grieving rituals and have opportunities to talk about the dead parent, but at present there is no evidence to support this view. The practical implication is that parents should probably follow their children's wishes (e.g. about going to the funeral), but should not put any pressure on the child (e.g. to talk when they do not wish to). Counselling may be harmful.

Many children's first experience of death is that of a pet. The death of a grandparent is a likely event in any child's life. Parents may have difficulty in supporting the child in mourning when they are finding it hard to cope with their own grief. Someone should take on the responsibility for answering the child's questions. Young children in particular have a very concrete view of death and may seem quite cold-blooded and curious about it. For example, they may ask questions at the graveside about what mummy will do in the coffin, or they may fail to understand the finality of death and ask when daddy is coming back. Such questions are quite appropriate in the context of a child's concept of death, but may be very difficult for bereaved relatives to handle.

Loss of a parent

The way in which a child responds to the death of a parent is influenced by several factors. These include the child's personality, grief at the loss, the effect on the child of the surviving parent's reaction (e.g. depression, irritability, dependence on the child) and the resulting changes in circumstances.

A bereaved child may need repeated explanations as to why her parent died. If she has an insecure attachment, her main concern may be abandonment by the surviving parent, and she may become excessively clingy. Family members may also need reassurance that apparent indifference often occurs, and that grief may resolve more quickly in children than in adults.

Loss of a sibling

The loss of a sibling is likely to cause sadness and loneliness in the surviving children, but parents should be aware that there may well be mixed feelings. A surviving sibling may feel a sense of pleasure at now being able to receive more exclusive attention from their parents. It is also common for a child to feel guilty that something she has said, thought or done may have caused the death of her sibling.

The parent's reaction to the loss will have a major impact on how the remaining children cope. If the parent is preoccupied with the dead child, the survivors may be deprived of love and attention. The parents may consciously or unconsciously blame the surviving children for being alive. Other reactions include becoming overprotective of a surviving child, or idealising the child that has died and setting impossible standards for those who remain.

Managing a child's bereavement

Explanation

Understanding the cause of death can help a child to cope with loss. Simple explanations about part of the body being too poorly for the doctors to fix, or discussions about ageing or accidents, can be adapted to the age of the child. If the cause of death is not clearly explained, there is a risk that children may feel that the death is their responsibility. Before death (e.g. with a chronic illness) children may also need adequate explanations, and the opportunity to visit the parent in hospital, even if this is not openly stated as a chance to say goodbye.

Mourning

Children should be given the option of sharing in the family's mourning process. This may involve religious ideas such as heaven, but it may be confusing for a child to be fobbed off with a phrase such as 'mummy has gone to heaven' in a family where this is not part of their religious belief. Young children view God and heaven in very concrete ways, and introducing abstract religious concepts may cause problems if the family themselves have no religious belief. Children should be encouraged to talk about the parent if they wish to do so, and should be provided with mementoes such as photographs or special objects.

Security

Following the loss of a parent, the mental health of the surviving parent and their ability to cope have a major impact on the emotional well-being of the children. If the main caregiver has died, then the child may need to build a relationship with a new carer, and it is important that this develops into a stable solid relationship to enable the child to feel secure. Children may attempt to look after the surviving parent, but while love and help should be accepted, the parent must make it clear who is caring and who is cared for. The parent may need help to re-establish their own support network.

Referral

Counselling is not usually necessary for bereaved children, provided that the surviving family members can help. If a child has major behavioural problems or symptoms of depression, then referral to a bereavement counsellor with experience of dealing with children, or to a child mental health service, may be appropriate.

Managing dying children

Primary care team members may be involved in supporting a terminally ill child and their family while the child dies at home. Depending on the locality, palliative care services, including perhaps a community paediatrician, social workers and a psychologist, may be available. In order to make the death as peaceful as possible, many issues may need to be addressed. Symptom control is obviously essential, and advice can be sought from specialist teams such as those from children's hospices if the general practitioner lacks experience in this area. Spending time talking to the parents (and the child, if appropriate) about their fears is invaluable, as is discussion of practical arrangements. There are several charities that can help to arrange for children's last wishes to be honoured.

How to discuss death with a child

It is important to take into account the child's age and developmental stage. It is usually best to allow the child to take the lead in any conversation, and only to discuss issues once they have been raised by the child. Attempts should be made to answer even the most difficult questions as directly and honestly as possible. Although most parents will be prepared to discuss their child's illness openly, many find it very difficult to talk to their child about his or her death. If the parent refuses to allow the subject to be discussed, health professionals will need to respect that decision while at the same time being as honest as possible with the child.

When a child has died

After the death of a child, the primary care team has a very important role in ensuring continuing care for the family, and especially in supporting parents and siblings who may suffer bereavement reactions.

Box 14.1:   Practice points for managing death, dying and bereavement

- Children's understanding of death varies greatly, mainly with age.
- Children's reactions to the death of others also vary greatly, and depend on many factors, including temperament, resilience and family reactions to the death.
- Members of the primary care team may have opportunities to facilitate children's recovery from the death of a loved one by:

  advising parents to allow their children to grieve in their own way
  helping with explanations of physical illness
  helping parents with their emotional needs
  ensuring that children have access to a nurturing adult in whom they can confide.

- The general practitioner may be able to support the family of a child who is dying at home by participating in the child's practical care.

References

1   Lansdown R and Benjamin G (1985) The development of the concept of death in children aged 5–9 years. *Child Care Health Dev.* **11**: 13–20.

2   Harrington R and Harrison L (1999) Unproven assumptions about the impact of bereavement in children. *J R Soc Med.* **92**: 230–3.

Further reading

Herbert M (1996) *Supporting Bereaved and Dying Children and Their Parents.* British Psychological Society, Leicester.

Reading materials for parents and children

There are many excellent children's books about death or bereavement that will enable children to discuss the subject and ask questions in a more neutral environment. Parents who find it difficult to discuss loss with their child may find such books a useful starting point. Local libraries usually have several such books in stock. The following list is just a selection.

Connolly M and Manahan R (1999) *It Isn't Easy.* Oxford University Press, Oxford. This is the story of a child whose brother has been killed in an accident. It follows him and his parents through their reactions and their feelings of sadness, anger and pain, and it shows how they begin to come to terms with what has happened. The book is intended for children aged four years and over.

Hughes S (1999) *Alfie and the Birthday Surprise.* Red Fox Paperbacks, London. Alfie's neighbour is sad about the death of his cat, so Alfie helps to prepare a party to cheer him up.

Perkins J and Morris L (1996) *Remembering my Brother* and *Remembering Mum*. A & C Black, London. These books aim to show the importance of talking about grief and loss, and remembering with love someone important who has died.

Varley S (1993) *Badger's Parting Gifts*. Picture Lions Paperbacks, London. This book tells the story of Old Badger's death. His friends realise all of the things he has given them during his life, by which they will remember him. The book is also available in several other languages.

CHAPTER FIFTEEN

Imaginary friends, voices and psychosis

Introduction

Adult mental health services are focused on major mental illness, such as schizophrenia and manic-depression, and the treatment of psychosis. Psychosis occurs in only a minority of clients under 18, so child mental health services are in contrast focused far more on problems of living.

Although much of medical education is taken up with differentiating the normal from the abnormal, defining psychosis is fraught with difficulty. For instance, defining a *delusion* as a belief that is not only false and irrefutable, but is also neither shared by others nor culturally acceptable, may be appropriate for most of the time for adults. However, can it be applied to a boy who believes that his transient wish that his younger sister would die led to her developing leukaemia? Similarly, defining a *hallucination* as a perception of something that seems real but which would not be accepted as real by anyone else works well enough for adults. However, young children do not make such a clear distinction between fantasy and reality, and for them their dreamed or imagined experiences may be far more real than the voice their mother is talking to on the telephone.

Assessment: when is it normal?

It may be most helpful to think of a *continuum* from what is clearly normal because it occurs so frequently, to what is clearly psychotic because it matches adult psychotic experience closely. It is worth emphasising that psychotic symptoms do not necessarily indicate mental illness as a cause, and that psychotic mental illness is exceedingly rare before puberty.

Imaginary friends are at the normal end of this continuum. Young children (and some adults) often endow soft toys and pets with human characteristics. For some, the imagined being is disembodied, and may be a close companion, confidant, playmate or commentator. The relationship may be kept secret, or it may be divulged to parents or other close associates. Our impression is that the advent of background television and particularly computer games has led to children talking about such friends less, and possibly also experiencing them less. Children are now more likely to talk about the hero of their most recent computer game or their favourite cartoon.

Children commonly experience *voices*. These are not necessarily indicative of disorder. Often they may be merely one part of the child's mind that expresses a different view from the rest (like the character Jiminy Cricket in *Pinocchio*). Table 15.1 lists some criteria for professionals to be more or less worried about children hearing voices.

Table 15.1:   How worried do you need to be about voices?

	Nearer to normal end of the continuum	*Nearer to psychotic end of the continuum*
Where is the voice?	Inside the head or inside the mind	Outside the head, as if someone else is really talking
Who is the voice?	A familiar imaginary figure	A frightening and unknown being
How many voices are there?	One	Several
Who are the voices talking to?	The child or young person	Each other
What are they saying?	Expressing a viewpoint; being a conscience	Telling the young person to kill himself or other people; talking about the young person; saying derogatory things about him
Emotional context	The child appears to accept the presence of the voice, and it is other people who are worried by it	The young person is scared and uncertain about the nature of these experiences. He may feel controlled by the beings he hears

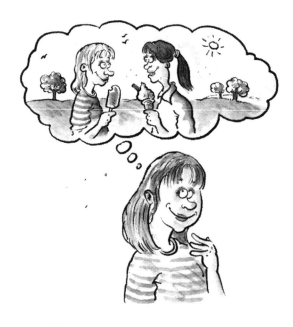

▼

Any history of abnormal experiences should consider *organic causes*, such as delirium during fever, or drug ingestion. This may involve prescribed drugs (e.g. dexamphetamine). A full enquiry about drug use should always be made, and a toxicology screen should be considered. *Visual hallucinations* are more likely to be due to an organic cause than auditory ones.

Another cause of auditory and visual hallucinations is *flashbacks*. These are recurrent memories of a traumatic experience. The experience may be any type of trauma, but sexual abuse is a particularly concerning example. The abuse may not have been disclosed, and the memories may have been partly suppressed. This can make management problematic (*see* Chapter 11, on childhood sexual abuse). In the past, such experiences have been regarded as 'borderline' between neurotic and psychotic. Vivid flashbacks with a realistic quality commonly occur in adults with borderline personality disorder, and they often seem to be linked to childhood abuse. We believe that using this terminology in those under 18 years of age leads to a fruitless debate about diagnostic categories. It is simpler to obtain as clear a description of the experience as possible, and to think of a flashback as one possible cause.

Approaching close to the psychotic end of the continuum are abnormal experiences in those with *autistic spectrum disorders*, especially Asperger's syndrome (*see* Chapter 5). Schizophrenia is said to be more common in this group of individuals. However, we believe that part of the increased incidence of psychotic symptoms is due to the difficulty in abstract thought that is characteristic of Asperger's syndrome. It may be particularly difficult at times for affected individuals to differentiate between internal and external events or between fantasy and reality in an age-appropriate way.

Finally, *schizophrenia* does occur in adolescence, and may present with truly psychotic phenomena, including auditory hallucinations with many of the features listed in the right-hand column of Table 15.1. It is not always easy to diagnose at first presentation, and both *depression* and *recreational drug use* are commoner causes of very similar symptoms.

Management and referral

Management is simple. The treatment of psychotic symptoms in young people (e.g. by medication) is not appropriate within primary care, so the only decision that needs to be made is whether or not the symptoms require further assessment. Those presentations that are clearly at the normal end of the continuum require reassurance, while those at the psychotic end, or for which there is significant doubt, require referral.

Case study 15.1

Paul, a nine-year-old boy, was brought to the general practitioner by his mother, who told the doctor that the headteacher had insisted that Paul must have a check-up. He had caused great consternation in school by climbing on to the first-floor banisters and then on to the ledge of the first-floor window, as if to jump out. He subsequently told his headteacher that a voice had told him to jump out of the window, and the headteacher wanted him referred for assessment. The general practitioner attempted to talk to Paul, but was unable to get more than a few words in reply. He agreed to refer him for assessment in view of the degree of anxiety engendered among all concerned.

The doctor received a report one month later. The child psychiatrist had elicited a clear description of the voice, as being a voice inside Paul's head expressing an idea of his own. The threat to jump from the window ledge had arisen immediately after a fight with another boy in his class, after which his class teacher had told him off. It seemed to the psychiatrist that Paul had wanted to create an effect.

The psychiatrist's report informed the general practitioner that the family were previously known to both the mental health services and Social Services as an impoverished family with three boys and a girl, all of whom had suffered behavioural problems. Paul was the eldest, and he seemed to elicit the most critical comments from his mother. The father was not prepared to become involved with the mental health services or Social Services, but there had never been sufficient evidence of harm to justify a child protection case conference. Family therapy had been tried unsuccessfully. Paul had had a few individual sessions and had been seen jointly with his mother intermittently over a period of several years, again without noticeable benefit. The psychiatrist asked the general practitioner to prescribe a trial of methylphenidate.

One week later the general practitioner reviewed the progress on methylphenidate, and Paul's mother reported that although it seemed to make no difference at home, his head-teacher had been happier with Paul's behaviour at school, and it was agreed to continue the drug at least in the short term.

Case study 15.2

Seven-year-old Oliver was brought to the general practitioner by his mother because she was concerned about his description of a friend called 'Fred' who would sometimes tell Oliver to do naughty things. The general practitioner suggested that Oliver could play with the toys in the corner of the consulting-room while he asked his mother some more questions about the background. Oliver was an only child, and his mother mentioned that he had had some difficulty in making friends at his local school. His access to television was limited, and he was not allowed computer games at home. The doctor then asked Oliver, in his mother's presence, about Fred. Oliver was quite clear that Fred was only pretend. He had known him for about three years (this was a surprise to his mother) and had had many conversations

continued opposite

with him. Sometimes Fred would suggest things that Oliver might do. Oliver was unwilling to admit that these might be his own ideas but, on the general practitioner's suggestion, he did reluctantly admit that they must come from inside his own head, since that is where Fred came from. Hearing this conversation seemed to reassure Oliver's mother, and the general practitioner suggested that there was nothing much wrong with her son. He suggested that Oliver should be allowed to mix more with children of his own age, and he suggested that she should explore the possibility of after-school clubs.

PART 3

Problems that may present in the first few years

CHAPTER SIXTEEN

Postnatal depression

Introduction

There is a substantial psychiatric morbidity associated with childbirth. At least 10% of women will have a major depressive episode in the year following childbirth. The risk is higher in the first three months than during the following nine months.[1] The subject is included in this book because of its proven effects on early mother–child interactions and on children's cognitive and social development.

In the postpartum period there are higher risks than at any other time in a woman's life of her suffering from a severe depressive illness, becoming psychotic, being referred to a psychiatrist and being admitted to a psychiatric hospital. The effects of untreated postnatal depression on the mother include difficulties with close relationships, social isolation and a 30% rate of continuance of maternal depression into the second year of the child's life.

Depressed mothers are less sensitive, less attentive and more critical of their infants.[2] The effects of untreated postnatal depression on children, compared to a control group, may include the following:

- impaired cognitive development from one year onwards
- less warmth and positive interaction between the child and their parent (in both directions)
- more insecure attachment, usually of the avoidant type
- behavioural difficulties from 18 months.

Aetiological theories

As yet there is no agreement about a hormonal basis for postnatal depression, although genetic studies suggest that biological factors must be relevant. Obstetric complications may increase the risk, but possibly only in those with a previous history of depressive disorder. A psychiatric history, particularly of depressive disorder, increases the risk, especially if the depression was postpartum. Social factors have been shown to increase the risk. These include stressful life events, unemployment, marital conflict and lack of personal support from spouse, family and friends. Childbirth is a major life event linked to many expectations that can lead to disappointment. Both partners have to adjust to the new baby and to the resulting changes in their relationship. Difficulties in making this adjustment may reveal cracks that were previously concealed. The very nature of the nuclear family can make it easy to become very isolated after childbirth. Factors related to the child are also important. For example, an irritable baby (who is difficult to handle), or a baby who is under- or over-aroused (who is unresponsive), increases the likelihood that his mother will subsequently become depressed.[3]

Assessment

Postnatal depression is often under-detected and under-treated. The symptoms can easily be overlooked and attributed to tiredness, sleepless nights and the demands of coping with a new baby. In addition, many mothers are reluctant to admit that they feel 'down', or are not really coping. Their answers to questions may be influenced by a strong desire to appear to be a capable mother.

First, look for the following symptoms of major depression:

- *cognitive* – a negative view of oneself, the world and the future
- *affective* – low mood, irritability, and possibly anxiety or agitation
- *behavioural* – loss of interest in life, poor concentration, social withdrawal, psychomotor retardation
- *biological* – poor appetite, weight loss, poor sleep, constipation, loss of libido.

Secondly, look for the following additional features:

- *guilt* – a mother may feel particularly guilty about experiencing despair at a time when she is supposed to be delighted with her new baby. She may conclude that she is a bad partner and mother
- *obsessional thoughts*
- *fears of harming the baby.*

Differential diagnosis

Postnatal depression must be distinguished from 'baby blues' (which commonly occur towards the end of the first week) and puerperal psychosis (which requires urgent psychiatric referral and treatment because of the risk to the baby) (*see* Table 16.1).

Table 16.1:   Causes of postpartum mood changes

Disorder	Prevalence (%)	Onset
Baby blues	50	3–7 days
Postnatal depression	10	0–12 months
Puerperal psychosis	0.1–0.2	1–4 weeks

Detection

Early detection is important. However, this cannot be achieved until the end of the first week or two, by which time the baby blues will have passed. Screening using the Edinburgh Postnatal Depression Scale[4] (*see* Box 16.1) has been shown to be an easy and reliable way of detecting postpartum depression. It involves a 10-item self-report questionnaire and has a high specificity and sensitivity. It has been both used and validated in clinical practice in primary care, and several studies have shown how easy it is for health visitors and general practitioners to use. Each question is scored from 0 to 3 according to increasing severity of the symptom concerned. Questions 1, 2 and 4 are scored 0–1–2–3, while questions 3, 5, 6, 7, 8, 9 and 10 are reverse scored 3–2–1–0. A score of 12 or higher indicates a need for further assessment. For ease of reference the Scale is repeated on one page at the end of this chapter.

Box 16.1:   The Edinburgh Postnatal Depression Scale

Name: ....
Date filled in: ...../...../.....
Baby's age: .... *weeks/months/years*

Cox JL, Holden JM and Sagovsky R (1987) Detection of postnatal depression: development of the ten-item Edinburgh Postnatal Depression Scale. *Br J Psychiatry.* **150**: 782–6.
[To protect copyright, this must be quoted on all reproduced copies.]

As you have recently had a baby, we would like to know how you are feeling. Please underline the answer that comes closest to how you have felt **in the past seven days** – not just how you feel today. Here is an example, already completed:

I have felt happy:
  Yes, all the time
  Yes, most of the time
  No, not very often
  No, not at all

This would mean 'I have felt happy for most of the time' during the past week. Please complete the other questions in the same way.

In the past seven days:

1 I have been able to laugh and see the funny side of things:
  As much as I always could
  Not quite so much now
  Definitely not so much now
  Not at all

2 I have looked forward with enjoyment to things:
  As much as I ever did
  Rather less than I used to
  Definitely less than I used to
  Hardly at all

continued overleaf

In the past seven days: (*continued*)

3 I have blamed myself unnecessarily when things went wrong:
Yes, most of the time
Yes, some of the time
Not very often
No, never

4 I have been anxious or worried for no good reason:
No, not at all
Hardly ever
Yes, sometimes
Yes, very often

5 I have felt scared or panicky for no very good reason:
Yes, quite a lot
Yes, sometimes
No, not much
No, not at all

6 Things have been getting on top of me:
Yes, most of the time I haven't been able to cope at all
Yes, sometimes I haven't been coping as well as usual
No, most of the time I have coped quite well
No, I have been coping as well as ever

7 I have been so unhappy that I have been having difficulty sleeping:
Yes, most of the time
Yes, sometimes
Not very often
No, not at all

8 I have felt sad or miserable:
Yes, most of the time
Yes, quite often
Not very often
No, not at all

9 I have been so unhappy that I have been crying:
Yes, most of the time
Yes, quite often
Only occasionally
No, never

10 The thought of harming myself has occurred to me:
Yes, quite often
Sometimes
Hardly ever
Never

Management[5]

Primary prevention

Antenatal classes and the fostering of social support may help to prevent postnatal depression, and should be widely available. A routine visit by the health visitor in the last trimester may help to encourage prospective mothers to attend antenatal and postnatal classes and form a relationship that may be invaluable later.

Secondary prevention of the effects on the child

Early detection of postnatal depression is essential. Despite increasing awareness of the extent and importance of postnatal depression, many cases remain undetected or inadequately treated.

Health visitors and general practitioners should not feel embarrassed about asking women how they are feeling and coping, particularly if they are tearful. Routine screening using the Edinburgh Postnatal Depression Scale should be carried out by the health visitor either during a routine home visit or when the baby has his or her development assessments. Asking about suicidal ideation and guilt may arouse strong feelings, but these questions are an essential part of the assessment, and women will feel a great sense of relief if they are able to share their concerns.

To our knowledge, the only antidepressant that has been studied in a controlled trial of postnatally depressed mothers is fluoxetine.[6] Both fluoxetine and brief psychological interventions are effective in the treatment of postnatal depression.[7,8] The manufacturers of fluoxetine and venlafaxine list lactation as a contraindication. There is also theoretical concern that the long half-life of fluoxetine may cause accumulation of the drug in the baby. However, it seems that all antidepressants are present in breast milk, although sertraline has been found not to affect serotonin metabolism in the infant.[9]

Lactating mothers are usually, quite appropriately, reluctant to give up breastfeeding. In practice, it is probably wisest to offer mothers the choice of a psychological intervention or antidepressants. If antidepressants are chosen, then a selective serotonin reuptake inhibitor (e.g. sertraline or citalopram) should probably be used, and the baby should be closely monitored for any changes in behaviour.

An intriguing suggestion is that of 'late sleep deprivation'.[10] In postnatally depressed women, mood was observed to improve after a night when sleep was confined to the period 9 p.m. to 1 a.m., and even more after a night of recovery sleep. This can be repeated at intervals of not less than once week. Alternatively, sleep deprivation due to a sleepless infant may be regarded as the cause of the depression, in which case a behavioural management programme for the baby's sleep may help the mother's depression.[11]

Health visitors can learn a variety of brief psychological interventions that are targeted directly at the depressive mood. An example is given in Box 16.2.

Box 16.2: A psychological therapy for postnatal depression

- This psychological treatment uses basic cognitive–behavioural skills[12] and active, reflective listening.[13] These techniques can be easily developed by health visitors, who may already use many of them as part of their routine contact with mothers of young children.
- The *initial session* lasts for one hour. The therapist allows the mother to describe her current circumstances and emotional state.
- *Subsequent sessions* last for 30 minutes each, and can be conducted fortnightly (giving a total of six sessions over a period of three months). The focus is on activity scheduling (e.g. taking the baby to the park, or going out socially), discussion of depressive thoughts, practical difficulties with managing the child, and relationship difficulties with the child, their partner or their extended family.

The risk to the child

Part of the management of a mother with postnatal depression involves thinking about the risk to the child. At the very least, the child will experience the mother as less available and responsive. Research has shown that this affects the child's emotional and cognitive development.[2] There may be more extreme risks to the child, particularly if the mother is so depressed that she is unable to care for the child effectively, or develops an intention to harm the child. Mothers will usually admit to this intention if asked about it. In this situation, advice should be sought as a matter of urgency from the local adult psychiatrist and children's Social Service department.

Referral

Indications for referral of a mother with postnatal depression to an adult psychiatrist are as follows:

• psychotic features or a past history of psychosis
• well-formed intentions to harm herself or the baby
• poor response to treatment.

Case study 16.1

Louise Atkinson, a 25-year-old first-time mother, came to see her general practitioner three weeks after the birth of her baby Gemma by vacuum delivery at 38 weeks' gestation. She had been advised by the hospital to have a repeat blood test and to check with the doctor to see whether she needed to remain on iron tablets.

When asked how she was getting along generally, Louise admitted to feeling very tired and lacking in energy. She was not sleeping very well, as Gemma was breastfeeding frequently through the night. Louise felt close to tears all the time, and panicky and unable to cope sometimes, particularly when she was alone at night. Her husband was a shift-worker who sometimes worked late evenings and sometimes worked nights. Louise was getting only three or four hours' sleep altogether, and during the day she felt physically and mentally exhausted, very forgetful, and had poor concentration and a poor appetite. She admitted to feeling frustrated with the new baby at times, but had not shouted at her, and had never for a moment considered smacking her.

On examination the doctor found Louise to be clinically anaemic, and therefore arranged for a blood count to be taken and asked her to come back in one week's time. In the mean time she met with the practice's health visitor to check whether she had completed a screen for postnatal depression with Louise, and whether she was happy that Gemma was not at any risk. The health visitor was concerned that Louise was depressed, but she was satisfied

continued opposite

that she was taking good care of Gemma. The doctor shared with the health visitor the information that Louise had suffered a previous bout of depression two years earlier, and had been treated with antidepressants.

The following week Louise was still feeling low and panicky at times. Her haemoglobin level was slightly reduced at 11.5 g/dL. She was still having to feed Gemma several times a night, yet Gemma was losing weight, apparently because she was getting inadequate amounts of milk. The doctor discussed the pros and cons of breastfeeding at length with Louise. She explained that, although breast milk was best for babies, in a developed country bottle-feeding was a very acceptable alternative. Apparently relieved to hear this, Louise decided, with the doctor's blessing, to switch to bottle-feeding. This would allow her husband to take his turn giving Gemma feeds during the night, at least on those nights when he was home. The doctor advised Louise to continue on iron tablets and told her that she wanted to review her again in a week when, if she was no better, they should consider a course of antidepressants.

One week later the situation was much improved. Gemma was taking milk much better from bottles and was putting on weight again. Louise had talked through her feelings with her husband, who was proving very helpful. She was constipated but was tolerating the iron and starting to feel more energetic. She remained rather forgetful and still had an erratic appetite, but she was no longer panicky, and only occasionally felt close to tears.

At review one week later, Louise was definitely improving, and she had more energy despite being up once or twice every night. She had had what seemed like a normal period and was feeling stronger physically as a result of taking the iron tablets. The doctor decided to avoid antidepressant treatment but to keep her under review for the next two months at least.

Box 16.3:   Practice points about postnatal depression

- It is often not recognised and is generally under-treated.
- Sufferers may have a need to conceal their symptoms.
- It can have significant long-term effects on both mother and child.
- Health visitors and general practitioners have an important role in assessment and treatment.
- Health visitors can give an effective brief psychological treatment.
- General practitioners can prescribe antidepressants that are effective and probably safe.
- Most cases can be managed in primary care and do not require referral.

Box 16.4:   A personal account of postnatal depression*

I was diagnosed as having postnatal depression when my son Louis was nine months old. My doctor and health visitor had been 'watching me' since his birth. My daughter Connie was nine years old at this time. I think, hindsight being 20/20 vision, that I had postnatal depression when *she* was born. However, I blamed most of my symptoms on an already failing first marriage. Fortunately, I am now in a very strong and happy marriage to my second husband, Pete.

I don't know whether there was one single reason for my depression, but I see it as a culmination of many factors, each of which on its own I would probably have been able to cope with. I had a happy and healthy pregnancy. Louis was 14 days overdue. He was induced, but went into fetal distress, and I was eventually given an emergency Caesarean section, which I was obviously not prepared for. Louis was a very colicky baby and cried a lot. He also had eczema, caused by a milk allergy, which took approximately four months to be diagnosed.

At five months old, he became very ill and we had the doctor out to him every day for a week. He was not improving, and eventually he was taken into hospital. The next morning, the consultant saw Louis and told me he suspected meningitis. Louis had to have a lumber puncture, and Pete had to hold him down while it was done. In fact, Louis did have viral meningitis, and was in hospital for a week. I stayed with him the whole time. He left hospital with gastroenteritis and we watched his weight plummet during the following two weeks.

It was when Louis recovered that my health began to deteriorate.

I felt that I was not the sort of person to whom this kind of thing happened. I am usually a strong person – the kind others turn to in times of crisis. Like most people, I had a fear of mental illness – of not being in control of my own mind.

I simply was not coping with life. For example, when our kitchen was Artexed, the man ripped our floor covering. Normally, I would not have paid him for the work, or would have negotiated some form of compensation. Due to the illness, I locked the children and myself in the living room and refused to talk to him. Pete was so taken aback by this behaviour that he simply paid the workman to get him out of the way so that he could calm me down.

I became very withdrawn and I would not leave the house unless it was really necessary. I couldn't answer the telephone. I would let the answering machine take the call, and maybe then pick the call up or get Pete to phone the person back later. Connie was in on this system. When she was at home, she would answer the telephone and tell the caller that I was unavailable.

Connie and I have always had a very close relationship. We spent five years on our own as a 'two family'. She has always been protective of me even when I really didn't need protecting. She will not have a bad word said against me, and frequently tells me I am the best or most cool mum.

During the depths of my depression, Connie and I almost swapped roles. She became very protective of me and would act as a cushion against the outside world. She became the parent and I the child. She grew up a lot in the first two years of Louis' life. Some of this must be due to the fact that she was no longer the one and only but now a big sister, and some must be due to her age – she was at an age when you switch from being a little girl to a

continued opposite

young lady. However, I do know that some of the explanation must have been living with me during my depression.

As a family we communicate well. We discuss most things openly, and Connie was a party to many discussions on how I was feeling and what others could do to help me. Her help was invaluable.

I could not go shopping alone, and still have problems in this area. I suffered from major panic attacks when out shopping, and I relied on my family to help me. Both Pete and Connie coached me through the panic attacks, standing with me and helping me to control my breathing. I still get panic attacks, mostly associated with shopping in town, but I am able to deal with them myself as they are far less severe than those I experienced initially.

I really hit an all-time low when my doctor told me I was clinically depressed. Until this point I was kidding myself that I was not that bad, even though I was suffering from some very severe symptoms. The main reason that I considered my depression not to be severe was because I felt no animosity towards Louis. I loved him from the moment he was laid in my arms. I thought that all mothers with postnatal depression rejected their babies. However, I learned from the other mothers whom I contacted through the locally run postnatal depression support group that this was far from true.

Looking at us now, I feel that as a family we have benefited from the depression. We are strong and definitely more understanding of illness in others.

As for the effect on Louis, I think everything that happens to a child goes towards developing their character. Louis is a happy, social child who interacts well with both adults and his peers. As I had returned to full-time working prior to my sick leave, he benefited from 9 months of my company, and his company made me strong at times when I might have gone to pieces on my own. After my sick leave I returned to work on a part-time basis, and this situation continues, so that Louis and I spend time together still. He is a 'mummy's boy', but no more so than other children whose mothers have not been through depression.

*We are indebted to Karen King of Worthing, West Sussex, for permission to publish this account of her own experience of postnatal depression.

Acknowledgements

We are grateful to Dr Jean Sherrington, Consultant in Adult Psychiatry, Sussex Weald and Downs NHS Trust, for helpful comments on clinical practice.

References

1   Cooper PJ and Murray L (1997) Prediction, detection and treatment of postnatal depression. *Arch Dis Child.* **77**: 97–9.

2   Murray L and Cooper PJ (1997) Effects of postnatal depression on infant development. *Arch Dis Child.* **77**: 99–101.

3   Murray L, Stanley C, Hooper R, King F and Fiori-Cowley A (1996) The role of infant factors in postnatal depression and mother–infant interactions. *Dev Med Child Neurol.* **38**: 109–19.

4   Cox JL, Holden JM and Sagovsky R (1987) Detection of postnatal depression: development of the ten-item Edinburgh Postnatal Depression Scale. *Br J Psychiatry.* **150**: 782–6.

5   Anon (2000) The management of postnatal depression. *Drug Ther Bull.* **38**: 33–7.

6   Appleby L, Warner R, Whitton A and Faragher B (1997) A controlled study of fluoxetine and cognitive-behavioural counselling in the treatment of postnatal depression. *BMJ.* **314**: 932–6.

7   Holden JM, Sagovsky R and Cox JL (1989) Counselling in a general practice setting: controlled study of health visitor intervention in treatment of postnatal depression. *BMJ.* **298**: 223–6.

8   Seeley S, Murray L and Cooper PJ (1996) The outcome for mothers and babies of health visitor intervention. *Health Visitor.* **69**: 135–8.

9   Epperson CN, Anderson GM and McDougle CJ (1997) Sertraline and breast feeding. *NEJM.* **336**: 1189–90.

10   Lamberg L (1999) Safety of antidepressant use in pregnant and nursing women. *JAMA.* **282**: 222–3.

11   Armstrong KL, Van Haeringen AR, Dadds MR and Cash R (1998) Sleep deprivation or postnatal depression in later infancy: separating the chicken from the egg. *J Paediatrics Child Health.* **34**: 260–2.

12   Hawton K, Salkovskis PM, Kirk J and Clark DM (1989) *Cognitive Behaviour Therapy for Psychiatric Problems.* Oxford University Press, Oxford.

13   Egan G (1997) *The Skilled Helper* (6e). International Thomson Publishing (Europe), Brooks Cole imprint, New York.

Organisations that can help

National Childbirth Trust, Alexandra House, Oldham Terrace, Acton, London W3 6NH (tel 020 8992 8637). Publishes pamphlets entitled *Postnatal Depression* (£2.95) and *Postnatal Depression Support* (£5.00).

Association for Postnatal Illness, 25 Jerdan Place, London SW6 1BE (tel 020 7386 0868).

Gingerbread, 49 Wellington Street, London WC2E 7BN (tel 020 7240 0953). A national network of local groups that provides single parents with support, friendship and social activities.

Twins and Multiple Births Association (TAMBA), (tel 01708 705219) (Tracey Harding). Helpline: 01732 868000 (6.00 p.m.–11.00 p.m., Mon–Fri; 10.00 a.m.–11.00 p.m., Sat–Sun). Supports families with twins, triplets or more through local Twins Clubs and specialist support groups.

National Newpin, Sutherland House, 35 Sutherland Square, Walworth, London SE17 3EE (tel 020 7703 6326).

Homestart UK, 2 Salisbury Road, Leicester LE1 7OR (tel 0116 233 9955).

Reading for parents

Cloutte P (1999) *Understanding Postnatal Depression.* MIND, London; website http://www.mind.org.uk/shopping/shop.asp?id=understanding.

Curham S (2000) *Antenatal and Postnatal Depression.* Vermilion, London.

Pitt B (1993) *Down with Gloom.* Gaskell Press and The Royal College of Psychiatrists, London.

Royal College of Psychiatrists (1997) *Postnatal Depression: Help is at Hand.* Royal College of Psychiatrists, London; website: http://www.rcpsych.ac.uk/public/help/pndep/dpn_frame.htm. The 'Help is at Hand' self-help leaflets 'may be duplicated and distributed free of charge as long as the Royal College of Psychiatrists is properly credited and no profit is gained from their use'.

Welford H (1998) *The National Childbirth Trust Book of Postnatal Depression.* Thorsons, Glasgow.

The Edinburgh Postnatal Depression Scale

Name: ....

Date filled in: ...../...../.....

Baby's age: .... *weeks/months/years*

Cox JL, Holden JM and Sagovsky R (1987)
Detection of postnatal depression:
development of the ten-item Edinburgh
Postnatal Depression Scale.
Br J Psychiatry. **150**: 782–6.
[To protect copyright, this must be quoted on all
reproduced copies.]

As you have recently had a baby, we would like to know how you are feeling. Please <u>underline</u> the answer that comes closest to how you have felt **in the past seven days** – not just how you feel today. Here is an example, already completed:

I have felt happy:
   Yes, all the time
   <u>Yes, most of the time</u>
   No, not very often
   No, not at all

This would mean 'I have felt happy for most of the time' during the past week. Please complete the other questions in the same way.

In the past seven days:

1 I have been able to laugh and see the funny side of things:
   As much as I always could
   Not quite so much now
   Definitely not so much now
   Not at all

2 I have looked forward with enjoyment to things:
   As much as I ever did
   Rather less than I used to
   Definitely less than I used to
   Hardly at all

3 I have blamed myself unnecessarily when things went wrong:
   Yes, most of the time
   Yes, some of the time
   Not very often
   No, never

4 I have been anxious or worried for no good reason:
   No, not at all
   Hardly ever
   Yes, sometimes
   Yes, very often

5 I have felt scared or panicky for no very good reason:
   Yes, quite a lot
   Yes, sometimes
   No, not much
   No, not at all

6 Things have been getting on top of me:
   Yes, most of the time I haven't been able to cope at all
   Yes, sometimes I haven't been coping as well as usual
   No, most of the time I have coped quite well
   No, I have been coping as well as ever

7 I have been so unhappy that I have been having difficulty sleeping:
   Yes, most of the time
   Yes, sometimes
   Not very often
   No, not at all

8 I have felt sad or miserable:
   Yes, most of the time
   Yes, quite often
   Not very often
   No, not at all

9 I have been so unhappy that I have been crying:
   Yes, most of the time
   Yes, quite often
   Only occasionally
   No, never

10 The thought of harming myself has occurred to me:
   Yes, quite often
   Sometimes
   Hardly ever
   Never

CHAPTER SEVENTEEN

Crying and colic

Introduction

Crying is one of the most powerful ways in which an infant can attract adult attention. It is part of the normal developmental process and serves several functions.

- It is a response to pain, and to physiological discomforts such as hunger.
- It is an expression of emotional distress, such as fear or anxiety.
- It is a means of communication with the caregiver, indicating a need to be met by them.

However functional it may be, crying – especially inconsolable crying that lasts for many hours – can be a cause of great distress to parents. Excessive crying is a common problem, and estimates of prevalence rates range from 14% to 35% of babies.[1,2]

Causes of crying

Three-month colic, persistent evening crying or evening fretting

It is difficult to provide a clear definition of *three-month colic*, and its aetiology is not fully understood. An alternative term is *persistent evening crying*. In general, it is accepted that colic is a pattern of inconsolable crying that occurs on a daily basis, often in the afternoon or evening, between about 3 and 14 weeks of age. Babies with colic tend to scream intensely for long periods, draw their legs up and look pale. Colic is a self-limiting condition that occurs in babies who are thriving and otherwise well.

More commonly and less severely, the baby grizzles during the evening but is pacified relatively easily by being carried around or taken for a car ride. This is often called *evening fretting*, and it probably reflects the baby's inability to soothe himself and therefore his reliance on caregivers to comfort him.

There are a number of theories about the causes of colic, none of which have been proven. One of the most popular, at least among lay people, is that it may be due to immaturity of the gut causing intestinal spasm. This theory is supported by the fact that antispasmodic drug therapy is the only medication that has been shown to have a therapeutic effect, and that premature babies who develop colic tend to do so within two weeks of the due date, regardless of gestation.

Hunger

One of the commonest reasons for frequent or near continual crying in a young baby is hunger. Weighing the baby and plotting their weight on a growth chart is a simple way to assess whether the baby is in fact being adequately nourished. On the other hand, mothers who breastfeed sometimes give up unnecessarily because they fear that their baby's crying is a sign of hunger when it is not.

Diet

The pattern of crying in formula-fed babies is different from that in breastfed babies.[3] Formula-fed babies cry more at two weeks of age, while breastfed babies cry more and sleep less at six weeks of age. Cow's-milk protein is often implicated in colic, but soya-based milks are not necessarily better – a hypoallergenic formula may be necessary.[4] Concerns have been expressed – with much anecdotal evidence – about substances transmitted in breast milk that may cause crying in the infant (e.g. cow's milk, caffeine, spices, brassicas, chocolate, beans).

Wind

Crying after a feed is often thought to be due to wind. According to this lay theory, it can be terminated by burping manoeuvres. A related theory is that wind can be caused by bottle-feeding from a teat with too large a hole, but clinical practice suggests that changing the teat size does not lead to a dramatic improvement.

Illness

Many parents feel that their inconsolably crying baby must be in pain and therefore ill. Colic will probably be implicated in the majority of these cases, and the child will be physically well. However, it is obviously important not to miss the less common causes of excessive crying, such as pain from acute infections (ear, nose and throat, or urinary tract) or from a strangulated inguinal hernia. Crying after a feed may be due to pain from gastro-oesophageal reflux, and this may be associated with unusual posturing of the baby's head and neck. There will usually (but not always) be a history of vomiting. If suspected, this possibility should be investigated by a paediatrician. A rare but extremely important condition is infantile seizures, in which the baby flexes the whole trunk in a salaam spasm and utters a brief cry. A child with possible infantile spasms should probably be referred as an emergency.

Birth complications and prematurity

The reputed Chinese aphorism 'difficult birth, difficult child' contains a grain of truth. Babies who have had complicated and traumatic deliveries have been shown to be more irritable and to cry more,[2] and this is also true of premature and low-birth-weight babies.[1] The nature of their cries is also reported to be high-pitched and irritating, and therefore more distressing to parents.

Temperament

Temperamental changes are associated with the amount and style of an infant's crying. Two temperamental groups that may cause particular problems are those babies who appear tense and dislike handling and stimulation, and active babies who seem to demand much attention and stimulation.

Maternal anxiety

It has been suggested that anxiety and tension in the mother may contribute to her baby's crying. A number of studies have shown that first babies cry more than second ones, but this may simply be a reflection of the fact that first-time mothers are often more aware of crying and less skilled at preventing it. It is also very difficult to separate cause from effect, as a mother whose baby cries inconsolably will tend to be more tense than one with a content infant.

Assessment

By the time the parents of a crying baby approach health professionals, they may have already received a vast amount of conflicting advice from friends and relatives, and they may well be feeling bewildered and inadequate. It is extremely important to allow them space to discuss their anxieties and to avoid appearing judgemental, if you are to maintain a therapeutic relationship.

The aim of assessment is to try to help the parents to see the problem in a systematic way, so that they can approach possible solutions in a logical fashion.

Approach to assessment

1 Consider medical problems.
   - Enquire about problems such as vomiting, poor weight gain and fits.
   - Plot the baby's length and weight on a centile chart.
   - Examine the ears and throat for infection.
   - Examine the abdomen for hernias.
   - Microscope a urine sample for white cells, and/or send it off for culture.
2 Obtain a detailed description of the crying.
   - Ask about the age at which crying started.
   - Were there any periods of improvement or deterioration?

- Is there a pattern to the crying (e.g. best and worst times of day, intensity and duration)?
- What methods have the parents used to try to control the crying?
- Which of these methods have been successful?

3 Consider the feeding pattern.
- Is the baby being breastfed or bottle-fed, or both?
- What is the quality of sucking?
- Note the length, volume and frequency of feeds.
- What is the relationship between crying and feeding?

4 Consider the sleeping pattern.
- What is the pattern of sleeping during the day and the night?
- What is the relationship between sleeping and feeding?

5 Consider psychosocial factors.
- What effect does the child's crying have on the parents?
- What do they fear may be wrong?
- What type of support is available for the mother from the father, the extended family or neighbours?

A crying diary

It may be difficult for parents to recall accurately the pattern of crying. It may seem to a stressed mother that her baby screams constantly, when in fact there are a number of screaming episodes which occur unpredictably throughout the day. It is often very helpful to ask the parents to fill in a diary for a few days in which they record accurate details of crying episodes (including time, duration, intensity, exacerbating or relieving factors and parents' responses), as well as sleeping and feeding patterns. This technique also has the advantage of saving a considerable amount of time in the consultation, if time constraints are an important factor.

Management

The majority of problems with crying babies are self-limiting and have no serious long-term consequences (although they may cause severe stress and distress within the family in the short term). In general, they lend themselves very well to management within the primary health care team. It is important that the general practitioner and health visitor discuss their approach to the problem, in order to prevent any inconsistencies that might confuse parents and undermine the team's credibility.

Table 17.1: Example of a crying diary

Day and date	Crying episode: beginning and ending times	How loud was it (on a scale of 0–5)?	Time of last sleep before crying	Time of last feed before crying	What did you do?	What made it better?	What made it worse?

Reassurance

Many parents of crying babies believe that the terrible wails must reflect a serious under-lying medical problem. They will be helped by perceiving that their worries have been taken seriously, and that the baby has been adequately examined. Examination is therefore important even if the doctor feels certain from the history that there is no physical problem.

For some parents, reassurance that there is nothing physically wrong with the baby, and that the crying will resolve spontaneously with no long-term ill effects, will be enough to solve the problem. For others, further advice on management is needed (see below).

In some cases (e.g. when a baby cries persistently during the day), the label of a 'difficult temperament' may be more helpful than that of 'three-month colic'. This takes the blame away from the parents without inferring any organic cause. This label is particularly useful for babies who also have sleeping and feeding problems (see Chapter 4 on temperament).

Routines

Experience at a 'crying clinic' where diaries were used suggested that, in some cases, relevant factors included a lack of routine or a lack of understanding by the parents of the baby's needs.[5] Providing simple clear advice on feeding (volume, timing and techniques) and sleeping patterns (settling routines and naps) seemed to help these parents. In another treatment trial,[6] parents were advised to go through the following check-list in response to the baby's crying.

- Could he be hungry?
- Does he want to suck (without being hungry)?
- Does he want to be held?
- Is he bored and wanting stimulation?
- Does he want to go to sleep?

Parents were advised to try each response for five minutes in turn, and not to worry about overfeeding or spoiling the baby. This resulted in a 70% improvement of the crying prob-lem. Both of these studies emphasised the value of diaries in assessment and providing feedback to parents and health professionals.

Specific interventions

Rhythmic movement

Rocking has been used to still crying babies for centuries, and it is often effective. A rate of around 60 rocks per minute seems to be most soothing (interestingly, this is the speed of comfortable rocking in a rocking-chair). Carrying the baby while walking at a rate of one step per second, pushing them in a pram or driving them in a car are also useful.

Soothing sound

Soft rhythmic singing in the form of lullabies is also a tried and tested method. It has been shown that continuous sound will decrease the arousal level of infants. Modern equivalents include tapes of womb music and white-noise emitters, or the sound of an electrical appliance such as a washing machine, hair dryer or vacuum cleaner.

Non-nutritive sucking

Allowing babies to suck is often an extremely effective way of comforting them, even if they are not hungry, and many babies seem to need to suck for far longer than is necessary for feeding. Many mothers instinctively allow this by offering the breast. However, promoting non-nutritive sucking by encouraging the baby to suck his hand or a dummy is also a potent calming method. A number of mothers and health professionals are anxious that the baby may become addicted to the dummy or harmed by its use. One of the main concerns expressed is that sucking a dummy will cause prominence of the front teeth. However, this only becomes a potential problem if the dummy is used excessively in older children (aged three years or above). The other concern is that using a dummy will delay a child's language or cognitive development. However, if the dummy is used only when the baby wants it, rather than to stop every cry – which might indeed inhibit communication – there is no evidence of long-term harm.

Position

Many babies seem to be happiest in a particular position. Some mothers find that constantly carrying the baby in a sling is very helpful. This may be due to a combination of movement, stimulation and proximity to the warmth and smell of the mother. Colicky babies are often more comfortable in a position that exerts gentle pressure on the abdomen – by lying the baby with his tummy over an arm, knee or pillow, or carrying the baby with his trunk slightly flexed. Tense babies like to be held firmly and not over-handled. They often respond well to being tightly wrapped in a sheet (a version of swaddling), whereas active babies generally prefer to be upright.

Stimulation level

In a similar vein, tense babies respond badly to over-stimulation, and it can be helpful to keep activities such as nappy changes, bathing and undressing to a minimum. Active babies appear to demand stimulation and like to be constantly on the move, so devices such as baby bouncers can be helpful, as can frequent walks, and access to mobiles, books and pictures.

Those babies who are unable to regulate their own level of arousal will cry excessively because they are tired and unable to settle themselves to sleep. It can be helpful to teach parents to recognise this, often by using diaries, so that, for example, rather than picking up the baby at the first moan, they wait several minutes to give him an opportunity to learn to settle himself. In general, reducing the level of stimulation has been found to be effective.[4]

Dietary interventions

Elimination of cow's-milk protein can improve colic in bottle-fed babies. A week's trial of a hypoallergenic formula can be used as a diagnostic test.[4] Substitution with soya milk is not reliable. Lactating mothers have also been advised to eliminate cow's-milk protein from their own diet for a week to see whether this relieves the baby's symptoms. It has been suggested that herbal teas such as camomile, fennel and balm mint may be calming. Supplementing the mother's diet with natural yoghurt bacterial cultures may also be helpful. (Professor David Candy, personal communication; an open trial of 'Yakult' supplementation in the diet of mothers breastfeeding babies with colic led to improvement in 15 of the first 17 babies treated.)

Medication

Many parents attempt to use medicines to soothe crying babies. The type most commonly used is gripe water, although there is no reliable research-based evidence to show that it works. In the past, dicyclomine (Merbentyl, an antispasmodic) was the most effective medication for colic. It is no longer recommended for babies under six months of age because of concern about rare respiratory and neurological side-effects. Infacol contains dimeticone, which is an antifoaming agent that is claimed to relieve flatulence, although its value is uncertain. If a crying baby is thought to be suffering from reflux, there may be some value in trying to thicken his feeds or use antacid preparations. In general, there is no clear research-based evidence that any of the currently available medicines are effective in crying babies.

Support

Any parent can be driven to desperation by an inconsolably crying baby, to the point of fearing that they may harm the child. In some cases, these feelings may be linked to memories of a difficult pregnancy, a painful labour or even an abusive childhood. It is also relevant to ask the parent of an apparently difficult baby about the symptoms of depression (*see* Chapter 16, on postnatal depression). In extreme situations, physical abuse may result, but this is usually confined to socially isolated families. It is essential to ensure that the parents are receiving enough support from each other, their extended family and their friends. The health visitor may be able to help by putting them in touch with a mother-and-baby group or a local postnatal group. Support from volunteers, some of whom may have been through similar difficulties, can be obtained through voluntary organisations such as Homestart, Sure-Start, Newpin, Crysis and the National Childbirth Trust.

Parents can be advised that if they reach a point at which they feel unable to cope with the crying, the best thing to do is put the baby in the safety of his cot, shut the door, go to another part of the house and, if possible, obtain help or support, even if this is only over the telephone. However, many parents feel too guilty to leave the child alone in this way, but may take on board advice that they must look after themselves in order to be able to cope with the baby's demands.

Referral

Babies with a serious underlying medical problem should be under the care of a paediatrician, and occasionally a paediatric assessment may be helpful in order to diffuse anxiety.

In some cases, a short break is necessary, in which case most paediatric wards will agree to admit the infant for observation. This also has the advantage of revealing patterns of family interaction and allowing a psychosocial assessment to be made.

There may be a risk of physical abuse to the child. This is more likely to occur in families who are unused to asking for help and who are socially isolated. If this is the case, then referral to Social Services should be considered.

Box 17.1:   Practice points for the management of excessive crying in infants

- The majority of infant crying is self-limiting and has no long-term sequelae.
- The management of infant crying is well suited to the primary healthcare team.
- Allow parents space to express their concerns, and listen to them carefully.
- Do not underestimate the stress that an inconsolably crying child can cause in a family.
- A diary may be very helpful to complete the assessment and to ascertain the impact of any interventions.
- As there is no single proven solution to the problem, be flexible and offer the parents a range of management options.
- Consider in particular:

    a one-week trial of substituting cow's-milk formula with hypoallergenic formula
    brainstorming a list of common-sense solutions (e.g. feeding, non-nutritive sucking, holding, rocking, hoovering, taking for a drive in the car, playing music)
    reducing stimulation, particularly for tense babies, and increasing stimulation for active babies.

- Ensure that appropriate support is available for parents.
- It is unusual for a child psychologist or other child mental health professional to be needed, as sympathetic listening, coupled with support and practical advice, is usually sufficient.
- Referral to a paediatrician may be necessary for social as well as medical reasons.
- Referral to Social Services may be necessary if the parents are so desperate and so socially isolated that abuse is a possible risk.

References

1   Butler NR and Golding J (1986) *From Birth to Five: A Study of Health and Behaviour in Britain's Five-Year-Olds*. Pergamon Press, London.

2   Thomas DB (1981) Aetiological associations in infantile colic: an hypothesis. *Austr Paediatr J.* **17**: 292–5.

3   Lucas A and St James-Roberts I (1998) Crying, fussing and colic behaviour in breast- and bottle-fed infants. *Early Hum Dev.* **53**: 9–18.

4   Lucassen PL, Assendelft WJ, Gubbels JW, van Eijk JT, van Geldrop WJ and Neven AK (1998) Effectiveness of treatments for infantile colic: systematic review. *BMJ.* **316**: 1563–9. [published erratum appears in *BMJ.* **317**: 171].

5   Pritchard P (1986) An infant crying clinic. *Health Visitor.* **59**: 375–7.

6   Taubman B (1984) Clinical trial of the treatment of colic by modification of parent–infant interaction. *Pediatrics.* **74**: 998–1003.

Further reading

Douglas J (1989) *Behaviour Problems in Young Children*. Routledge, London.

Support groups

Crysis, London WC1N 3XX (tel 0207 404 5011).

Homestart UK, 2 Salisbury Road, Leicester LE1 7OR (tel 0116 233 9955).

National Childbirth Trust, Alexandra House, Oldham Terrace, Acton, London W3 6NH (tel 0208 992 8637).

National Newpin, Sutherland House, 35 Sutherland Square, Walworth, London SE17 3EE (tel 020 7703 6326).

CHAPTER EIGHTEEN

Feeding problems in pre-school children

Introduction

Feeding problems in pre-school children are extremely common. At any time, about 10% of young children will demonstrate some problem with food refusal, and studies have suggested that one third of five-year-olds have a mild to moderate eating problem.[1] The vast majority of these children are thriving and will outgrow their feeding problem with no long-term ill effects.

Assessment

When a parent presents with a problem related to feeding, a thorough assessment of the situation is essential.

History

The following information should be obtained.

History of the presenting complaint

What exactly is worrying the mother? Is the child faddy, refusing food, not eating at the table or behaving unacceptably? Is there real concern that the child is not thriving?

An account of a typical meal

Do meals occur at a regular time with a reliable pattern? Which foods is the child being offered and how large are the portions? Do the family sit down and eat to provide an example, or are there multiple distractions such as people coming and going, or confusing commands being given? What is the duration of the meal? Is there a sense of rush? Are the parents coercive, tending to be punitive in their handling of the child and noting all that the child does wrong? How does the child behave? Can anyone feed the child successfully?

Parental expectations and attitudes towards food

Are there unrealistic expectations of the amount of food that a small child requires? What conscious or unconscious views are held by the parents (e.g. 'Babies should be fat', 'Food equals love' or 'The plate must always be clean')? Is there criticism from grand-parents? Are there parental memories of battles over food as children?

Dietary history

When was the child weaned from breast milk/from bottled milk/on to solids? What are the child's food likes and dislikes? Does the child drink a lot of milk or sugary drinks? Does the child eat between meals? (Parents often initially deny this, but close questioning may reveal considerable amounts of snacks and sweets being offered to make up for refused meals.) Do other family members give the child sweets and food (perhaps clandestinely)?

Developmental history

Speech delay can sometimes be associated with feeding problems, and so can general developmental delay. Feeding may be one of several behaviour problems.

Medical history

Is there any suggestion of an organic cause of failure to thrive (e.g. chronic illness or malabsorption)? Is the child on any medication that may suppress their appetite?

Family and social history

Were there similar problems in other family members? Have there been any recent traumatic events which may have triggered these problems (e.g. the arrival of a new sibling, maternal depression, departure of a partner or loss of a grandparent)?

Examination

The majority of children who present with feeding disorders are physically normal and thriving, but a small percentage may have rare medical problems. It is important not to miss these few children who may be genuinely failing to thrive. It is also important to provide informed reassurance to the majority of parents whose children are growing normally. The child's weight and height should always be plotted on a centile chart and an explanation given to the parents, ideally with previous readings for comparison.

A general medical examination should assess nutritional status and ensure that the palate is intact.

Food diary

It is often very helpful to ask the mother to fill in a food diary (*see* Table 18.1) for a few days. All food eaten should be recorded, so as well as meals the diary should include snacks such as sweets, crisps and biscuits. It is also important to include food that is refused and information about mealtime behaviour. As well as providing useful information for the health professional, such a diary is often reassuring to the mother, who may realise that her child is eating more than she had realised. It also provides an opportunity to give simple common-sense advice about nutrition and behaviour, which may be all that is necessary.

Observation of a meal

If it is possible to observe a meal in person or to watch a video of mealtimes recorded by the family, much useful information can be obtained. This may not be possible for a busy general practitioner, but a visit by a health visitor could be timed to coincide with a meal. If a video recording is used, it can also be played back to the parent to illustrate the interactions that occur. For instance, if the child refuses food, and this produces a strong reaction from the parent, the child is likely to continue this behaviour.

Specific problems and their treatment

Weaning problems

Babies are commonly weaned from a milk-only diet to one that includes solids at around four to six months of age. Introducing solids at this stage seems to be important for the full development of chewing skills, and if the introduction of solids is delayed until much later, lumpy food may be rejected or vomited. There is also some evidence to suggest that presenting a range of foods and tastes between four and six months, and persisting in re-offering a refused food at subsequent meals, is important for preventing the development of faddiness.[2]

Problems that are commonly seen at this time include the following.

Reluctance to give up breast or bottle

The age at which parents want their babies to give up breast- or bottle-feeding varies very widely. One of the most important points to ensure is that the mother is clear about her

Table 18.1: Example of a food diary

Day	Food eaten at breakfast	What happened at breakfast?	Snacks and drinks	Food eaten at lunch	What happened at lunch?	Snacks and drinks	Food eaten at tea	What happened at tea?	Snacks and drinks
Monday									
Tuesday									
Wednesday									
Thursday									
Friday									
Saturday									
Sunday									

motivation rather than ambivalent. Various conflicting factors may affect the mother's decision (e.g. cultural or family influences, and the need of a child to have a comfort suck).

In general, a gradual but firm approach works best, with a limit established on the number of feeds rather than continual demand feeding. It can help to discuss how to do this and to offer suggestions for alternative comforting (e.g. giving drinks in a teacher-beaker, allowing finger-sucking or providing a teddy or blanket). Once a routine has been established, the mother gradually decreases feeds by reducing the number per day and at the same time increasing other sources of fluid. It is important to stress that once a feed has been dropped it should not be re-established in a moment of weakness.

Reluctance to chew lumps

This problem often develops if solids have been introduced too late, so primary health care teams can usefully offer important preventive advice to new parents about the timing of weaning. The problem can also sometimes be related to an episode when a child has choked or vomited on a lump and has subsequently developed a fear of a repeat episode (aversive conditioning). If a child will only take puréed food, then a gradual introduction of texture is best, adding substances such as flour, rice or potato until the food reaches the texture of mashed potato. Finger foods can also be introduced – licking spreads or jam off bread or biscuits can be a first step towards solids. Similarly, those babies who will only take commercially produced puréed baby foods can have gradually increased amounts of puréed home cooking added.

If the child seems to be afraid of food or overly fastidious, then encouraging him to touch and play with food without any expectation of eating it should reduce such tensions and may increase his interest. If a child seems to have little idea of how to chew, it can help if the parent demonstrates chewing and biting. Games that encourage the child to develop oral musculature can also help (e.g. blowing through a straw into water, blowing bubbles or licking honey off the lips).

In extreme cases of failure to manage solid foods, referral to a speech and language therapist for a specialist assessment of oral–motor function may be necessary.

Food refusal

At around the age of 9 to 15 months many children start to refuse food offered to them on a spoon. This is commonly associated with extreme faddiness. Such behaviour occurs in about 10% of children,[3] who nearly all manage to thrive but who are a cause of great concern to their parents. This problem may be due to coercive or rushed feeding by the parent at a time when the child is developing a new-found sense of self. The child therefore asserts his autonomy by closing his mouth and turning away.

The first step in managing children who refuse food is to make a detailed assessment of the problem, including a food diary, and to check that the child is physically well and thriving. This enables the health professional to reassure the parent that the child is growing normally, and to offer simple practical advice. Most of these children are being offered snacks between meals, usually because the parents are anxious about their nutritional status. The first step is therefore to forbid all food between meals (including sweets, crisps and sugary drinks).

The next step is to offer straightforward advice about meals. These management tips can be given to parents to act as reminders (*see* Box 18.1, which can be photocopied and stuck to the refrigerator).

Box 18.1:   Management tips for food refusal

Your child must not be given *any* food, sweets, snacks or sweet drinks between meals.
Offer a range of food in small portions.
Offer meals without putting any pressure on the child to eat.
Eat with your child if possible.
Remove food without comment after 20 minutes if it has not been eaten.
Praise the child if any food is eaten.
Avoid the consumption of too many drinks at the table.
Do not fuss about irrelevancies such as the order of courses, finger feeding and messiness.
Remember that there must be *no* snacks *between meals*, however little your child eats at the table.

Other feeding problems

Unacceptable mealtime behaviour

The parent may have no concerns about the child's nutritional intake, but may feel that there are major problems with regard to discipline at mealtimes. This includes situations where the child refuses to sit at table, meals become protracted episodes, or parents alternate between cajoling and force-feeding the child. The child may refuse food that is offered, knowing that the parent will then offer a more attractive alternative. In all of these cases, the child is controlling the situation and being rewarded with prolonged adult attention, as well as other advantages such as more attractive food or extra playing time.

All of these problems can be dealt with using simple behavioural techniques such as removing attention for the unwanted behaviour (i.e. not eating), and providing encouragement for desired behaviours (i.e. sitting at table, eating what is offered). In general terms the parent agrees to make no comment if the child refuses food, and to reward acceptable behaviour with praise and attention. It is also helpful if the parents model the desired behaviour by sitting at the table and eating with the child. A reward can be offered if the child behaves well, and it is important to stress that the parent should not reward food refusal by offering more tempting foods.

Pica

This is defined as eating substances that are not normally regarded as food, and it should not be confused with mouthing, which is a normal developmental stage. A number of toddlers go through a (usually brief) phase of experimenting with eating unpleasant substances. Advice on home safety and removal of toxic substances is an important part of child health surveillance at this time. A common point of contact with the primary health care team occurs following ingestion of a potentially toxic substance. As well as offering appropriate advice on acute management (often following consultation with the local poisons unit), it is useful to reinforce the home safety message.

The other group who may be affected are older children, usually boys, who gain status among their friends by eating disgusting substances. Although such behaviour is rarely harmful, it can be difficult to prevent. Advice about other ways of handling these challenges may be helpful!

Pica may be associated with developmental delay or iron deficiency, and if old paint is being ingested there is a risk of lead poisoning. If the pica seems to be particularly persistent, these possibilities should be considered.

Rumination

Rumination is defined as the repeated regurgitation and re-chewing of food without associated gastrointestinal or other medical disorder, such as oesophageal reflux.[4] It is rare but serious, because of its association with failure to thrive. It is often associated with developmental delay, particularly in older children. It can be difficult to distinguish at first from the possetting seen in normal infants, but vomiting may be so frequent and copious as to leave a noxious odour and a demoralised parent. If the symptom persists for longer than a month, and the amount brought up appears sufficient to cause poor growth, a period of observation on a paediatric ward should be requested.

Referral

Referral to a paediatrician should be considered if the child's weight is below the third centile or there is a fall across centiles. The failure to thrive may have an organic cause. Alternatively, if weight gain is easy to establish in hospital, with repeated weight loss at home, a non-organic cause is more likely.

It is tempting to dismiss all behavioural feeding problems as unimportant unless they are associated with failure to thrive. For the parent, a child's refusal to eat as expected may cause endless anguish. However, once such habits have become established, they can be very difficult to shift. If treatment is to be successful, it should probably be completed before the age of six years, and ideally before school entry. The earlier a behavioural approach is adopted along the lines described above, the more likely it is to be success-ful. In most cases, this can be supervised by the health visitor. Occasionally, various combinations of dietitian, clinical psychologist and speech and language therapist may be necessary. Above the age of six years it is unlikely that any psychological intervention will be successful. It may then be wisest to wait until the child is old enough to want to change his own diet (Dr Bryan Lask, personal communication).

Case study 18.1

Daniel, aged seven years, had a long history of feeding problems. He still had three or four bottles of milk at night. His mother, Jacqui, was distressed not only about her lack of sleep, but also by his failure to eat normally during the day. His growth had always been satis-factory. In fact, he was slightly overweight for his height, his mother was very overweight, and his maternal grandmother, who had lived with them, had died unexpectedly from the complications of obesity when Daniel was five years old.

Daniel had already been referred by his health visitor to a specialist service at the age of four, following intensive input from her before then. His behavioural problems did not im-prove much following Jacqui's attendance at a parenting group. She still found it impossible not to give in to him. His behaviour worsened after his grandmother's death, and subsequently after an exacerbation of his stepfather's Crohn's disease. When Daniel reached six years of age, the consultant child psychiatrist said that he could not help him any more.

The general practitioner insisted that someone must make another attempt. A clinical nurse specialist with a particular interest in feeding disorders saw Daniel and his mother. She arranged with a consultant paediatrician for an admission to the children's ward for one week. Here Daniel was deprived of bottles of milk. He was observed to be clingy when Jacqui was on the ward, but perfectly happy when she was not there. When he returned home, Jacqui succeeded in restricting him to one or two bottles of milk per day at most. She no longer needed to get up for him at night, although she still complained about his behaviour.

Box 18.2:   Practice points about feeding problems

• Feeding problems are extremely common in pre-school children.
• It is essential to plot the child's weight and height on a centile chart.
• Food diaries can be helpful in assessment of food intake and the parents' behavioural responses.
• Simple behavioural programmes, using differential attention for desired and undesired behaviours, can be very effective.
• Early detection and advice during routine chid health surveillance can prevent problems from developing.

References

1   Butler NR and Golding J (eds) (1986) *From Birth to Five: a Study of Health and Behaviour in Britain's Five-Year-Olds.* Pergamon Press, London.

2   Illingworth RS and Lister J (1964) The critical or sensitive period with specific reference to certain feeding problems in infants and children. *J Paediatrics.* **65**: 839–48.

3   Richman N, Stevenson J and Graham PJ (1982) *Pre-school to School: a Behavioural Study.* Academic Press, London.

4   American Psychiatric Association (1994) *Diagnostic and Statistical Manual of Mental Disorders.* American Psychiatric Association, Washington, DC.

CHAPTER NINETEEN

Sleep problems

Introduction

Sleep problems are extremely common in young children, and the stress that chronic sleep deprivation may impose on parents can be very great. However, the majority of these children will grow out of their sleep problem with no long-term ill effects.

The pattern of infant sleep differs from that of adults, with more than one sleep–wake cycle occurring in each 24-hour period. This adapts over the first two years to about eight hours' sleep at night with an afternoon nap, which is gradually dropped in the pre-school years. As with adults, there is wide variation in sleep requirements.

The basic structure of sleep with rapid-eye-movement and non-rapid-eye-movement patterns is established in the first year. Children dream extensively during rapid-eye-movement sleep, and nightmares are common in primary school children. It is also import-ant to note that all small children wake during the night, but usually settle themselves back to sleep, so their parents are unaware that they have woken. Those children who are unable to settle themselves will cry and disturb their parents, so are referred to imprecisely as night wakers.

Assessment

As with any behavioural problem, accurate assessment of the situation is essential (asking what happens and when). It is important to find out exactly what the parent feels is the problem.

You should also enquire about issues such as:

- bedtime routines
- excessive daytime sleep
- tiredness in parents
- power struggles with the child
- lack of support or undermining by a partner or grandparents
- parents' concerns about the effect of sleeplessness on the child.

It is also important to ask about the use of drugs such as salbutamol or methylphenidate. It is worth conducting an examination for relevant physical conditions, such as itchy eczema, asthma with night cough, otitis media or obstructive sleep apnoea due to large tonsils.

A clear problem may emerge at this stage that responds well to simple advice. Parents can be reassured that loss of sleep will make the child tired, but will have no long-term effects on growth, and is likely to resolve eventually, with few consequences for later life.

The next stage is to establish the nature of the child's sleep pattern. The best way to build up an accurate picture of this is to ask one of the parents to keep a sleep diary for a week. A typical example is shown in Table 19.1.

The diary can also include extra information such as which parent takes charge, and more details about bedtime routines. It is very important to establish that the parent understands exactly how to fill in the diary, and the reasons for its use. Depending on the information obtained from the diary, it may be possible either to offer simple advice to resolve the problem, or to implement a specific behavioural programme.

Management

Prevention

When primary health care team members come into contact with pre-school children and their families as part of routine child health surveillance, it may be worth asking about sleep. In this way problems may be detected at an early stage, before they have become entrenched. It can also provide an opportunity to offer simple preventative advice (e.g. about the importance of establishing good bedtime routines, and the value of ensuring that young children are sometimes put down in a cot and allowed to get used to settling themselves to sleep).

Specific sleep problems

Failure to settle

About one in six pre-school children are described as having difficulty in settling to sleep in the evening. There is a variety of possible reasons for this, including the following:

* lack of a bedtime routine or a regular time for going to bed
* being 'hyped up' by exciting evening activities
* separation anxiety due to insecure attachment
* fear of sleep or bed because of an unpleasant bedroom, nightmares or sexual abuse
* being allowed to sleep too late in the morning or too long in the afternoon, so that the sleep–wake cycle becomes out of phase with that of the parents
* having a difficult temperament, with poorly established circadian rhythms.

Some of these problems may be revealed by a sleep diary and may respond to simple advice. For all children it is wise to set a bedtime and to establish a bedtime ritual with a

Table 19.1: Example of a sleep diary

Day and date	What time did the child wake up?	Did the child need wakening?	What was the child's mood on waking?	Times and duration of daytime naps	Bedtime routines	What time was the child told to go to bed?	What time did the child go to sleep?	Parents' actions at child's bedtime	Times and duration of night-time waking	Parents' responses to child waking
Monday										
Tuesday										
Wednesday										
Thursday										
Friday										
Saturday										
Sunday										

fixed progression of events leading up to bedtime, such as bathing, drinking hot milk, brushing teeth and listening to a story. This cues in a small child, who cannot tell the time, to the approach of bedtime. The idea is that the child will be relaxed enough on getting into bed to at least lie quietly, even if they do not go to sleep. It is also important to limit in advance calls for more attention, such as demands for extra drinks. Advise the parents to ensure that the bedroom is comfortable and conducive to sleep (e.g. with a night-light, fresh air, quietude and an appropriate temperature). Having soft toys in the cot, and a tape-recorder playing lullabies or a story, may also help. The child's task is to fall asleep on his own, and the parents' task is to help him to learn how to do this.

If this basic approach fails, then further measures will be needed. First consider whether the parents are exhausted and at their wit's end. If this is the case, then it may be worth considering sedating the child for one or two weeks. Appropriate sedatives are listed in the formulary (*see* Chapter 39). Sedation will not change a child's long-term sleep patterns, but it will allow the parents to recover from their sleep deprivation, and should enable them to start a programme of behavioural treatment.

Once the parents are feeling strong enough, there are two different approaches to consider:

* gradual management
* leaving the child to cry.

Gradual management (controlled crying)

This technique is more acceptable to many parents than leaving their child to scream for long periods. It may take slightly longer, but is just as effective and often less traumatic.

Many parents will report that they have tried controlled crying before but it did not work. Closer questioning usually reveals that they could not bear the screaming and gave up too soon. It is vital to stress to parents before they start to use this technique that the screaming will get worse before it gets better, and that they should not be tempted to give up in the middle of the treatment programme, as this will merely convey to the child that if he screams for long enough the parents will give in. Both parents must agree to use the technique, employing it properly and supporting each other. It is worth advising parents to warn neighbours so that they will not be anxious about their reaction. The parents *must explain to the child what is going to happen.*

The procedure is as follows.

1   A parent settles the child briefly, *stopping short of him falling asleep,* and leaves the room. The bedroom door is left ajar.
2   The parent does not return for five minutes unless the child gets out of bed, in which case she returns to him and tells him that she will shut the bedroom door if he gets out of bed again.
3   After five minutes, she returns to the child and settles him briefly (for about two minutes) and then leaves the room again. *She must leave the room before he falls asleep.*

4   Ten minutes later, she returns and settles him briefly again.
5   Fifteen minutes later, she visits the child again, and she subsequently visits at 15-minute intervals until the child is asleep. She must always leave the room before the child falls asleep, as the object of the exercise is to help the child to learn how to fall asleep on his own. All she has to do is quieten him.
6   After the first night, the intervals are increased by 5 minutes (i.e. 10 minutes to the first settle, then 15 minutes, then 20 minutes, etc.) (*see* Table 19.2).
7   Most children will be settling well by the end of a week. The problem will nearly always have resolved before 45-minute timings are reached.

Sometimes the situation deteriorates to such an extent that the child is entirely unable to settle alone, and the parent spends enormous amounts of time in the child's room, often sitting or lying by the cot or holding the child until he falls asleep. In these cases, the aim is for *very gradual change*. The parents must gradually encourage the child to sleep alone. Initially the child lies in the cot or bed with a parent just touching them. Over the course of several evenings the parent slowly moves away, first sitting on a chair by the bed, then moving the chair gradually nearer the door, until eventually she is outside the room. The parent should be encouraged to have something to do other than paying attention to the child, such as reading, knitting or listening to music. If the parent has been singing to the child for hours, she should be encouraged to hum more and more softly each evening.

Table 19.2:   Helping a child to fall asleep alone

Time to wait before going in to the child (minutes)

Day	First time	Second time	Third and subsequent times
1	5	10	15
2	10	15	20
3	15	20	25
4	20	25	30
5	25	30	35
6	30	35	40
7	35	40	45

Letting the child cry

This is a quick solution if the parents can manage it, but many parents find it an extremely stressful technique. Some children become so upset that they vomit, which necessitates adult attention in order to clean up, and defeats the purpose of the exercise. As with the previous approach, the parents should agree about the details of the technique, prepare a suitable environment and warn the neighbours. The parents *must explain to the child what is going to happen*. Once the child has been kissed goodnight, he should lie quietly in his bed and wait until he falls asleep, as they are not going to come in to him when he cries.

The procedure is as follows.

1   The child should not be able to get out of the door, but should be able to reassure himself that the parents are still around and have not deserted him. A chain on the door or a stair-gate in the doorway is a useful ploy.
2   The parents need to let the child know that they are still around. They should be urged to talk, sing, wash up noisily or have the radio or television switched on. This is in contrast to the usual parental practice of creeping around silently 'to let him get to sleep'.
3   The parents must have something to do apart from listening to the screams or they will not be able to stand it.
4   The total duration of crying before sleep should be recorded on a chart.
5   Both parents must understand that the crying will *get worse before it subsides*. This is an example of the *extinction burst* – any behaviour that is intended to attract attention, or which is perpetuated by social reinforcement, will initially intensify if attention is withdrawn. If the parents can last out for the first four nights, the crying will then gradually subside. The record that is kept on the chart will show this more clearly than the recollections of fraught and somewhat guilty parents.
6   Next morning the child can be praised for going to sleep on his own, and given a reward if a reward system has been set up.

As mentioned above, for the child who repeatedly comes out of his bedroom once well settled, a physical barrier such as a stair-gate or a door chain can be useful, as this will keep the child in his room without him feeling closed in. It is also possible to use a reward system, breaking down the task into small steps and rewarding each step. For example, the first step might be coming no further than the top of the stairs, the next step might be coming no further than the bedroom doorway, and the next might be staying quiet. The aim is to have the child lying quietly in bed ready for sleep. This can often be more realistic than setting the goal of a particular time of sleep onset.

Reward systems can be used in other ways, especially for children over three years old. A chart for stars or stickers can be used, or a string next to the bed to hold beads. The rewards should be given for completing set tasks. Examples include (in order of difficulty) getting into bed without fuss, staying quietly in bed for at least three minutes while the mother goes downstairs, and staying quietly in bed for ten minutes. Once a behaviour has been established for a week, a new task is set and the colour or nature of the reward is changed.

Night waking

This is really a failure to settle back to sleep after ordinary waking at night. Approximately 50% of night wakers will be found to have a problem settling to sleep in the evening when a careful history is taken. In these cases, the settling problem should be dealt with first, and this may solve the night-time problem.

If the child falls asleep easily in the evening when there is light from the landing and noise from the television, but finds it difficult to settle when he wakes at night and it is dark and silent, it may be worth trying to duplicate the calming conditions at night.

The initial approach is to attempt to settle the child, leaving the room before he falls asleep, or firmly returning him to bed if he comes into the parents' room. If this fails, then a gradual approach, as described earlier for settling to sleep, should be used. It is worth remembering that it is much more difficult to leave a child to scream in the middle of the night, and it is even more important to have warned the neighbours in advance.

Parasomnias

Nightmares

Dreams and nightmares occur during rapid-eye-movement sleep. It is not clear at what age children start to have nightmares, but it may well be before they are able to talk well enough to describe them. Nightmares definitely occur during the second year of life, and are common between the ages of three and ten years. Few children do not experience nightmares at some stage, often triggered by something that is seen on television or experienced during the day. The parents can be reassured that the occasional nightmare is quite normal and not a sign of emotional disturbance.

Children who are suffering from nightmares will cry out or wake and be obviously frightened. They will remember parts of the nightmare, and can often describe the dream to their parents, either at the time or the following morning. They may be frightened to go back to sleep in case the nightmare recurs. The management of the problem consists of going quickly to the child, then holding and reassuring him until he slips back to sleep (note that this is the opposite of the gradual withdrawal recommended above). Providing a night-light or comforting toy may also be helpful. As nightmares often occur at a time in the child's development when he is questioning the world around him, it may be worth checking whether the child is asking questions about death or other potentially worrying topics, and then providing explanations that he can understand. If nightmares occur frequently, or if there is a recurrent theme, the parents may need more encouragement to explore their child's fears. Drawing pictures or playing imaginative games may be easier for the child than talking. A clear history of trauma, such as a road traffic accident, is an obvious explanation for nightmares. The clinician should also consider the possibility of parent-inflicted trauma, such as sexual abuse or domestic violence.

Night terrors

Children with night terrors may also cry out and appear to wake, so how do night terrors differ from nightmares? The differences are shown in Table 19.3. Night terrors occur either in deep sleep, or when there is a rapid shift from deep to very light sleep, which can result in an effective overshoot into an extremely aroused state. The child looks as if he is having a terrible experience, often screaming and appearing terrified, with wide open eyes. He may be mumbling incoherently. It is not possible to get any account of the content of the experience from the child. If the parents can do so, then it is more likely to be a nightmare. The child appears to be awake but is not, and will usually fall into a calm sleep after a few minutes if left alone. In contrast to nightmares, the child will have no memory of the episode in the morning.

Table 19.3:   The difference between nightmares and night terrors

	Nightmares	*Night terrors*
Timing	Second half of the night's sleep	First half of the night's sleep
Type of sleep	Rapid eye movement	Deep (phase IV)
Content	Scary dream	Unknowable

Night terrors probably occur in less than 5% of children. They often run in families, and can occur in children of varying ages. They do not indicate any underlying psychological problem, although the authors have seen them occur in children who are stressed for a variety of reasons.

The most important aspect of *management* is to reassure the parents by giving accurate information and explaining that the child will grow out of this behaviour. Night terrors are frightening to watch, and parents need to be told that the child is asleep and will come to no harm. Parents should be advised not to try to waken the child.

If the night terrors are occurring frequently, they can be very disruptive to the family. In such cases, *anticipatory waking* can be used, but only if they occur at roughly the same time each night. The child is woken about half an hour before the expected onset, and allowed to go back to sleep after a few minutes. This changes the pattern of the sleep stages, and often has the effect of abolishing the problem, sometimes after as short a period as one week.

In the unlikely event of night terrors occurring excessively and being resistant to anticipatory waking, they can be abolished by using small doses (starting with 1 mg) of diazepam at bedtime, as benzodiazepines inhibit stage IV sleep (*see* formulary in Chapter 39). A short course lasting one week only is recommended.

Sleep-walking

Sleep-walking occurs at a similar stage of sleep to night terrors. It is common, particularly in school-age children, and there is often a family history. The relevance of sleep-walking is that it is potentially dangerous. It is worth checking that bedroom windows and outside doors are locked. There is no point in waking a sleep-walking child, as he will have no memory of the event in the morning. *Management* consists of reassuring the parents that the sleep-walking does not imply an underlying psychological problem, and ensuring the child's safety. During the sleep-walking episode the child should be gently steered back to bed, and the whole episode should be played down. Anticipatory waking or even benzodiazepine suppression can be tried if the problem is frequent.

Sleep problems in older children and adolescents

Initial insomnia in older children and adolescents may be related to anxiety or depression. *Middle insomnia* is rather more specific for depression. A specific anxiety about sleep may be related to separation anxiety, fears about sexual abuse, or wishing to protect the mother from violence by the father. As with younger children, a frightening event may cause post-traumatic stress, with anxiety or nightmares. Insomnia may also be due to drugs – either prescribed (e.g. salbutamol) or bought from friends (e.g. amphetamines). Excessive coffee drinking may also be a cause.

Many teenagers seem to need more sleep than they can easily obtain, and prefer evenings to mornings. They seem to be geared to a 25-hour day, so gradually become nocturnal if left to their own devices. This is not usually a problem for teenagers who are attending school or work regularly, but in others it may be. *Management* is more successful if bedtimes are moved forwards rather than backwards. For instance, you could advise moving a 4 a.m. bedtime on by two hours every day during a holiday period. This should lead to a 10 p.m. bedtime after nine days.

Box 19.1:   Practice points for sleep management

- Assessment is important. This may include a careful history, examination and a sleep diary.
- Failure to settle should be tackled before night waking.
- Behavioural methods work very well for both of these problems in small children. The choice is between:

    gradual management or
    leaving the child to cry.

- Night terrors can be managed by anticipatory waking.
- Nocturnal teenagers who want to be able to get up in the morning should move their bedtime forwards rather than backwards.

CHAPTER TWENTY

Breath-holding

Introduction

There are two types of breath-holding attack, namely blue and white. Most start at between six and 18 months of age, and disappear by six years.

Blue (cyanotic) spells

These are found in babies and toddlers and are common, affecting up to 5% of children. They appear to run in families. A typical blue spell is precipitated by frustration, rage or pain. After a few yells, at the end of an expiration, furious crying halts and gives way to determined closure of the glottis, which blocks inspiration. This leads quickly to cyanosis followed by loss of consciousness. The child may become rigid, and may occasionally show a few clonic movements. Recovery is swift and complete. The differences from epilepsy include a clear precipitant (usually being thwarted), the occurrence of forceful crying and then cyanosis before loss of consciousness, and the absence of post-ictal drowsiness.

White (pallid) spells

These are different. Following surprise, pain or mild injury (e.g. bumping the head in a fall while learning to walk), the first experience of an adult bath, or a new taste, the child becomes limp and apnoeic. Robust crying does not precede apnoea, the breath is not clearly held in expiration, nor is cyanosis very prominent. The child's state reflects the effect of a high vagal tone, with bradycardia or even asystole. (Children who have pallid breath-holding attacks are particularly sensitive to eyeball pressure, which may cause prolonged asystole.) An anoxic seizure may follow. When explaining the episode to parents, it is probably better not to use the term 'seizure' or 'epilepsy', but rather to talk about 'the heart rate going very slowly'. The risk of epilepsy is no greater than that in the general population, but there is an increased incidence of later syncope in response to pain or surprise. Recovery is swift and uneventful, except in the case of a seizure, in which case some drowsiness may follow.

Management

In theory, breath-holding attacks can be diagnosed by history alone, but an EEG can be helpful if the history is unclear, provided that it is skilfully interpreted. Other investigations are of no help.

Treatment essentially consists of reassurance, but this never works unless an adequate explanation is given. Parents usually want to know whether breath-holding is dangerous (it is not, and brain damage does not occur), whether it is epilepsy (it is least confusing to say no) and whether it may turn into persistent seizures (it does not). The parents may also ask for advice on how to terminate attacks when they occur.

Doing nothing at all works. It is worth emphasising that the child should be protected from harm during the brief spell of unconsciousness. Flicking drops of cold water in the child's face may help (it is not necessary to drench them with a tumblerful).

Although it is difficult to ignore breath-holding attacks, it is important to encourage the parents not to be manipulated, once they are convinced that the child will come to no harm. Becoming anxiously over-protective may lead to greater difficulties with regard to limit-setting in the future.

When to refer

If there is a clear history of classic blue breath-holding attacks, referral should not be necessary. However, the history is not always as clear as in textbooks, and it may be more difficult to give authoritative reassurance about white attacks than about blue. A paediatric opinion may provide the additional conviction that is necessary. Referral should also be made in the presence of other conditions (e.g. developmental delay or other causes of seizures).

Box 20.1:   Practice points for breath-holding attacks

- Take a careful history.
- Paediatric referral may be necessary if the history is unclear.
- If the history is clear:
    explain how unserious the condition is
    prescribe minimal intervention
    advise against giving in to what is effectively a tantrum.

CHAPTER TWENTY ONE

Head-banging and body-rocking

Introduction

Parents may come to see you to complain about these behaviours and others that are essentially normal. To be able to reassure them effectively, it is best to have a few simple facts at your fingertips, and also to know when reassurance is inappropriate.

Head-banging and body-rocking are examples of stereotypies – that is, spontaneous repetitive movement patterns that occur in young children, apparently without purpose. The child moves his head or torso rhythmically in a back-and-forth motion. The behaviours are most likely to occur when the child is asleep, drowsy or preparing to go to sleep. They are more common in children with mental retardation or autism. There may be an association between head-banging, attention-deficit hyperactivity disorder and ear, nose and throat problems.[1] In normal children, the peak age of onset for both behaviours is about nine months. By the age of three to six years, motor stereotypies occur in 3–4% of normal children, compared to approximately 25% for thumb-sucking and nail-biting.[2] Other behaviours that are seen in normal children include hair-twisting and face-pulling.[3]

Assessment

From the history, find out what is upsetting the parent. For instance, is there a fear that the child will harm himself, or a belief that the stereotypy is a sign of abnormal development? There is no evidence that any harm is done by these movements. It is worth ensuring that an adequate developmental check has been made, and arranging one if this is not the case. If the behaviour is frequent and persistent, it may be worth searching more rigorously for a developmental problem.

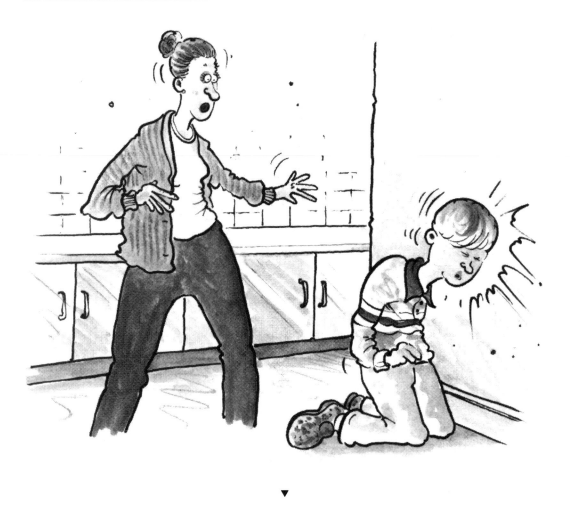

Management

The parents should be supported in ignoring these behaviours. Distracting the child with alternative and incompatible activities may also be effective. Children eventually grow out of stereotypies,[4] with or without specific treatment.

Referral

If reassurance fails, or you remain uncertain whether there really is some developmental problem, then referral is probably worthwhile, usually to a developmental paediatrician.

<hr>

Box 21.1: Practice points for head-banging and other repetitive behaviours

- The best management usually consists of informed reassurance.
- Check for developmental problems, especially global developmental delay or autism.
- If parental anxiety proves to be intractable, or if there is doubt about the child's development, refer the case.

References

1 Simonds JF and Parraga H (1984) Sleep behaviors and disorders in children and adolescents evaluated at psychiatric clinics. *J Dev Behav Pediatrics.* **5**: 6–10.

2 Foster LG (1998) Nervous habits and stereotyped behaviors in preschool children. *J Am Acad Child Adolesc Psychiatry.* **37**: 711–17.

3 Troster H (1994) Prevalence and functions of stereotyped behaviors in non-handicapped children in residential care. *J Abnorm Child Psychol.* **22**: 79–97.

4 Abe K, Oda N and Amatomi M (1984) Natural history and predictive significance of head-banging, head-rolling and breath-holding spells. *Dev Med Child Neurol.* **26**: 644–8.

PART 4

Problems that may present in school-age children

CHAPTER TWENTY TWO

Attention-deficit hyperactivity disorder

Introduction

There is an overlap between disorders of behaviour and disorders that affect levels of attention and activity. Pure hyperkinetic disorder affects 1–2% of primary school children, but complaints of inattentive restlessness may be made of up to 20% of children.[1] In community surveys, hyperkinetic symptoms (attention deficit, hyperactivity and impulsivity) pre-date the appearance of behaviour problems, and are therefore regarded as a major risk factor. They are potentially treatable, probably most effectively at the age of six or seven years, by a combination of medication and behavioural techniques (see below), but the public health and resource implications of this are only just beginning to be recognised in the UK.

'*Hyperkinetic disorder*' is the World Health Organisation term, which has therefore been the description of choice in Europe, while '*attention-deficit hyperactivity disorder*' is the American term, which is also used in Australia and many other parts of the world, and is usually abbreviated to 'ADHD'. Hyperkinetic disorder is a stricter category, and therefore applies to fewer children than attention-deficit hyperactivity disorder. Many parents seem to prefer 'ADHD', perhaps because much of the literature available for parents uses the American terminology. Because of this, we shall use the term 'attention-deficit hyper-activity disorder' in most of what follows.

General practitioners in some health authorities are currently discouraged from prescribing for attention-deficit hyperactivity disorder. This is partly because two of the medications used are controlled drugs, and partly because it was impossible to prescribe these in general practice until 1995. Since then, the number of children on medication has risen, and continues to rise, so that it will be necessary to relax the guidelines which suggest that medication should only be prescribed by specialists. In our opinion, it would be a better use of resources, and more convenient for families, if general practitioners took over the repeat prescribing and monitoring of children who have been assessed, diagnosed and stabilised on medication by a specialist. Eventually it might be possible for prescriptions to be initiated in primary care. School doctors are in an especially good position to make an initial assessment, as they have ready access to information from the child's teachers. With this in mind, we shall describe the assessment and treatment of attention-deficit hyperactivity disorder as it might be conducted in primary care or the school medical service.

Assessment

As with many diagnoses in psychiatry, there is no diagnostic test for attention-deficit hyperactivity disorder. It is a *syndrome complex*. The diagnosis is made by checking off symptoms on a list. It is also not an 'all-or-nothing' diagnosis, but a spectrum.

The *symptoms* in hyperkinetic disorder are grouped into three clusters, namely attention deficit, hyperactivity and impulsivity (*see* Box 22.1). These diagnostic criteria are based on the ICD-10 criteria.[2] They are very similar to the DSM-IV criteria.[3] With sufficient of each, a child will justify the label, provided that functional impairment is directly attributable to this. When interpreting these criteria, it is essential to compare the child's behaviour with that of a normal child of the same developmental age. Many two- and three-year-olds are normally overactive and have a short attention span, but this does not mean that they have this disorder. It is easier to make judgements of the criteria in children over the age of four years.

In attention-deficit hyperactivity disorder, there are two main differences that lead to the diagnosis being more inclusive than hyperkinetic disorder. First, hyperactivity and impulsivity are grouped together – a child must have six of the combined nine symptoms. It is easier to satisfy this one criterion than to satisfy the two criteria for hyperactivity *and* impulsivity. Secondly, children in North America are given a diagnosis if they have *only* attention deficit or *only* hyperactivity/impulsivity. This is more controversial in the UK. When in doubt, it is probably justifiable to commence a trial of medication if both the parents and the school are keen.

Box 22.1:   Diagnostic criteria for attention-deficit hyperactivity disorder

The child should have six or more of the following nine symptoms of *inattention*:

* failure to pay close attention to detail, so frequently makes careless mistakes
* difficulty in concentrating on tasks or play activities
* failure to listen when spoken to directly
* failure to follow through on instructions and finish tasks
* lack of organisation
* reluctance to start tasks that require concentration
* loses items that are necessary to complete tasks
* distracted by irrelevant activity
* forgetful in daily activities.

continued opposite

The child should have three or more of the following five symptoms of *hyperactivity*:

- fidgets
- cannot remain seated
- inappropriate running or climbing
- noisy
- being 'on the go' or often acting as if 'driven by a motor'.

The child should have one or more of the following four symptoms of *impulsivity*:

- blurts out answers before questions have been completed
- failure to wait in turn
- interrupts or intrudes on others' conversations or games
- talks constantly.

There must be some impairment of functioning both at home and at school, which must affect either academic achievement or family functioning.

The symptoms must have started before the age of seven years.

The symptoms cannot be accounted for by depression or anxiety.

Unfortunately for the busy general practitioner, *behaviour in the clinic is not a good indicator* of the diagnosis. Most children with attention-deficit hyperactivity disorder behave well for short periods of time (30–45 minutes) in a strange environment, particularly if provided with novel toys or a supply of adult attention. In contrast, *descriptions of behaviour in school* provided by teachers *can* be a very good indicator of the diagnosis. Although parents who are good historians will give an accurate account of what the teacher has said to them, it is more reliable to obtain the information directly, preferably by sending the questionnaire shown in Box 22.2, or by asking the same questions in a telephone call to the class teacher. The questionnaire can be given to the parent to give to the class teacher, and they can later return it to the doctor.

A useful adjunct to diagnosis is the 10-item Conner's parent questionnaire[4] (*see* Box 22.3). The scoring is 0–1–2–3 for each item, giving a maximum total score of 30. A score of 20 or higher is indicative either of a child who is liable to have attention-deficit hyperactivity disorder, or of parents who hold many negative beliefs about their child.

A similar 10-item teacher's questionnaire can be used in school. The scoring is the same, except that scores of 15 or higher should be regarded as compatible with a diagnosis. Teachers tend to be more objective in their judgements than parents.

Comorbidity can be a source of confusion, as a large variety of conditions may coexist with attention-deficit hyperactivity disorder. This is partly because this situation offends the 'Occam's razor'-like principle that is taught in medical school – never to use two diagnoses when one will do. In fact, comorbidity is common in attention-deficit

Box 22.2:   Questionnaire for teachers

Child's name: ....   Date form filled in: ..../......./.......

Academic progress
Estimated ability: below average/average/above average
School performance: underachieving/appropriate/overstriving

Special education needs
Any difficulties with: reading/spelling/writing/language
Any other educational difficulties?
What special provision is received?   type of help/hours per week

Levels of activity and concentration
Attention span compared to other   better/the same/less/a lot less
   children in class
Distractibility   yes/no
Repeatedly standing up or wandering around   yes/no
Fidgeting   yes/no
Ability to follow instructions   none at all/simple only/adequate
Interrupts others   yes/no
Tendency to do things without thinking   yes/no
   (impulsivity)
Organisational skills   above average/average/poor
Frustration tolerance   above average/average/poor

Behaviour
In the classroom
In the playground
At dinner time

Relationships with peers

Relationships with adults

Emotional development
Response to praise   anxiety/withdrawal/self-confidence/
                                  low self-esteem

Temperamental characteristics and adaptability

Parental involvement with the school

Any other comments

Box 22.3:   Short Conner's parent questionnaire

Child's name: ....   Date form filled in: ..../......./.......

Instructions: Place a tick in the column which best applies to your child's behaviour in the last month

Behaviour	How frequent?			
	Not at all	*Just a little*	*Pretty much*	*Very much*
Excitable, impulsive				
Cries easily or often				
Restless in the 'squirmy' sense (fidgety)				
Restless, always 'up and on the go'				
Destructive				
Fails to finish things				
Distractibility or attention span a problem				
Mood changes quickly and drastically				
Easily frustrated in efforts				
Disturbs other children				
Cries easily or often				

hyperactivity disorder, the most likely candidate being some form of behaviour disorder. In the past, this has resulted in attention-deficit hyperactivity disorder being misdiagnosed as conduct disorder or oppositional defiant disorder. There is a strong association between the two groups of conditions, but research clearly demonstrates they are two distinct dimensions.

Attention-deficit hyperactivity disorder uncomplicated by behaviour problems can be seen in five- to seven-year-olds, and this presents a golden opportunity for the prevention of later behavioural problems. The latter are likely if there is impairment of classroom functioning, even if there is no effect on family relationships. In adolescents, the secondary effects of untreated attention-deficit hyperactivity disorder may be well entrenched, with conduct disorder and delinquency causing major management difficulties.

Other comorbid conditions include learning difficulties, which may be generalised or specific. Specific learning difficulties include dyslexia (specific delay in reading and/or spelling and/or writing), language disorder, autistic spectrum disorder, dyspraxia (motor incoordination or clumsiness)[22.1] and Tourette's or tic disorder[22.2] (*see* Figure 22.1).

Box 22.4:   Short Conner's teacher questionnaire

Child's name: ....   Date form filled in: ..../......./.......

Place a tick in the column which best applies to the child.

	Degree of activity			
Observation	*Not at all*	*Just a little*	*Pretty much*	*Very much*
Constantly fidgeting				
Demands must be met immediately, easily frustrated				
Restless or overactive				
Excitable, impulsive				
Inattentive, easily distracted				
Fails to finish tasks that have been started, short attention span				
Disturbs other children				
Mood changes quickly and dramatically				
Destructive				
Excessive demands for teacher's attention				

The *differential diagnosis* includes the following.

- *Anxiety*. This can be worsened by the stimulant medication that is often used to treat attention-deficit hyperactivity disorder.
- *Depression* can cause confusion, especially in adolescents, as it can mimic the effects of attention-deficit hyperactivity disorder. Both attention-deficit hyperactivity disorder and depression can be masked by conduct disorder, which may improve when either the depression or the attention-deficit hyperactivity disorder is effectively medicated.
- *Drugs* (e.g. anticonvulsants, antihistamines or beta-agonists) can cause a picture similar to attention-deficit hyperactivity disorder.
- A rare psychiatric disorder that mimics attention-deficit hyperactivity disorder is *disinhibited attachment disorder*. It is seen mainly in children who have had a series of disrupted foster or adoptive placements, or who have not had the opportunity to develop healthy attachment relationships in their family of origin. In theory, the behavioural problems that these children present are driven solely by their severely disorganised attachments. In practice, many of them have medical problems as well, and it is sometimes worth trying medication.

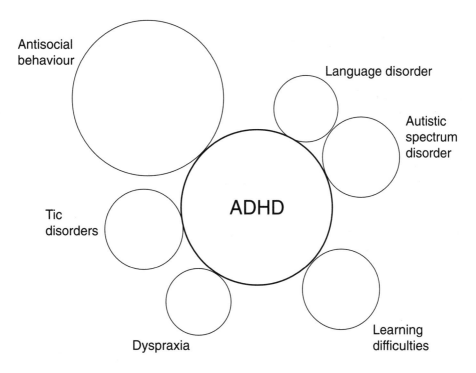

Figure 22.1:   Cormorbidity with ADHD.

Treatment by dietary manipulation

Many parents believe that diet is a factor in their child's behaviour or hyperactivity. Some of them are definitely right about this, but it is not clear how many.

Many children respond to caffeine-containing beverages (e.g. 'Coca-Cola') by becoming more boisterous. Some children also become more active in response to asthma treatments (e.g. salbutamol). The mechanisms underlying these reactions are presumably pharmacological responses.

A number of children appear to respond with worsening behaviour or increased hyperactivity to food dyes such as tartrazine and food preservatives such as benzoate. Some children also seem to respond to other foods in this way. The mechanism for this reaction is not yet understood. Although this used to be called 'food allergy', it is not like other forms of allergy, and is presumably due to a chemical effect rather than an immunological one.

Unfortunately, there is no way of telling which foods produce this type of reaction in an individual child other than by trying the child on a diet for which a certain food is excluded, to see whether the behaviour improves, and then reintroducing it in order to see whether the behaviour returns. Neither skin-prick tests, blood tests for specific IgE nor hair analysis have any predictive value. The best guide is therefore if the child seems worse on a particular food, and better when they are trying to avoid it. Exclusion diets are not as simple as this, as a child may be sensitive to several different foods. In addition to any suspected foods, it is probably sensible also to try to avoid colourings and preservatives.

For a proper trial of dietary manipulation, it is essential to refer the child to a paediatric dietitian. Excluding multiple foods can be dangerous, and children have been known to stop growing adequately, or to develop nutritional deficiencies. Other problems with exclusion diets include the problems for the child and parents in complying with them, and the added expense.

There are reports that some children with attention-deficit hyperactivity disorder have low blood zinc levels.[5] There is also evidence of essential fatty acid deficiency in children with attention-deficit hyperactivity disorder,[6] and supplementation may be helpful.[7] Although dietary supplementation with vitamins or fatty acids such as evening primrose oil[22.3] is usually safe, zinc supplementation can be potentially dangerous unless supervised. It is important to ensure that the parents are not endangering their child's health or their own finances by excessive use of remedies for which they have to pay.

Treatment options

After an assessment, some parents may want to try dietary manipulation or behavioural management (see below) first. Recent evidence suggests that the best medication regime is more effective than the best behavioural regime, and that combined treatment has no benefit over medication.[8] Stimulant medication is also likely to have larger effects than dietary manipulation. It is therefore a matter of whether parents want to expose their children to the risks of medication. It is worth pointing out that methylphenidate has been used on children since the 1950s, and we are familiar with both the short- and long-term side-effects of this drug. Give the parents a list (see below). It is important that the parents feel that they have the time to make this choice themselves, and that the they have sufficient information to enable them to do so. We sometimes suggest that they should not just take our word for it, but go away and find out information from other sources, such as friends, the Internet or libraries. They should be given contact telephone numbers for local or national support groups as soon as the diagnosis has been suggested.[22.4]

Treatment with medication

Parents should be given the option of a *trial of medication*. If they agree to this, the child should be given some information directly. For instance, you could say 'I am giving you a tablet that *may* help you with your schoolwork, by helping you to sit still and get on with it'. This trial of medication should last for a few weeks. The exact duration will depend on how long it takes to titrate to the optimum dose, and the convenience of follow-up appointments.

The dose should be *titrated* by starting at a low dose and working up to a high dose, with advice to reduce the dose if side-effects occur. There are many ways of doing this, and much depends on personal preference. A regime that we use for younger children is to start with a single after-breakfast dose of 5 mg and work up at weekly intervals to 20 mg. Once the best morning dose is found (often 10 mg), then a mid-day or after-lunch dose can be added, which can be the same or less. Children over ten years of age can usually start with 10 mg of methylphenidate. For teenagers, it may be better to start with a three times daily dose, since this is likely to be the most effective regime. One tablet (10 mg) three times per day (at approximately four hourly intervals, often at 8 a.m., 12 p.m. and 4 p.m.) can be increased after a week to two tablets (20 mg) three times per day.

The same principles can be applied to dexamphetamine. The small number of children under six years who are treated with this drug can start with dexamphetamine or methylphenidate 2.5 mg. (Dexamphetamine is licensed for this and methylphenidate is not, but we find methylphenidate to be more effective and less prone to side-effects.)

It is important to advise the parents that, on a single or twice daily dose, the benefits of stimulants will normally have worn off by the time the child gets home from school. The parents therefore have to cope with the same behaviours as before treatment in the evenings. A three times daily dose may delay sleep onset to an unacceptable degree in younger children.

The trial of medication should be monitored both by the parents and by the school. Comments from the child about the effect of the tablets, and any side-effects, are also very useful.

Parents should be given a list of *side-effects* to be alert for (*see* overleaf).

It is important to check the child's height and weight before starting stimulant medication, using an adequate stadiometer and reliable scales, and to plot the values on a growth chart. Height and weight should be measured again at approximately six-monthly intervals or else termly at school, as long as medication continues. The parents can be reassured that research has shown that the final height of the child is not affected.[9] The growth spurts of some adolescents appear to be delayed, but this is thought to be due to the underlying condition rather than to the medication.

The effects on sleep can be very troublesome. Really late bedtimes can be disruptive for the family, or make the child tired the next day, and adjustment of the medication may be necessary, such as omitting the last dose, or adding clonidine. Occasionally, an afternoon or early evening dose may improve the bedtime problem.

Tics can also be troublesome if they occur. Affected children usually have a history of some tics preceding the medication and/or a family history. It is thought that the tic disorder emerges earlier than it otherwise would, due to the stimulant medication. The tics may not improve when the stimulant medication is stopped.

A few children develop hallucinations on stimulants, particularly with dexamphetamine. These are usually visual and sometimes tactile. They can be quite distressing, but are usually due to the dose being too high.

Box 22.5:   Side-effects of stimulant medication

Frequent side-effects:
- *loss of appetite*, which can result in weight loss or increasing thinness; height is not affected
- *postponement of sleep onset time at night* – once asleep, children will usually sleep well.

Less frequent side-effects (may be due to an excessive dose, or an over-rapid increase in dose):
- headaches
- dizziness
- tummy pains
- nausea
- nervousness
- tearfulness
- anxiety
- drowsiness or an excessively calm state may occur, which is usually reversed once the dosage is reduced
- tics (twitches, jerks, nervous habits)
- hallucinations (seeing things).

It may be worth giving parents a check-list of side-effects to fill in and bring back with them the next time they come to see you (*see* Box 22.6).

Box 22.6:   Side-effects check-list

Reduced appetite	Headaches
Difficulty in getting to sleep	Dizziness
Nightmares	Drowsiness
Stares a lot or daydreams	Unusually happy
Talks less with others	Sad or unhappy
Uninterested in others	Tearful
Stomach-ache	Anxious
Feeling sick	Bites fingernails
Irritable	Tics or nervous twitches

Contraindications

- *Epilepsy* is a relative contraindication. The consensus view is that dexamphetamine is less likely to lower the seizure threshold than methylphenidate.
- Known *tic disorder* is also a relative rather than an absolute contraindication, but tics are likely to worsen considerably with stimulants, which should therefore probably not be given unless adequate medication is provided for the tics first.

- *Anxiety* is likely to worsen if stimulants are given. Depending on the clinical picture, it may be preferable to use psychological treatments for the anxiety initially, or to use anxiolytic medication such as imipramine as a treatment for the attention-deficit hyperactivity disorder and the anxiety.
- *Chaotic households* may not be able to keep the tablets safe. If there is a suspicion that street drugs are used, it is probably wiser to avoid stimulants, as they are likely to be sold on the black market rather than given to the child.

Use of stimulant medication (methylphenidate and dexamphetamine)

Our experience is that most parents are very responsible about the use of medication. First, most parents show a healthy reluctance to put any of their children on regular medication. Secondly, they can be entrusted with the responsibility for adjusting the dose of the medication, provided that the principles are clearly explained and guidelines are written down. The optimum dose cannot be determined by age or weight, so it has to be worked out for each child individually by a process of trial and error. Parents soon become experts on their own child.

Methylphenidate is our first choice, because it is most often effective and is available in three strengths: 5 mg, 10 mg and 20 mg. A second choice, dexamphetamine, is in our experience slightly more likely to cause side-effects, and is available only in 5 mg tablets. Both appear to last for three to four hours, although the rebound effect on sleep can occur 10 to 12 hours after the last dose.

The maximum daily dosage of methylphenidate is 60 mg. However, some children may need higher doses.

Other medications

The main alternative to stimulants is still a tricyclic antidepressant. The preferred drug according to the literature is *imipramine*. This is slightly more stimulating than amitriptyline. The dose varies widely, but the same principles should be used, starting with a low dose (e.g. of 12.5 mg in 2.5 ml of imipramine, or 10 mg in 5 ml of amitriptyline) and gradually increasing it. These antidepressants have their own list of side-effects, including drowsiness, dry mouth, constipation and the risk of overdose (*see* Chapter 39). Newer antidepressants (i.e. selective serotonin reuptake inhibitors) do not seem to be as effective.

Clonidine can be very useful. It can be prescribed on its own, but it seems to be more useful as an adjunct to methylphenidate. It can either be given at the same time as the methylphenidate (when it seems to have a synergistic effect), or as a single night-time dose, one to three hours before bed-time, when it seems to help children settle for bed. The starting dose is usually 25 micrograms per dose, which can be increased gradually to 100 micrograms for children under ten years of age, and 200 micrograms for older children. Clonidine is particularly useful in children with a tic disorder, although sometimes the tics do not respond to it. Side-effects include the following:

- drowsiness (which is usually helpful)
- dizziness (due to lowered blood pressure, which should be measured before and after treatment, particularly if the total dose is 100 micrograms or higher)
- depression (with high doses only)
- bad dreams and a restless night in a few children, which renders it useless in such cases.

There is controversy about the safety of clonidine when given simultaneously with methylphenidate. This arises from three case reports from North America of deaths in children. For all three cases there were alternative explanations, such as the presence of congenital heart disease. As yet there seems to be no clinical consensus.[10] It would be wise to leave the simultaneous prescription of methylphenidate and clonidine to specialists. However, this caveat does not apply to the use of methylphenidate during the day and clonidine at night (Professor Eric Taylor, personal communication).

A large number of other drugs have been tried, including risperidone, which has been shown to be effective in the treatment of conduct disorder.[11] Bupropion (Zyban), which is chemically related to antidepressants, and controlled release methylphenidate (Concerta) can be used in a single daily dose to improve compliance in adolescents.

Combinations of drugs are also often used. The combination of stimulants and tricyclics is said to be risky because the blood levels of tricyclic compound are increased by the stimulant, but otherwise a stimulant during the day and a sedative at night seems to be a logical combination.

Monitoring of medication

The *first follow-up appointment* should be after the initial trial period. Telephone contact may be necessary during this time (and parents can be encouraged to telephone with any queries). At follow-up, it is usually clear whether or not the drug is working. Although a repeat of the Conner's parent's (and teacher's) questionnaires can be useful, it is not essential, because there is usually either a dramatic initial response or very little change. The child's view of what the tablets are doing is important. It is also very important to obtain the school's opinion, either directly or from the parents. Because the tablets are given mainly to cover the school day, there may be an improvement at school but not at home (sometimes the evenings at home are worse, because of withdrawal from the tablets). Occasionally, an improvement is seen at home but not at school.

It is also important to enquire about *side-effects*. Specific enquiries should be made about appetite and sleep.

If the balance of evidence suggests that there is a significant *improvement*, then the medication should probably be continued. If the side-effects are acceptable, then there is no need to change the medication, and a distant follow-up appointment can be given (e.g. for six months). If the side-effects are unacceptable, then another similar medication should be tried for a similar trial period.

If there is *little evidence of improvement* at home or at school, then the first step is to check compliance. If you can be confident that the parents are giving the medication to the child, and that the child is swallowing the tablets, then the medication should be stopped. It is important to review the diagnosis before prescribing an alternative, as it is easy to get things wrong the first time – for instance, misdiagnosing anxiety, or giving too much weight to the mother's history and not enough to that of other informants. If the diagnosis still seems to be correct after review, then it is definitely worth trying another medication. For instance, some children respond dramatically to dexamphetamine, despite showing no improvement with methylphenidate.

Subsequent follow-up appointments, if these are intended only to monitor medication, must be judged according to the response. In straightforward cases, the third appointment can be after an interval of six months, and the child can then be seen annually.

Comorbid conditions need to be treated. They are frequently a reason for referral. Teenagers are often particularly difficult to treat successfully, as conduct disorder (which may well be a consequence, at least in part, of untreated attention-deficit hyperactivity disorder) can dominate the clinical picture, and is unlikely to respond to medication or behavioural management.

Monitoring of height and weight may reveal inadequate weight gain. This is probably due to a combination of reduced appetite and increased metabolic rate. A common pattern is for weight to decrease for the first two or three months, and then follow a slightly lower centile than before. A more worrying pattern is for the weight to show little significant change, while the height follows its centile, so that the child becomes thinner as he gets taller. The remedy is simple: an increase in calorie intake – but weight-conscious parents who discourage eating at bedtime find this surprisingly difficult.

- The child should have as large a breakfast as possible, but the main opportunity for increasing calorie intake is in the evening. Lunch is hardly eaten, since the appetite is at its most suppressed at that time. Many children have a full evening meal, and then want to snack throughout the evening. This should be encouraged. If these snacks are sufficiently nutritious, then the calorie intake should normally be sufficient to allow adequate weight gain. Bowls of cereal are particularly valuable, and peanut butter or other sandwiches are also a popular choice. It is important to check that the child is given his own supply of full-cream milk, as the family may normally drink semi-skimmed milk.
- Suggest as many 'drug holidays' as possible. Keeping the child off medication for weekends, half-term and school holidays may enable him to eat enough to catch up in weight. This regime does not reduce the effectiveness of the tablets on school days. On the contrary, it appears to enhance it.
- Refer the child to a paediatric dietician, who may suggest that you prescribe food supplements.

Difficulty in getting to sleep at a reasonable hour is another common clinical problem. This can be dealt with by adjusting the medication in a variety of ways (e.g. reducing the dose or altering the timing of stimulants, or adding clonidine).

The worsening (or apparent onset) of *tics* is a less common clinical problem, but one that causes significant management difficulties. Stimulants often need to be stopped, and medication for tics may be necessary. However, both can be given together. The emergence of tics would be a good reason for referral.

Stopping medication

Parents often ask *how long the medication will need to continue*. Without a crystal ball, it is impossible to predict this. We know that there are some adults with attention-deficit hyperactivity disorder (not yet served well by the health service), but that many affected children will grow out of the condition as teenagers. One estimate is that 30% of affected children will continue to have the condition as adults, but the implications of this are beyond the scope of this book. In practice, the medication should only be continued as long as there is definite evidence of benefit that outweighs the disadvantages of any side-effects.

Drug treatment holidays are often recommended. This may be for several reasons. The most important is probably to ensure that the child really is worse off without the drug than with it. They can also help with weight gain. Some children may only need to be on medication on school days, and not during weekends, half-term or holidays, except at times when their parents want them to be particularly focused and calm. Some parents are reluctant to allow their children to have drug holidays, as they say their behaviour is so awful whenever a dose is forgotten. However, the effects may be different if a long wash-out period is allowed (this may be at least two days if the dose is high). The school summer holidays are the most easily tolerated, as it is usually possible to find outside activities that are sufficiently stimulating for the child. A period of two weeks is recommended. There is no need to tail off the dose. In contrast, clonidine and tricyclic antidepressants are best reduced gradually, at least if they have been used for over six months.

It is usually clear when a decision to stop medication altogether is appropriate. However, many of those children who show an initial response need to continue for an uncertain number of years. This has implications for service provision, because of the large numbers of follow-up appointments that are necessary.

Treatment by modifying parental reactions to the child's behaviour

It used to be said that *behavioural management should be tried before medication*, but it has now become clear that, in general, medication is more effective than behavioural interventions.[13] Clinical practice suggests that behavioural interventions may work better in the presence of optimal medication.

Parents often feel a great sense of relief on being told that their child has a 'medical' condition, as this removes any blame from them. In many cases it gives parents the confidence to be more effective in managing their child's difficult behaviour, even if they choose not to use medication.

Many parents are aware of basic behavioural techniques, and can adapt these to the particular problems presented by a child with attention-deficit hyperactivity disorder. The parents of younger children may be able to obtain sufficient help from their health visitor. However, some will need more help, and these should be referred to a local child psychologist or clinical nurse specialist (tier 2). Some may also require attention to issues within the family, such as difficulties between the child and a step-parent, or differences in management style between the parents. Such cases may require referral to a multi-disciplinary team (tier 3).

Some of the behavioural management of children with attention-deficit hyperactivity disorder can be undertaken in primary care by a trained health visitor or other interested professional. As a brief synopsis of what this involves, we shall include some *core principles to behavioural management* here. These could be shared with parents who are adept at using written materials to change their parenting practices. Other parents will need help in interpreting them and carrying them out. (The percipient reader will note that many of these principles are similar to those described in Chapter 38 on teaching behavioural techniques.)

Before applying these principles, it is helpful to have a *functional analysis* of the behavioural problems presented. This means being clear about what circumstances lead to the behaviour, and what reactions the behaviour provokes in others. An ABC chart (*see* p. 74) would be one way of conducting this functional analysis. For instance, a child with disruptive behaviour in the classroom or at home may be inadvertently rewarded by being given more teacher or parent time than other children. This indicates that a fresh approach to the problem may be required, such as finding a more secluded part of the classroom in which the child can work, or ensuring that they receive positive attention in a structured way.

Behavioural management of a child with attention-deficit hyperactivity disorder can be very time-consuming, and it may require much attention to detail. If successfully combined with optimal medication, it can transform the life of the child and their family, and noticeably improve the child's ability to benefit from their schooling.

Core principles of behavioural management

Inattention

Poor concentration and distractibility can be helped by environmental manipulation. This may mean providing a structure that helps the child to cope with tasks more easily, where 'structure' refers to the space around the child, the time he is expected to take, and the amount and frequency of attention that he receives. Attention should be as positive or rewarding as possible (e.g. joining in with the play activity, or praising any small achievement).

- Provide an environment in which there is a minimum of distraction, at least for parts of the day (e.g. a small room with few objects, or a table facing the corner of the class-room). For this to work, there needs to be predictable times when social contact occurs (with the teacher, non-teaching assistant, or other children). This principle can also be applied at home to help with particular tasks (e.g. homework or creative play).
- Break down tasks into the smallest possible components, and make sure that all tasks are achievable, by setting standards that are appropriate for the child (e.g. with regard to the amount and accuracy of work, or the amount of mess allowed).
- Provide a suitable time frame. It is unrealistic to expect a child with attention-deficit hyperactivity disorder to persevere with one task for a long period. Allow brief spells of time to be spent on the task.
- Reward each task or sub-task when it has been completed, half completed or attempted, at every opportunity – usually with labelled praise (*see* below).
- Try to build up the duration of concentration gradually, step by step.
- If you cannot provide continual adult attention, try to find stimulating activities that the child can engage in on his own or with other children.
- Cards or posters with lists of rules and goals may be useful. They can be displayed on the wall of the child's room at home, or on his desk at school. Cards can be used to prompt desired behaviours, such as tidying up, and to provide a time frame, such as for five minutes after homework or playing.

General behaviour and compliance

Techniques for behavioural management are the same as for other children of the same age, but it is often much more difficult to make the techniques effective.

- List the child's positive attributes.
- What would you like him to be able to achieve?
- Consider the difficulties that his condition causes for him. Think how much more he is achieving than other children without attention-deficit hyperactivity disorder when he completes even a simple task.
- Think about how negatively he makes you feel.
- Think how poorly he must view himself.
- Try to help him to feel better about himself whenever possible. Praise should be frequent, reinforced by eye contact and other non-verbal cues, and labelled. For instance, 'I really like that drawing of a car you've done – it looks so powerful!' or 'Thank

you for tidying up straight away after you finished that game' [hug]. Labelled praise should be the main reward.

- Make sure that all praise and rewards are immediate.
- If you use tangible rewards, such as points systems or presents, vary them frequently.
- Try to find opportunities for doing things together which you both enjoy. Ten minutes a day spent playing together is enough to make a difference, although it can seem very difficult to find this time.
- When giving commands, gain the child's attention by making eye contact and persuading him to stop what he is doing and listen to you. Make requests simple and specific, so that he knows exactly what he has to do. It may help to ask him to repeat what you have asked him to do. Avoid sequences of commands, vague commands, or giving several commands at once. Wait for ten seconds for him to comply, and praise him immediately when he does.
- If he does not comply, remember that it does not help to blame yourself or him for this. Blame the attention-deficit hyperactivity disorder!
- Using more punishments than rewards may make things worse.
- Co-ordination between strategies at home and at school makes both more effective.
- Set up routines for certain behaviours on certain days. For instance, one sequence of activities is needed for getting up and going to school, and a different one for the weekend. Prompt cards may help with these routines.

Impulsivity

A lack of inhibition may be the central problem in attention-deficit hyperactivity disorder. It is also one of the most difficult aspects of the disorder to manage. It is not easy to teach greater awareness and problem-solving, but it can be done. Carrying out this process can be a challenge, so think of ways of keeping the child on the task, such as frequent rewards, and only doing a small part at a time.

- Encourage the child to talk about his thoughts, plans and strategies for doing things. For instance, if he is good at computer games, ask him to talk through exactly what he does. Then try talking through what happened recently in the playground, or with a sibling or a friend at home.
- Define a problem (e.g. getting into fights in the playground, getting frustrated when the computer game does not go right, not being able to do more than five minutes of homework a night).
- Encourage him to think how this made him feel.
- Encourage him to think how this made the other person or people in the situation feel.
- Discuss with him the reasons for feelings, and how one event may lead to another over time.

- Brainstorm a number of alternative solutions. Some of these may be daft, but do not rule out any solutions yet. Together you could note down good and daft ideas on paper, or on a computer. This is easier to do if it is in concrete form, but once the child has got used to the process, you can forget the paper or the computer, and do it just by talking, and then eventually he can do it on his own just by thinking. For instance, you could have a rule of thumb to think of three alternatives, and then decide which one seems best.
- Discuss each possible solution, and think about how it might make things different, or what the consequences might be.
- Choose one of the possible solutions, and make a plan based on this for what the child will do the next time the same situation arises.
- Rehearse it.
- Encourage the child to think before he acts next time the problem situation arises – at any rate for long enough to apply the new solution (although this is easier said than done).
- Check whether he has carried out this plan. If he has not, continue to encourage him until he does. If he has carried it out, go through it with him as soon as possible afterwards in order to review how he has coped. You may need to go through the problem-solving process several times to find a really successful strategy.

Referral

At present it is not generally recommended that general practitioners should initiate medication for attention-deficit hyperactivity disorder, but it is acceptable in some areas for maintenance prescriptions and monitoring to be undertaken in primary care for those children who have been assessed by a specialist. The specialist is usually an interested child psychiatrist (not all are), a paediatrician who takes a special interest (most do not) or a school medical officer (usually one who has been trained by a child psychiatrist or paediatrician with a special interest).

At the time of writing, in most parts of the UK all cases of suspected attention-deficit hyperactivity disorder have to be referred to a specialist, at least for the initial assessment and trial of medication. In the future, it should be possible for general practitioners to initiate treatment themselves for straightforward cases. Referral will still be necessary for cases with complex comorbidity and for those that require time-consuming behavioural management.

Box 22.7:   Practice points for children who may have attention-deficit hyper-activity disorder

- The diagnosis should be based mainly on information from the parents and the school, although observation of the child may help.
- There is extensive comorbidity, which may include:

    oppositional defiant disorder or conduct disorder
    specific learning difficulties
    dyspraxia (clumsiness)
    language disorder
    autistic spectrum disorder
    tic disorder or Tourette's syndrome.

- The parents may prefer dietary or behavioural management to the use of medication.
- Individually tailored medication has been shown to be superior to other interventions.
- The best age at which to start stimulant medication is between five and eight years.
- Most parents are very good at monitoring and adjusting medication appropriately.

Notes

22.1   One particular combination of conditions is known as *'DAMP'* – disorders of attention, motor control and perception. These children have features of attention-deficit hyper-activity disorder, dyspraxia and other specific learning impairments or autistic features (affecting perception). This new term has superseded the now outmoded term 'minimal brain dysfunction'. See Landgren M, Kjellman B and Gillberg C (1998) Attention deficit disorder with developmental coordination disorders. *Arch Dis Child.* **79**: 207–12.

22.2   Another combination of conditions includes Tourette's disorder, ADHD and obsessive-compulsive symptoms (*see* Chapter 32 on tics).

22.3   Efamol – a preparation of essential fatty acids – is prescribable as gamolenic acid or Epogam (both licensed for treatment of eczema).

22.4   Two national groups are the ADD/ADHD Family Support Group UK, 93 Avon Road, Devizes, Wiltshire SN10 1PT (tel 01380 726710) and LADDER (The National Learning and Attention Deficit Disorders Association), PO Box 700, Wolverhampton WV3 7YY, but local groups are constantly being set up.

References

1   Williams R, Richardson G, Kurtz Z *et al.* (1995) The definition, epidemiology and nature of child and adolescent mental health problems and disorders. In: Health Advisory Service (ed.) *Child and Adolescent Mental Health Services: Together We Stand.* HMSO, London.

2 World Health Organisation (1993) *The ICD-10 Classification of Mental and Behavioural Disorders: Diagnostic Criteria for Research.* World Health Organization, Geneva.

3 American Psychiatric Association (1994) *Diagnostic and Statistical Manual of Mental Disorders.* American Psychiatric Association, Washington, DC.

4 Conners K (1973) Rating scales for use in drug studies with children. *Psychopharmacol Bull Special Issue Pharmacother Child.* **9**: 24–84.

5 Bekaroglu M, Aslan Y, Gedik Y *et al.* (1996) Relationships between serum free fatty acids and zinc, and attention-deficit hyperactivity disorder: a research note. *J Child Psychol Psychiatry Allied Discip.* **37**: 225–7.

6 Burgess JR, Stevens L, Zhang W and Peck L (2000) Long-chain polyunsaturated fatty acids in children with attention-deficit hyperactivity disorder. *Am J Clin Nutr.* **71(Supplement 1)**: 327S–30S.

7 Aman MG, Mitchell EA and Turbott SH (1987) The effects of essential fatty acid supplementation by Efamol in hyperactive children. *J Abnorm Child Psychol.* **15**: 75–90.

8 (1999) A 14-month randomized clinical trial of treatment strategies for attention-deficit hyperactivity disorder. The MTA Cooperative Group Multimodal Treatment Study of Children with ADHD. *Arch Gen Psychiatry.* **56**: 1073–86.

9 Spencer T, Biederman J and Wilens T (1998) Growth deficits in children with attention deficit hyperactivity disorder. *Pediatrics.* **102**: 501–6.

10 Wilens TE, Spencer TJ, Swanson JM, Connor DF and Cantwell D (1999) Combining methylphenidate and clonidine: a clinically sound medication option. *J Am Acad Child Adolesc Psychiatry.* **38**: 614–19.

11 Findling RL, McNamara NK, Branicky LA, Schlucter MD, Lemon E and Blumer JL (2000) A double-blind pilot study of risperidone in the treatment of conduct disorder. *J Am Acad Child Adolesc Psychiatry.* **39**: 509–16.

12 Conners CK, Casat CD, Gualtieri CT *et al.* (1996) Bupropion hydrochloride in attention deficit disorder with hyperactivity. *J Am Acad Child Adolesc Psychiatry.* **35**: 1314–21.

13 Taylor E (1999) Development of clinical services for attention-deficit hyperactivity disorder. *Arch Gen Psychiatry.* **56**: 1097–9.

Further information

ADDNet UK has a useful website, with links to others, at http://www.web-tv.co.uk/.

Books for parents

Green C and Chee K (1997) *Understanding ADHD.* Vermilion, London. A favourite among parents by the popular North American author of *Toddler Taming.*

Kewley G and Hollingworth G (1999) *Attention-Deficit Hyperactivity Disorder.* LAC Press, Horsham. This fact-packed account is written by an Australian paediatrician who has set up a private clinic in the south of England.

Mental Health Foundation (2000) *All About ADHD*. Mental Health Foundation, London. A small booklet that provides convenient basic information, available for £1 from The Mental Health Foundation, 20/21 Cornwall Terrace, London NW1 4QL (tel 020 7535 7400; fax 020 7535 7474); e-mail mhf@mhf.org.uk; website www.mhf.org.uk.

Taylor E (1997) *Understanding your Hyperactive Child: the Essential Guide for Parents*. Vermilion, London. A book full of information by the leading UK authority on the subject.

Books for children and adolescents

Gordon M (1991) *I Would If I Could: A Teenager's Guide to ADHD and Hyperactivity*. Atlantic Books.

Nadeau KG, Dixon EB and Rose J (1997) *Learning to Slow Down and Pay Attention*. Magination Press, Washington, DC. This book is aimed at children aged 8–12 years, and uses cartoons, games, activities and graphics to offer children a variety of coping strategies.

Acknowledgement

We are grateful to Mrs Ann Kimber, clinical child psychologist, for designing an earlier version of the questionnaire that appears in Box 22.2.

CHAPTER TWENTY THREE

Specific and generalised learning disability

Introduction and definitions

Learning disability refers to a generalised impairment in intellectual functioning of a long-standing nature. It is usually associated with impaired functioning in the domains of social and self-help skills. In the UK it used to be referred to as *mental handicap*. In the USA the term *mental retardation* is still used. All three terms are roughly synonymous with levels of intellectual functioning at least two standard deviations below the population mean. The educational term *learning difficulty* is roughly synonymous with the above, but has a different set of sub-classifications. The rationale for the current terminology is as follows.

- It focuses on important interventions, particularly educational ones.
- It avoids the term '*mental*' with its connotation of mental illness (which most people with learning disability do not have), and therefore carries less stigma.
- It avoids the assumption of immutable handicap.
- This is how affected individuals like to be referred to.

Generalised and specific learning difficulty

Generalised learning disability is usually diagnosed when the intelligence quotient (IQ) is less than 70. This applies to approximately 2–3% of the population. *Specific* learning disability (also known as specific learning difficulty or specific developmental delay) is usually diagnosed when there is a particular skill deficit in relation to the child's overall IQ. Examples include expressive language disorder (*see* Chapter 5 on language disorders), specific difficulties with writing (*dysgraphia*), specific difficulties with mathematics (*dyscalculia*) and specific literacy difficulties, usually with a combination of delays in reading, spelling and writing (*dyslexia*).

Medical and educational terminology

In medical terminology, learning disability may be *mild* (in the IQ range 50–70), *moderate* (35–50), *severe* (20–35) or *profound* (below 20). There is confusion here between medical and educational terms. The medical term *mild learning disability* corresponds to the educational term *moderate learning difficulties* (IQ 50–70; affects approximately 2% of the population). The educational term *severe learning difficulties* covers the remaining categories, with an IQ of below 50 (roughly 3.5 per 1000). Thus there are special schools for pupils with moderate learning difficulties and for those with severe learning difficulties (and some for both).

Aetiology

Mild (IQ 50–70) and moderate-to-profound (IQ < 50) learning disability have differing causes and implications. Intellectual functioning in people with mild learning disability is on a continuum with those of normal IQ, as it is the thick part of the tail of the normal distribution. Individuals with mild learning disability often have one or more of the following:

* a family history of below average intelligence (sometimes with assortative mating)
* socio-economic deprivation
* parental neglect and/or abuse.

The tapering end of the tail of the normal distribution consists of individuals with moderate-to-profound learning disability. In contrast to the above group, their parents are usually of average intellectual ability. The children usually have a specific cause of their marked intellectual impairment, which may be:[1]

* a chromosomal abnormality, such as Down's syndrome, that may manifest with characteristic dysmorphic features (40%)
* a specific genetic abnormality that affects brain development adversely, such as fragile X syndrome (15%)
* an abnormality of pregnancy or the perinatal period such as congenital infection, fetal alcohol syndrome or birth trauma (10%)
* postnatal causes such as head injury (10%)
* undetermined (25%) – this is the group with which many parents find it most difficult to come to terms.

Assessment and management

Parents of children with moderate-to-profound learning disability may deal principally with specialist services, but may turn to primary care when they are dissatisfied with the help they are receiving, or at an earlier stage if they require referral. Parents of children with mild learning disability or specific learning difficulties may suffer from a lack of recognition of their child's needs, or a shortfall in provision, or both. It is therefore helpful in primary care to have some idea of the types of difficulties that such children and their parents may experience.

Family effects

Parents may need assistance in working through their grief about having a child with a disability. Initial *denial* is a universal coping mechanism, but may slow down this process at times. Denial or anxiety may make it difficult for parents to hear or understand the explanations that are given at the time of first diagnosis. Parents require frequent repetition and elaboration of suitable information as their understanding develops.

Subsequently, realising the lifelong burden, parents may become increasingly aware of their child's difficulties. Intellectually, this may help them to cope. However, emotionally it may be quite a burden (*chronic sorrow*). They often experience fluctuations in mood, linked to the degree of acceptance of their child's disability. Events that rekindle awareness of their child's differences from others, and their loss of the anticipated and hoped for ideal child, may in particular cause a recurrence of sorrow. At these times further help is often needed. Sympathetic support and basic practical advice may often be sufficient (*see* below).

Rates of parental and sibling *emotional disturbance*, and of family disharmony and fragmentation, are increased. It is important to consider the effect of the child's state on siblings, the parents as individuals and the parents as a couple. To what extent are their practical and emotional needs being met?

A particularly difficult time for families often occurs when the disabled child reaches the age when other people's children are thinking about *leaving home*, for college, university or full-time employment. Fortunately, special education is a statutory responsibility of local education authorities until the individual is 19 years old. Even so, there is often a gap in provision around this age. Parents may become acutely concerned about the young person's capacity for independence, and about who will ensure that he is cared for when they are too old to look after him. There is frequently psychological conflict within the individual's and parents' minds between the need for continuing dependence and support on the one hand, and the drive towards independence and autonomy on the other.

Social effects

The social complications of having a child with learning disabilities may include a loss of earnings (due to having to care for the child), restricted opportunities to leave the home and social isolation.

Parents can be given practical support in several ways.

- Social Services may be able to provide respite foster care to allow parents and siblings to have a break. This is also helpful in that it educates the individual with learning disability about different living arrangements and routines, thereby encouraging greater flexibility of lifestyle.
- A number of allowances and benefits are available. Parents may need assistance (e.g. from the Citizens' Advice Bureau) to explore what is available.
- Parent support groups can be invaluable, but are not suitable for everyone.
- Other voluntary organisations have a patchy distribution, but are often able to fill the gaps in need that are left by statutory organisations.

It is important to be aware of your local provision and to recruit assistance from child mental health, developmental paediatric and educational services and Social Services, as well as from the private and voluntary sector.

Educational effects

Parents often find that they have to fight hard to get their children's needs met. It is a sad truth that, in a randomly rationed welfare state, parents who are able to persist in fighting for their child's needs in an assertive and articulate way will get those needs met in the end, whereas other parents may not. *Parental rights* are built into the laws pertaining to educational and social welfare provision. Children who have a statement of special educational needs are most likely to receive the type of education to which they are entitled, but even they may need parental pressure at the time of the annual review to ensure that such provision remains appropriate.

Children with *less florid problems* may be less likely to receive appropriate extra help in school, although there is wide variation between different education authorities, and between different schools within the same education authority. A frequent example is dyslexia (as defined above), which is so common that most education authorities do not have the funds to supply sufficient remedial teaching for children with this condition. Parents require ongoing support to sustain pressure on local authorities to give their child optimal help. However, there is much excellent special education provision within the public sector – indeed parents often realise that such provision is far better than any that is available within the private sector.

Behavioural effects

Children with all varieties of learning disability are at increased risk of developing behaviour that is challenging for their parents and teachers. Attention-deficit hyperactivity disorder is a component of this. There may also be language and socialisation difficulties and rigid adherence to sameness or routine – autistic features become more common with decreasing intelligence. At the severe end of the spectrum, self-injury may be an issue. Impulsive violent outbursts of verbal or physical aggression may often lead to the kind of anxiety in carers that makes children feel even more out of control.

Behavioural challenges can be managed by the same behavioural principles that are used for children of more average intelligence. Components of attention-deficit hyperactivity disorder or autism may render behavioural strategies in general less effective, although they still play a crucial role in management. Young people with learning disability have also been shown to be able to benefit from more traditional individual or group psychotherapy, as well as occasionally from the judicious use of selected medications.

Box 23.1:   Theory points for learning disability

- Medical and educational IQ bands have different names.
- The causes of mild learning difficulty are mainly familial or environmental.
- The causes of moderate-to-profound learning disability are mainly genetic or traumatic.
- Parents may experience major difficulties in adjusting to a child with learning disability. Initially denial may impede management, and subsequently chronic sorrow may require ongoing support.
- Effective interventions include social, educational, behavioural and pharmacological approaches.

Referral

Services for children with learning disability are even patchier than child mental health services in general. They may be linked to community paediatrics, to the services for adults with learning disability or to the child and adolescent mental health service, and sometimes they are not owned by anyone. This makes it difficult to generalise about whom to refer to. In addition to specialisms within the health service, Social Services have a duty to provide for children defined as being 'in need' (Children Act 1989), which should include all children with moderate-to-profound learning disability and some children with mild learning disability.

Referral for behavioural problems that do not respond to straightforward measures is best made to a clinical psychologist, clinical nurse specialist or psychiatrist working in whatever service is responsible locally. Referral for carer relief (e.g. respite foster care, or a sessional worker to take the child out) should be made to Social Services, as should requests for further advice on welfare benefits and local support groups. Parents who are concerned about a possible recurrence in any future children should be directed without hesitation to a consultant clinical geneticist. The understanding of genetic contributions to disease and disability is progressing fast, and there are now numerous recognised genetic causes of learning disability, many of them familial. Family therapy may be needed for some families whose adjustment goes off course or gets 'stuck'. The development of a new identity following the arrival of a member with a disability is a family affair, but it may require external facilitation. Individual psychotherapy should be considered for children with learning disabilities for the same indications as in children with normal intelligence. Low IQ is not a barrier to successful psychotherapy.

Case study 23.1

Lucy was at a special school for children with moderate learning difficulties. At the age of eight years, she described imaginary miniature people in the lock of her bedroom door. They were talking both to each other (but not about her) and to her. Her mother was anxious that she was developing schizophrenia, since her maternal grandfather had had this diagnosis. Her general practitioner referred her to a child psychiatrist. After a detailed assessment over several sessions, involving other members of his team, he decided this was not schizophrenia, but an elaboration of imaginary friends, combined with an emotional disorder. It was noted that Lucy found it easier to talk to women than to men. The parents were helped to see that the mother was inadvertently encouraging Lucy's repeated mentioning of the voices by responding to them with heightened anxiety.

Over the next two years, Lucy continued to have behavioural outbursts, and was occasionally violent towards her older sister. Her general practitioner saw her mother regularly, and sometimes saw both parents together, to offer a sympathetic ear and practical advice. The parents obtained disability living allowance, and used the money to go on family outings. Eventually they complained that they were having great difficulty in coping with Lucy's behaviour, and the general practitioner referred Lucy to Social Services for respite foster care. Before a foster carer could be found, Lucy disclosed to her class teacher that she had been sexually abused by a previous foster carer four years earlier. Social Services were informed. Individual psychotherapeutic help was arranged for Lucy, as she appeared to be willing to talk about the abuse, and was having recurrent nightmares about it.

Case study 23.2

David, aged ten years, had been struggling ever since school entry to keep up with the school curriculum. His parents believed that he was dyslexic. Although his class teacher acknowledged that he was behind with reading, and even more so with spelling, she implied that he was not trying hard enough, and refused to use the term 'dyslexia'. He seemed to manage well in mathematics, science and art lessons, but had difficulty in writing up his experiments. His parents were particularly concerned about how he would manage in secondary school. The general practitioner wrote to the school to ask them to request the educational psychologist to see David. The school did not reply to the general practitioner, but told the parents that there was not enough 'educational psychology time' to go round. The general practitioner then referred David to the local child and adolescent mental health service, which replied that they did not deal with problems that occurred exclusively in the school setting.

continued opposite

The general practitioner then persuaded the parents to continue pressing for extra help for their son. They consulted the Parent Partnership Officer of the local education authority. Armed with information about their rights as parents, they visited their Member of Parliament, who wrote a letter to the director of education in support of David being at least assessed. David was then seen by the school's educational psychologist, who confirmed that David did have a specific literacy disability, and advised the school to provide extra help. This they did, but the help was not sufficient to stop David falling further behind during the next six months. The parents eventually took the education authority to tribunal, representing themselves, and won the right for David to have a statement of educational needs. Although it was by then too late for David to get any help in primary school, he did at least receive specialised teaching from the start of secondary school.

Box 23.2: Practice points for children with learning disability

- Parents may rely on the general practitioner or health visitor for support.
- This help may need to be ongoing throughout the child's life span.
- There may be a heightened need for support at times of crisis, such as:
    just after diagnosis
    when the full implications are sinking in
    when behavioural problems seem to be overwhelming
    when educational needs are not being met
    when the family needs a break in order to be able to cope
    when formal education is coming to an end
    when the parents die

Acknowledgements

We are indebted to Dr Jeremy Turk for advice on the details of this chapter.

Reference

1 Graham PJ, Verhulst FC and Turk J (1999) *Child Psychiatry: A Developmental Approach*. Oxford University Press, Oxford.

CHAPTER TWENTY FOUR

Bullying

Introduction

Definition

Bullying by children is the intentional, unprovoked abuse of power by one child or more in order to inflict pain on or cause distress to another child on repeated occasions. It can be either physical or psychological, or both. It can take a variety of forms, from teasing or name-calling (the commonest) to hitting or kicking, stealing money or possessions, telling nasty stories or rumours and social ostracism.[1]

Bullying, although common, must be considered unacceptable. It is unprovoked, repeated, involves an imbalance of power between the children involved and always causes distress to the recipient – unlike playful activities. It is a covert activity that is concealed from teachers and parents, and it can be regarded as a form of abuse (peer abuse).

Distinguishing between bullying and normal play

Many children are involved in teasing and/or fighting with their peers. However, children are able to distinguish rough-and-tumble play from bullying. In playful fighting or teasing, playful intent is signalled by laughing and smiling, no hurt is inflicted, all of the parties enjoy it and the participants stay together until it is over. In contrast, children describe bullying as occurring when children 'gang up' on a single child who is weaker than them, subjected to this treatment regularly and upset by it. Children view bullying as aggression for no reason, and even non-participant observers find it upsetting.

Prevalence

Bullying occurs in most schools and all age groups. Questionnaire estimates suggest that roughly one in four primary school children and one in ten secondary school children are bullied at least once a term, and that 10% of primary school pupils and 4% of secondary school pupils are bullied at least once a week.[2] Some children are both bullies and victims.

Children with obvious medical conditions, physical peculiarities or special needs may be especially vulnerable to bullying. For example, having a stammer or red hair may lead to victimisation. Bullying is a source of distress and may be particularly prevalent among children seeing doctors, either being the cause of the problem, or even being a consequence of the child seeing the doctor. Victims may present in primary care with psychosomatic symptoms,[3] and both bullies and victims may present with depression.[4] Parents are often unaware of the problem, and teachers frequently deny that it occurs.[5]

Bullying is not just distressing for the victim at the time. Victims may suffer from poor school performance, social anxiety and isolation, all of which may predispose to relationship problems and depression in adult life. Bullies often show other forms of antisocial behaviour, and are more likely to become delinquent and have criminal records as adults.

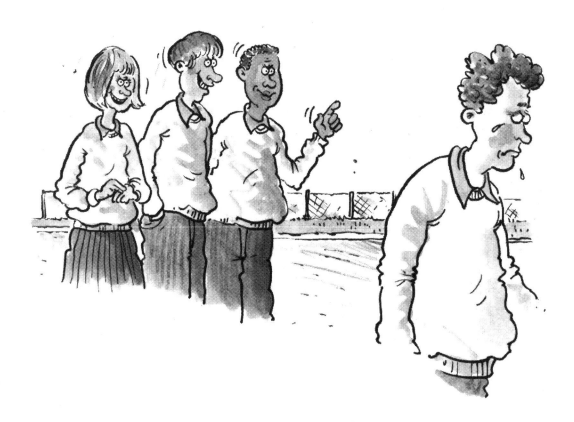

▼

Assessment: when should you consider it?

Children who are the victims of bullying usually suffer in silence. Certain signs and symptoms may indicate that a child is being bullied. These may not always be apparent, and other problems may be the superficial presentation (*see* Box 24.1).

Box 24.1:   Ways in which bullying may present

Requests to be driven to school
Fear of walking to or from school
Change of route to school
Unwillingness to go to school
School refusal or truancy
Poor school performance
Unexplained cuts/scratches/bruises
'Loss' of books/possessions/pocket money
Comes home extremely hungry (because dinner money has been taken)
Asks for or steals money (to pay the bully)
Refuses to say what is wrong
Cries himself to sleep and has nightmares
Withdrawn, distressed and stops eating
Depression
Deliberate self-harm or (attempted) suicide
Recurrent abdominal pain
Headaches
Other somatic symptoms

Ask the child directly, either alone or with their parents, whether they have been bullied. Children may not have the same definition of bullying as you, so simply asking 'Have you been bullied?' may not be enough. Try something more specific, such as 'Does anyone call you names?' or 'Is anyone at school horrid to you?'. Even if the child says no, maintain a high degree of suspicion. It is important to remember that bullying, like other forms of abuse, can present in a wide variety of ways.

Management

Once a bullying problem is suspected or has been discovered, it must be taken seriously and not dismissed as part of growing up or as a passing phase. Bullying can be successfully tackled as a *whole school problem*. Although it may sometimes be helpful to develop strategies with the child to be more assertive or to ignore more effectively, bullying is unlikely to stop unless it is dealt with by the school. If you do not have time to put pressure on teachers yourself, encourage the parents to do so on their child's behalf.

Advise the parents that bullying is common, and that victims feel helpless and require adult help to sort out the problem. The child must feel able to tell his parents and teachers about it. This means that firstly he must be believed, secondly he must believe that the teachers will do something effective about the bullying, and thirdly he must not be further victimised by the bullies because he has talked about them. For a teacher to say 'Don't tell tales' or 'Bullying does not happen in our school' is of no help to the child at all. Many parents need little prompting to be assertive about this issue. However, some may require detailed guidance. They should start with the class teacher or head of year, and then go higher, to the headteacher or governors if necessary. They may need to demand to see the school's bullying policy, and provide the school with some of the publications listed below, and they may need to persist in badgering the school until something effective is done. Schools are beholden to parents to maintain the welfare of their children, and parents sometimes need to remind schools that they are parenting their children during the day.

Common-sense measures may also be necessary. If bullying occurs on an unsupervised school bus, the parents may need to explore alternative means of travelling to school. Victims can be taught how to deal with specific incidents. For instance, it may be safer to go to school with a friend, to avoid isolated areas of the school, and not to take valuable items into school.

Referral

Bullying should be dealt with by the school. Some parents may be more assertive than others in putting pressure on their child's school to deal with the problem. On occasion, it may be necessary to involve the school's educational welfare officer or the school doctor. Depending on local circumstances, the school's educational psychologist or school counsellor may also be helpful. Most schools have a head of pastoral care who should be responsible for the school's bullying policy.

Referral to a paediatrician may be necessary if there is doubt about the relevance of somatic symptoms. Emotional or behavioural symptoms may need referral to a child and adolescent mental health service in their own right. However, the bullying will not stop because a child's name is on a waiting-list. Measures to reduce the extent and frequency of bullying must be implemented as soon as the bullying comes to light, otherwise the child's feeling of hopelessness will be compounded. A general practitioner who is the first professional to hear of a child's plight is therefore in a key position to initiate an effective response.

Case study 24.1

Billy Tonks, aged ten years, was brought by his parents to see their general practitioner as an extra case to be fitted in at the end of morning surgery. Billy's father had taken the morning off work in order to accompany the boy and his mother to see the doctor. Billy had not gone to school that morning because of severe stomach pains, which had been occurring very frequently in recent weeks. Each time his mother kept him away from school the pain had disappeared by mid-morning.

On enquiry, the doctor discovered that Billy had recently changed schools, since when he had become rather bad-tempered in the evening, displaying tantrums which he seemed to have grown out of in the past, and he had even started bed-wetting again – a problem that had previously been successfully overcome when he was eight years old.

The doctor decided to explore the idea that Billy might have suffered from the change of school, and asked him in his parents' presence whether he was happy at his new school. It was not clear whether Billy's grunt in reply was a yes or a no. Billy became slightly more talkative when he was asked about his friends, and he told the doctor that he still had friends near his home, but that he had made no new friends at his new school. The doctor asked Billy directly whether he was being bullied and he denied this, although his mother interrupted to say that they had suspected this and had already asked him about it. The doctor asked whether anyone had been calling him names, and Billy revealed that this was happening both on the school bus and in the playground, but that his teachers were not aware of it. Billy would not say what the names were, but it was apparent to the doctor that he found them difficult to ignore and at times upsetting.

The doctor wrote a note for Billy's parents to take to the school, pointing out that they had evidence of bullying, and insisting that there must be more supervision in the playground and on the bus. The doctor arranged to see the parents three weeks later.

At follow-up, the parents revealed that they had had a number of meetings with Billy's headteacher. Billy had given the names of the main culprits, and the school had agreed a plan which helped Billy to feel able to go to a lunchtime supervisor if he was called names, so that the situation could be dealt with immediately and appropriately. The situation on the school bus was proving more difficult to deal with, as there were no adults on the bus apart from the driver.

At further follow-up four weeks later, Billy seemed happier, and his bed-wetting, abdominal pain and temper tantrums had all more or less disappeared. Billy's father had altered his working timetable so that he was able to drive Billy to school in the morning. Billy was getting a lift home from a friend of his mother's in the afternoon.

Box 24.2:   Practice points for managing bullying

- Always think of bullying when there are:

    difficulties related to school attendance
    somatic symptoms occurring on school mornings or
    general unhappiness.
- Enquiry needs to be more than just asking 'Are you being bullied?'
- It is the responsibility of the school to sort out bullying problems.
- Encourage parents to put pressure on teachers to help their child.
- Only involve other professionals if this does not succeed.

References

1   Dawkins J (1995) Bullying in schools: doctors' responsibilities. *BMJ.* **310**: 274–5.

2   Whitney I and Smith PK (1993) A survey of the nature and extent of bullying in junior/ middle and secondary schools. *Educ Res.* **35**: 3–25.

3   Forero R, McLellan L, Rissel C and Bauman A (1999) Bullying behaviour and psychological health among school students in New South Wales, Australia: cross-sectional survey. *BMJ.* **319**: 344–8.

4   Kaltialo-Heino K, Rimpela M, Marttunen M, Rimpela A and Rantanen P (1999) Bullying, depression and suicidal ideation in Finnish adolescents: school survey. *BMJ.* **319**: 348–51.

5   Dawkins J (1995) Bullying in schools. *BMJ.* **310**: 1536.

Further sources of information

Children may telephone **Childline** free on 0800 1111. This organisation also publishes a useful booklet: MacLeod M and Morris S (1996) *Why Me? Children Talking to Childline about Bullying,* available from Childline, Freepost 1111, London N1 OBR; website http://www.Childline.org.uk

Kidscape, 2 Grosvenor Gardens, London SW1W ODH (tel 020 7730 3300). This organisation produces a useful leaflet, *Stop Bullying*, and also provides advice, runs training courses and produces other helpful booklets and information about bullying.

Royal College of Psychiatrists (1999) *The Emotional Cost of Bullying.* **Mental Health and Growing Up Factsheets.** No 19. Available from the Royal College of Psychiatrists, 17 Belgrave Square, London SW1X 8PG (tel 020 7235 2351 ext 146; fax 020 7245 1231); e-mail booksales@rcpsych.ac.uk; website http://www.rcpsych.ac.uk/pub/pubsfs.htm

Department for Education and Employment (1994) *Bullying: Don't Suffer in Silence. An Anti-Bullying Pack for Schools.* HMSO, London.

The **Anti-Bullying Campaign for Parents and Children**, 10 Borough High Street, London SE1 9QQ (tel 020 7378 1448). This organisation provides telephone advice and support.

CHAPTER TWENTY FIVE

Enuresis

Introduction

Enuresis can be defined as the involuntary passage of urine in the absence of significant physical abnormality. There is some debate about the age at which wetting should be considered abnormal. In general, 24-hour urinary continence is achieved by three to four years, but 10% of five-year-olds, 5% of ten-year-olds and 2% of teenagers still have enuresis.

In view of these facts, clinicians vary with regard to the age at which they start treatment. In general, children are actively treated at around the age of six or seven years, but it is possible to treat children as young as four if the problem is causing major distress to the family.

Enuresis may be nocturnal (night-time) or diurnal (daytime or day- and night-time). Much nocturnal enuresis seems to be due to delay in the maturation of the bladder and associated neural pathways.[1]

Enuresis can also be classified as primary enuresis, which is present from birth, and secondary enuresis, which occurs after a significant period of dryness. Primary enuresis is more likely to have a serious underlying cause.

Aetiology

Genetic factors

A positive family history is the strongest predictor of enuresis – 75% of children who wet will have a first-degree relative who had enuretic problems as a child. The likelihood of wetting is directly related to the closeness of the relationship, with monozygotic twins both demonstrating enuresis twice as often as dizygotic twins. Genetic factors are more important in determining the occurrence of primary enuresis, but family attitudes to bed-wetting may be as important as genetic factors.

Physical factors

- *Urinary tract infections* are particularly associated with secondary enuresis. There is also an association between daytime wetting and bacteriuria.
- *Developmental delay.* Many enuretics are thought to show isolated developmental delay in acquiring bladder control at night. These children often show other areas of specific developmental delay (e.g. in motor control or speech). There is also a predictable association of enuresis with generalised learning disability.
- *Polyuria* may be secondary to diabetes mellitus, diabetes insipidus or renal tubular disease.
- *Faecal retention* may cause enuresis as well as soiling, probably due to pressure on the bladder.
- *Small functional bladder capacity* has been particularly associated with diurnal enuresis.
- *Structural abnormalities of the urinary tract*, which can sometimes be quite subtle, can cause enuresis (usually daytime enuresis), often in the form of stress or urgency incontinence.
- Minor degrees of *spina bifida*, affecting just the sacral nerves, can be a cause of enuresis, and may sometimes go undetected.

It might be expected that seizures would cause enuresis, but children with epilepsy are no more likely to suffer from enuresis than those without. Many parents think that their children suffer from enuresis because they sleep so deeply. Studies have not confirmed this, and it seems that bed-wetting can occur in any phase of sleep other than rapid-eye-movement sleep.

Emotional factors

Bed-wetting can occur as a response to acute stress such as birth of a new sibling, parental divorce or starting a new school. If this is the case, it is more likely to be secondary enuresis, and this tends to be self-limiting. Enuresis may also occur in response to chronic stress such as an unhappy relationship between the parents, domestic violence or sexual abuse. In this case, the picture is often less clear and the enuresis may be primary, suggesting that the chronic stress interferes with the normal developmental process of acquiring dryness. Social factors may also have an impact on enuresis (e.g. impoverished conditions, multiple stresses affecting the parents, having to share beds, or difficulties in washing bed linen).

Assessment

History

The following questions need to be asked.

- What is the 24-hour pattern of micturition?
- What is the lifetime history of bowel and bladder control?
- Are there any associated physical problems, such as dysuria, excessive thirst, faecal soiling, or specific or general developmental delay?
- Are there associated emotional or behavioural problems?
- Is there a family history of enuresis?
- Is there any relationship to life events?
- What are the social conditions, especially the sleeping arrangements?
- What are the attitudes of the parents and the child to the wetting?
- What interventions have been tried so far?

Examination

This is usually normal but it may assure the parents that the problem is being taken seriously. Examine the abdomen to exclude palpable bladder or faeces, look at the genitalia, and test sacral sensation to exclude sacral spina bifida.

Investigation

A midstream urine specimen should be screened for sugar, protein and infection. If the history or examination suggests more significant disease, then the child should be referred to a paediatrician for further investigation.

Management of nocturnal enuresis

Assuming that treatable physical causes have been excluded, the following treatment programme is helpful for most children.

Reassurance

The family should be told that bed-wetting is very common. The child may not know that at least one other person in his class (on average) will have the same problem, and it is often very reassuring to realise that others are affected, too. If there is a family history, the fact that the affected individual grew out of the problem eventually may also be reassuring. An explanation that the child cannot help bed-wetting, and that the problem is probably due to delayed maturation of the bladder, is also useful.

Minimise inconvenience and complications

Simple practical advice such as using plastic mattress covers and nylon sheets that dry more easily may minimise the inconvenience to the family. It is useful to check that the child is washed each morning, so that he does not go to school smelling of urine, and to treat any urinary dermatitis with a barrier cream. Lifting the child to the toilet before the parents go to bed may reduce the amount of urine that is leaked later. Evening fluid restriction is sometimes advised, although it probably does not prevent bed-wetting.

The parents' response to the bed-wetting may be making the problem worse. It is important that they do not punish the child for wet nights or make him feel guilty or ashamed. Conversely, if the child is allowed to come into the parents' bed when he wets, or is given a great deal of attention, the family may be inadvertently providing positive reinforcement for the behaviour.

In general, a calm matter-of-fact approach is best, with the child helping to strip and remake the bed. No comment should be passed after wet nights, but dry nights should be rewarded with exaggerated approval.

The decision as to whether further treatment is indicated will depend very much on the age of the child and how much distress is being caused to the family. The argument for not treating children under five or six years of age is that a proportion of them will stop bed-wetting spontaneously in any case, and that some of the methods used, such as alarms sounding at night, may frighten very young children. However, children as young as four years can be treated if it is felt to be appropriate for the particular situation.

Reward charts

A simple chart can be drawn by parents showing the days of the week, and if the child has a dry bed a star or special sticker is awarded and stuck onto the chart the next morning. It is essential that the parents are enthusiastic about the chart, as their praise and encouragement when a dry night is achieved are as important an incentive for the child as the star or sticker. If the child has three consecutive dry nights, a gold star or special sticker can be used. It must be stressed to parents that, once awarded, stickers cannot be removed, and that black marks must not be given for wet nights. It is also possible to use other rewards that may be more motivating, such as a surprise bag containing small treats, when a dry night is achieved.

The effect of these charts will be rapid if they are going to work, and the motivation of children and parents is highest during the first few weeks. Such programmes should not in general be continued unaltered for more than six weeks at the most. Regular review is essential. If there has been no effect by three weeks, the parents should be questioned to ensure that the technique is being used properly, and if there is no obvious reason for the failure the chart should be discontinued and other methods considered. Around 20% of children will stop wetting with the use of a diary alone, and approximately one-third will stop wetting if rewards are given in addition.

Enuresis alarms

These alarms work on the principle that when the child starts to wet, the urine completes an electrical circuit and sounds an alarm that wakes the child. The theory as to why this method works is that the child is conditioned to associate relaxation of the bladder sphincter with waking up.

Alarms are not available on prescription but can be bought by parents. Alternatively, most paediatric departments have alarms available for loan, as do some health centres.

There are a number of different types of alarm.[25.1] The most commonly used type consists of a small buzzer that is fixed to the child's night-clothes and attached to a sensor containing two electrodes, which is put inside an absorbent pad. The pad is then placed inside the child's underpants. The first few drops of urine complete the circuit, sounding the alarm and waking the child, who should get up, go to the lavatory to finish urinating and then change the bed and reset the alarm with the help of his parents. Dry beds should be rewarded with a star on a chart, since if this reward technique is used in addition to the alarm it provides reinforcement as well as a record. The progress of the family should be monitored closely with regular reviews and checks to ensure that the equipment is functioning correctly. The parents are usually told to stop using the alarm after 14 to 21 dry nights, but they are warned of the risk of relapse. It is extremely important that both the parents and the child understand exactly how the alarm works and the ways in which the child could stop it working. The device is so designed that it cannot give the child an electric shock.

It is not essential to use the alarm every single night. In fact, there is some evidence to suggest that intermittent use may decrease the risk of relapse. Another way of reducing the relapse rate is to use a technique known as *overlearning* once the child is managing to stay dry at night. A glass of water is drunk before going to bed, and it is explained to the child that although he may have a few wet beds, this technique will teach his bladder to hold larger volumes. Once he is dry again, two glasses are given with the same explanation, and when he is dry again both the alarm and the bedtime drink are discontinued at the same time.

Family members need to be very motivated to make an alarm work. If the parents just turn off the alarm and leave the child without changing the bed, he has no opportunity to learn, and the parents will complain that the alarm is not working. When reviewing progress or lack of it, it is important to ask detailed questions about how the alarm is being used. There may also be technical problems with the equipment, such as the alarm sounding at the wrong time. Parents should be told to contact the clinician the next day if this occurs. Common problems are low batteries and holes in the separating sheets. The alarm will also sound if the separating sheet has been allowed to dry without being washed.

In general, enuresis alarms are a very safe and effective way of dealing with bed-wetting. Studies have shown that about 80% of children become dry within two to three months of starting to use the alarms, although there is a relapse rate of about 20% after finishing treatment. If the child relapses, the alarm can be reinstated until the child becomes dry again, and further relapses after this are then very unusual.

Drug treatment

Several medications will stop bed-wetting in the short term. They have all been shown to have a very high relapse rate when discontinued. They cannot therefore be regarded as an effective treatment when used alone. There may well be situations when short-term use is justified (e.g. for a child who is embarrassed to go away on school camp). Occasionally their long-term use may be justified (e.g. in teenagers for whom all other treatments have been tried, and who are very unsettled by the symptom).

Imipramine at a dose of 25–50 mg at night will be effective in most children. It is important to warn parents about the overdose risk, especially to younger siblings, and of the possibility of sleep disturbance and anticholinergic side-effects such as a dry mouth and blurred vision.

Desmopressin is a synthetic antidiuretic hormone analogue that can be given intra-nasally or in tablet form at a dose of 200 micrograms at night for children over five years (and preferably over seven years of age). Short-term use is more appropriate, as discussed above, and the drug should be withdrawn for at least one week if it is used for three months. Parents should be warned to avoid fluid overload, and to stop the desmopressin if the child has diarrhoea and vomiting, because of the risk of hyponatraemic convulsions.

Box 25.1:   Summary of the management of nocturnal enuresis

- Noctorunal enuresis is common.
- 'Delayed bladder maturation' is a useful explanation.
- A diary on its own can be effective.
- A calm non-punitive approach with rewards for dry nights has a high success rate.
- Drug treatments can be helpful in the short term or in intractable cases.

Management of diurnal enuresis

Diurnal enuresis is more common in girls. If children develop daytime wetting after having been dry, it is important to rule out urinary infection and to consider the fact that bladder sensation can be reduced if a child is preoccupied (e.g. by worry). If the child is deliberately wetting in various places in the house, this suggests an emotional disturbance.

Children who have never been dry by day appear to suffer from passing urine frequently and with great urgency. The urgency tends to be unpredictable and to come on suddenly. Some girls try to control this by applying pressure to their perineum, either by holding it or by sitting on their foot. It is thought that the problem may be related to a small functional bladder capacity or to incomplete voiding.

A diary may be helpful for identifying the pattern of wetting. Alternatively, admission to a paediatric ward may quickly reveal the nature of the problem and enable treatment to be commenced under supervised conditions. This of course requires paediatric referral.

Initial treatment can focus on the parent regularly reminding the child to go to the lavatory, and then gradually letting the child take over responsibility for remembering. Once the child can recognise the sensation of wanting to pass urine, the interval between reminders can be gradually lengthened, the aim being to increase bladder capacity and decrease frequency.

In older children, enuresis alarms such as those described in the section on nocturnal enuresis section can also be used. These can act either as an intermittent buzzer to remind the child to go to the lavatory, or more successfully to alarm at the start of wetting.

Medication has not been shown to be effective in diurnal enuresis.

Box 25.2:   Summary of the management of diurnal enuresis

- Diurnal enuresis is more heterogeneous than nocturnal enuresis.
- It is worth searching harder for physical causes.
- A large proportion of children respond to bladder retraining. This involves regular reminders, which are then gradually spaced out.

Referral

Paediatric referral may be necessary for investigation, particularly in cases of diurnal enuresis. If an emotional cause is suggested by the history, referral to a child and adolescent health service may be useful, but nocturnal enuresis will respond to a behavioural programme whoever supervises it. If you have a local enuresis clinic, this may be more appropriate. Failure to respond to any treatment option may be an indication for prolonged medication, particularly in teenagers, or for referral to an appropriate specialist.

Case study 25.1

Simon, aged eight years, was brought by his mother Trudy to the health centre. The family was new to the practice. Trudy explained to the doctor that Simon had started wetting the bed at night again at the age of eight. On enquiry, it emerged that Simon's parents had separated and he had recently moved house and school.

The doctor advised that the wetting would probably cease in a few months, as it was probably due to emotional upset, and that no specific treatment should be necessary. He suggested investing in a plastic mattress cover, and he stressed that on no account should Trudy become upset with Simon if she found that he had wet the bed. He asked them to return in one month for review.

Trudy returned with Simon two weeks later, saying that she was extremely upset about all the wet sheets, and she had found that she could not stop herself shouting at Simon sometimes. The doctor wondered if Trudy was depressed, but decided not to pursue this possibility at this time, as he sensed that Trudy might perceive this as a suggestion that Simon's problems were her fault. He prescribed four weeks of desmopressin treatment and once again asked Trudy and Simon to return in one month.

At follow-up four weeks later, Trudy seemed to be much calmer, and Simon's bed-wetting had not been as frequent. The doctor took advantage of the improved relationship with Trudy to discuss keeping a diary, changing the sheets calmly, and praising Simon for dry nights. He also mentioned that the next step might be to try rewarding Simon for dry nights with his favourite swap cards, and he assured Trudy that there were other steps that could be taken if necessary. He asked her to come back and see him on her own.

The following week Trudy was able to talk to the doctor about the separation from her husband and how difficult it had been for her. The doctor concluded that she was moderately depressed, and he made a referral to the practice counsellor.

At follow-up three weeks later, Simon's bed-wetting had ceased and Trudy reported that her first session with the counsellor had been helpful.

Notes

25.1   The Enuresis Resource and Information Centre's website is a useful source of information: http://www.enuresis.org.uk/. Their address is 34 Old School House, Britannia Road, Kingswood, Bristol BS15 8DB (tel 0117 960 3060).

Reference

1   Lister-Sharp D, O'Meara S, Bradley M and Sheldon TA (1997) *A Systematic Review of the Effectiveness of Interventions for Managing Childhood Nocturnal Enuresis.* NHS Centre for Reviews and Dissemination, University of York, York.

CHAPTER TWENTY SIX

Faecal soiling/ encopresis

Introduction and definitions

Encopresis can be defined as repeated voluntary or involuntary defecation in inappropriate places, occurring in children aged four years or older on a regular basis for at least one month. *Faecal incontinence* usually implies that the passage of stool is involuntary. The prevalence of the disorder decreases with age, and it is commoner in boys (by a factor of three to four) and in children with enuresis (percentages are 1.5% for seven- to eight-year-olds and 0.8% for ten- to twelve-year-olds. *Constipation* refers to difficulty or delay in passing stool. *Faecal soiling* is the passage of faeces, often loose, into clothing in association with chronic constipation.

Types of encopresis

Chronic constipation with overflow

This is by far the commonest cause of faecal incontinence. The child becomes constipated for a variety of reasons, and the impacted faeces then block and distend the rectum, impairing anal tone and faecal retention. Stool, which may be of any consistency, leaks around the mass. Parents often fail to realise that the child is constipated, as the stool may be runny or normal.

Secondary psychological problems may result from this that have in the past been viewed as primary. For instance, the child may be so ashamed of his soiled underwear that he hides it in drawers, at the back of a cupboard or under the bed, where a parent may find it unexpectedly. Parents may (quite understandably) become exasperated, and find it impossible not to be angry with the child (and often also themselves) about the smell and the mess. The self-esteem of the scapegoated child plummets further, and the whole family sinks into a slough of despondency.

Primary faecal incontinence

Some children never achieve faecal continence, and this can be due to a variety of reasons. The child may never have been trained appropriately, or he may have developmental delay, so that his mental age is too young for continence.

Secondary faecal incontinence

Children who have achieved bowel control may relapse. This is often a response to a stressful event such as the birth of a sibling. Less commonly, chronic diarrhoea, or steatorrhoea due to malabsorption, may cause intermittent soiling.

Voluntary encopresis

A small number of children with serious emotional problems will intentionally pass formed stools, or smear them, in places chosen so as to distress their parents (e.g. on sheets or walls), and may even write insults with fingers covered in faeces.

Assessment

History

Enquire about *common causes* of chronic constipation.

- An anal fissure that causes pain on defecation may result in a vicious cycle, with the child retaining stools through fear of pain. Rectal loading in itself may cause a fissure.
- Fear of the lavatory or of passing a stool may result from punitive potty training, or from an unpleasant toilet that is cold, dark or smelly, or from a frightening incident such as slipping into the toilet bowl.[26.1]
- A diet that is low in fibre or fluid can cause chronic constipation.
- A battle of wills between the child and his parents may lead to the child refusing to use the lavatory.
- Medical causes of constipation in childhood include hypothyroidism, neurological disorders, Hirschsprung's disease, chronic renal failure and anal stenosis. A history of delayed passage of meconium (more than 48 hours after birth) or constipation from the first few days of life is suggestive of organic disease.
- Drugs (e.g. imipramine and oxybutynin) can also cause constipation.
- Developmental delay or learning difficulties may be associated with delayed attainment of bowel control, and sometimes with stool smearing, which may be exploratory in nature.

Obtain a *description of soiling behaviour*. What are the child's words for 'faeces' and 'lavatory'? Has the child ever been continent? When and how did soiling start? How often does it occur? What happens? Are there associated physical symptoms, such as abdominal pain, anal pain or wetting? Are there associated emotional or behavioural problems? What are the parents' attitudes to the child? What have they done about the problem so far?

Examination

The child's weight and height should be plotted on a centile chart. Palpate the abdomen for faecal masses, and check the anus for visible fissures (many may be invisible). Rectal examination used to be fashionable, but is not a good test for constipation, and it can be unpleasant for the child. Constipation can be assessed by a plain abdominal X-ray, but an X-ray 72 hours after the ingestion of radio-opaque markers is more informative (Professor David Candy, personal communication). This is a more satisfactory test for constipation than rectal examination, and it provides a useful visual aid for further discussion with the family. It also enables discrimination between faecal soiling and other forms of encopresis.

Management and referral

Faced with a child who is soiling, it is probably safest to assume initially that he is constipated. First, you are most likely to be correct (estimates vary from 70% to 90%). Secondly, suggesting an organic cause will relieve the parents and child of blame, and so enable them to tackle the problem with renewed vigour. For parents who refuse to believe that their child may be constipated, even after an explanation of how likely this is, a plain abdominal X-ray might help to convince them. If this is equivocal, then it may be best to refer the child to an interested paediatrician before commencing laxative treatment.

The management procedure can be summarised as follows.

1   If you decide to manage the problem yourself, first *explain* to the child and his parents how soiling occurs. Draw a diagram of the rectum with a large stool inside stretching the walls apart (*see* Figure 26.1). Explain how the usual message to the brain from a full rectum telling the child to do a poo either does not happen, or may happen all the time. Explain how this causes poor sphincter control and leakage, and why the leaked stool is often not as hard as the rectal mass. For younger children, talking of an external cause such as the 'poo monster' may help the child enormously. He then has to work out how to defeat the poo monster, rather than feeling that all the smell and mess is his own fault.

2   Second, *empty the child's rectum*. This is sometimes more difficult than it sounds. Start with oral laxatives (*see* Chapter 39). Lactulose has the advantage of being both a stool-bulking agent and an osmotic laxative, and it is generally well tolerated by children. Docusate is both a stool softener and a mildly stimulating agent. Senna

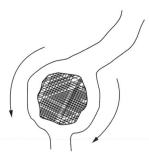

Figure 26.1:   Impacted stool in the rectum – it may be difficult for solid faeces to get past this.

should be used in addition to one of these if defecation is infrequent. A stronger alternative is sodium picosulphate. In severe cases, when the stool is irretrievably impacted, a polythene glycol-based laxative can be used (Norgine (Movicol); not licensed for children). If oral laxatives fail, then you can refer to a paediatrician for possible enemas. The last resort is manual evacuation under general anaesthetic.

3   Third, *maintain soft stool.* The child should be on a high-fibre diet with large amounts of fruit, vegetables and if possible wholemeal bread, as well as plenty of fluid. It is also important to continue laxatives (children usually require adult doses). Because the rectal tone has diminished, it will fill up again if given a chance. Therefore laxatives should be continued for at least six months. A good sign of recovery is when the child starts to regain sensation and can tell that he needs to defecate.

4   Advise the parents to restart a simple *toilet training programme*, the basis of which is encouraging the child to sit on the toilet regularly, usually three or four times a day for five minutes, mainly after meals. The parent should remain close by to prevent the child feeling 'banished'. Praise and/or rewards should be given initially for this (note that rewarding for cleanliness will encourage retention and could prolong the problem). The experience should be made as pleasant as possible, with toys, tapes or stories available. Any stool passed in the lavatory can be a source of extra praise or rewards, and any accidents should be simply ignored (as punishment will definitely prolong the problem). A chart can be used, with stickers or stars, but is not essential. The problem with such charts is keeping the child interested for as long as it takes for rectal tone to return to normal. Back-up incentives may be needed (e.g. for keeping up the pattern of sitting for two weeks).

5   *Predict relapse.* There are a number of reasons why such a treatment programme may fail. One of the commonest is failure to clear the rectum completely initially or to keep it empty. Close monitoring is important to maintain a positive attitude in the family, and to detect any setbacks quickly. Faecal retention in school may be due to unpleasant toilets, and accidents in school may lead to bullying. You may need to enlist the support of the child's school in ensuring that the child can sit on the toilet after lunch. Inform the parents that relapse is likely, but make sure that they have the

strategies to cope with it, such as an increase in laxative dose and a renewed level of encouragement for regular toileting.

6   If this programme runs into major difficulties, *refer to a paediatrician*. Although a child mental health service can be very helpful, it is essential to assess and treat constipation first.

In the absence of constipation, consider developmental delay or learning difficulty, and then search harder for possible social or emotional reasons. Advise the parents to improve lavatories that are inconvenient or frightening for the child. Ask about recent stresses in the child's life. If these are time-limited, common sense and sympathy may be the best option, with review after a month or two. Consider instituting a behavioural toileting programme as described above. Those few children who deposit or smear stool require specialist management. Often such children have other indicators of emotional disturbance, and may be known to Social Services. Even with this group, it is wisest to assess for constipation and developmental problems, and they should be seen by a paediatrician before being referred to a child mental health service.

Box 26.1:   Practice points on faecal soiling

*   Faecal soiling can cause considerable distress to both the child and his parents. Be sympathetic and attentive to the problem.
*   The majority of children who are seen have chronic constipation, even without a history or examination to confirm this.
*   Appropriate treatment of constipation is essential.
*   A simple behavioural programme can be added.
*   Long-term follow-up is needed.

Case study 26.1

The health visitor asked to see the general practitioner between appointments in order to discuss Joe Baines. The health visitor knew the family well, as she had visited Joe's mother Tiffany after the birth of all three of her children. Joe, the oldest child, had started school recently, and the school nurse had let the health visitor know that Joe was soiling his underwear during the school day. The health visitor had assessed the situation and considered that Joe was constipated, and asked the doctor to prescribe lactulose 10 mL twice daily, which she did, with instructions to increase the dose until a soft, regular stool was obtained.

The health visitor asked Joe about his poos, and he was reluctant to say much, but he did say that the toilets at school were dark and smelly, and he was being teased about being smelly himself. The health visitor agreed with Tiffany on a three times daily sitting programme,

continued overleaf

and she communicated the plan to the school nurse. The nurse negotiated an arrangement for Joe to use the staff toilet after his lunch break. She also recruited one of the dinner ladies to help Joe to go to the toilet and praise him for staying there.

The health visitor initially met with Tiffany every two weeks to review progress. The soiling at school resolved quickly, but there were occasional lightly soiled pants found in the laundry basket at home. The health visitor outlined a behavioural programme with Tiffany, using stickers as rewards for clean days. She discovered that Tiffany had stopped giving Joe the lactulose after the first prescription ran out, and she therefore obtained a repeat prescription.

After two months, all was well, and Joe said that he was bored with all the regular sitting on the toilet, which was therefore reduced to once daily. The health visitor reported to the doctor that she would maintain monthly contact with the family for a few months.

Six months later, the health visitor was able to report that Joe had a regular toileting habit. There had been some transient soiling after Joe's younger sister was in hospital for a week, during which time he was looked after by his grandmother. However, there had been no recurrence of soiling for three months.

Acknowledgements

We are indebted to Professor David Candy, paediatric gastroenterologist, for his comments on an earlier draft of this chapter.

Notes

26.1   W. H. Auden expressed this succinctly in one of his shorter poems:
         Avatory, avatory, avatory
         The baby fell down the lavatory.

CHAPTER TWENTY SEVEN

Obsessive-compulsive disorder

Definition

There is a continuum from normal obsessional behaviour and adherence to routines to a disorder marked by maladaptive obsessional thoughts and compulsive behaviours.

For instance, most children are comforted by rituals such as a predictable sequence of events at bedtime (e.g. pyjamas, brushing teeth, story) or avoiding the cracks in pavements (monsters might come up through them!). The use of rituals, or adherence to obsessions, becomes more prominent when a child is under stress. This should be regarded as a normal childhood defence against anxiety.

In contrast, repetitive behaviours or rituals that interfere with everyday life are abnormal. They are often fuelled by anxiety. *Obsessions* are recurring thoughts that are intrusive, repetitive and associated with urges, known as *compulsions*, to do certain things (e.g. checking, washing, counting, or lining things up). Acting out these urges reduces the anxiety and makes the thoughts 'go away', so that a vicious circle is set up. The reduction in anxiety reinforces the obsessions and compulsions, which therefore continue. The child and his parents often find it easier to give in to the compulsions, sometimes leading to quite absurd situations.

Case study 27.1

A girl became anxious about contracting infectious diseases. She developed a fear of contaminating her hands with germs from other people. This fear became a recurring thought, which assumed an overriding importance. Because of this, she repeatedly washed her hands or cleaned the house. She would not touch other people, and insisted on eating only food that she had prepared herself.

Assessment

A careful history is important, to ascertain if possible the nature of the thoughts and a clear account of the behaviours. Often the child will go to great lengths to avoid certain situations. The parents may underestimate how often the compulsive behaviours occur, and keeping a diary can be a very useful initial step.

There is often a prominent component of anxiety. The *differential diagnosis* includes tic disorder (*see* Chapter 32) and Asperger's syndrome (*see* Chapter 5). It is worth taking a careful history of themes, as these differ in the three conditions. The obsessions in pure obsessive-compulsive disorder tend to be with contamination, dirt, germs, being neat and clean, fear of something going wrong, or hypochondriasis. The corresponding compulsions are mainly concerned with cleaning, washing or checking that things are all right (e.g. that there are no monsters under the bed). Themes in Tourette's syndrome tend to concern symmetry, violence, religion or sex, whereas compulsions are concerned with forced touching, checking that things are 'just right', 'evening up' for symmetry, counting, ordering, repeating and self-damage. In Asperger's syndrome the compulsions observed are more of the nature of a need for routine and a repetitive adherence to certain interests, which tend to be centred around facts. Examples include the collection of bar codes, endlessly poring over maps, or exclusively reading the Guinness book of records. Another distinguishing characteristic of true obsessive-compulsive disorder is that the symptoms are generally egodystonic (subjectively uncomfortable), whereas in tic disorder and autistic spectrum disorder they are egosyntonic (subjectively comfortable).

Family factors may sometimes be relevant. For instance, a child may discover that his parents' response to his compulsive behaviour is the only time when they work together as parents. If there is a weakening marital relationship, then the symptoms may serve the valuable function of keeping his parents together.

Referral

Children with obsessive-compulsive disorder should be referred sooner rather than later. Parents often come for help quite late in the development of the condition. If you are unsure whether the symptoms are transitory, then it may be worth keeping the situation under review for a while before deciding upon referral.

Behavioural treatments are effective, particularly if combined with family therapy. However, they are time-consuming and require appropriate experience, so management within primary care is inadvisable. Selective serotonin reuptake inhibitors do work in that they lead to a reduction in anxiety and associated symptoms, but they are not usually recommended as the sole treatment.

Box 27.1:   Practice points about obsessive-compulsive disorder

- The diagnosis is based on a careful history from the child and parents, supplemented if necessary by a diary.
- Consider the function of the symptoms (e.g. in reducing anxiety, or in the effect they have on other family members).
- Refer the child if it is clear that the obsessions and compulsions lie outside the normal range and are causing impairment.

CHAPTER TWENTY EIGHT

Anxiety, worry, fears and phobias

Definitions

Anxiety exists along a continuum from normal to abnormal – that is, there is no clear cut-off point separating abnormal and normal anxiety. Anxiety is *abnormal* when it affects the child's ability to participate in expected age-appropriate social and academic activities – in other words, when it causes distress and dysfunction. Pathological anxiety may be *specific* (related to a single object or situation) or *generalised*.

Anxiety may occur continuously or in discrete bursts, such as *panic attacks*. These are clusters of extreme symptoms, often including prominent autonomic arousal (*see* Box 28.1), and usually provoked by a particular trigger or triggers. The autonomic symptoms are often misinterpreted, (e.g. as a sign of going mad or dying) and lead to further anxiety, setting up a vicious circle.

Box 28.1: Autonomic symptoms that can occur during a panic attack

Sweating
Tremor, shaking
Palpitations, pounding heart
Shortness of breath or a smothering feeling (usually due to breathing too fast)
A choking feeling
Chest pain or discomfort
A dry mouth
Butterflies in the tummy or nausea
Dizziness; feeling faint, unsteady or light-headed
Pins and needles (paraesthesiae)
Feeling cold or hot all over
Going pale
Feeling unreal (derealisation) or detached from oneself (depersonalisation)

Worry is the cognitive component of anxiety – repetitive thoughts about what might happen. The other components of anxiety are *behavioural, emotional* and *somatic*. For instance, an anxious child may be clingy, restless or obsessional, avoidant or fearful of new situations, and may have autonomic bodily changes or vague symptoms such as stomach-ache or headaches.

A developmental perspective

As children develop, the things that frighten them change. In young infants, sensory experiences (e.g. loud sounds or being dropped) may generate fear. The fear is evidenced by the startle response and other movements.

Separation anxiety starts at about nine months of age and subsides gradually by four or five years. It is manifested by clinginess, fear of strangers, and distress when an attachment figure leaves. These behaviours are more apparent in unfamiliar circumstances, when the child is ill or tired, and when there is an insecure attachment.

Isolated *fears* (e.g. of the dark, spiders or monsters) are common in young children. *Phobias* are specific fears that have become maladaptive. For example, everyone is rightly apprehensive about wasps, but a child who refuses to go into the garden at all during the summer due to fear of being stung by a wasp could be said to suffer from a wasp phobia.

As children grow older, they become more concerned about their appearance and performance and about what others think of them. Such fears are influenced by the *context* in which they occur. For instance, parental responses to a child's fears may either reinforce or reduce that child's anxiety, and a child's fears about appearance may be exacerbated by name-calling.

In some cases, a child's anxiety reflects parental anxiety, most commonly maternal anxiety or depression.

Assessment

Consider the developmental age of the child. Are their fears or anxiety age-appropriate? Is the child in a situation in which you would expect any reasonable person to be anxious (e.g. another child has been murdered in the next street)? Is the anxiety causing the child any distress or interfering with his functioning? Are there symptoms of depression as well as anxiety?

In the case of panic attacks, it is important to enquire about the underlying fear, which is sometimes difficult to identify (it may be too frightening even to think about). Common underlying fears include fear of going mad, making a fool of oneself in public, and dying.

How are other family members responding to the anxiety? Are they inadvertently reinforcing it, either by giving in to it or by repeatedly offering reassurance? Are they helping the child manage it effectively by insisting that he follows through with feared tasks (e.g. getting to school, or staying in his bedroom on his own)?

You must decide whether the symptoms are pathological or appropriate in the child's circumstances and understandable for his age. For example, a four-year-old who starts primary school, finds it difficult to fit in, and then freezes on stage during a school play should not be regarded as in any way abnormal.

Treatment

If the symptoms are appropriate, then all that is needed is parental reassurance. If you consider the symptoms pathological, then you should try to help the parents to manage their child's anxiety in different ways.

Many parents give in to the child's fears either by supporting avoidance tactics, or by offering such frequent reassurance that this maintains the anxiety. It is therefore important to encourage the parents to help the child to experience whatever it is he is avoiding. This is necessary to help him to learn to manage his anxiety or overcome his fears. Warn the parents that the anxiety will initially become a great deal worse if it is confronted, and the child may become distressed (e.g. with crying or stomach-ache). This will not last, and it will lessen as the child is increasingly able to tolerate experiencing the source of the anxiety. Examples include a fear of meeting new people, or of going to school, and similar principles apply to the management of school refusal (*see* Chapter 29 on school refusal). The exposure to the feared situation may be sudden (*flooding*) or consist of a series of small steps (*graded hierarchy*), in either case with help from the parents to enable the child to negotiate each stage.

In some circumstances, anxiety may benefit from medication. Performance anxiety can be appropriately treated with single doses of propranolol (10–40 mg) as needed. Initial insomnia due to worries or anxiety may respond well to small doses of a sedative tricyclic antidepressant such as amitriptyline (10–50 mg). More generalised anxiety responds well to selective serotonin reuptake inhibitors. (The distinction between anxiety and depression is not always clear-cut.)

Case study 28.1

James, an eight-year-old boy, was brought to the general practitioner by his mother with a complaint that he was unreasonably afraid of cats. This problem had come to a head because the day before he had seen a cat on the pavement, broken away from his mother's hand and run into the road in order to get away from the animal. His mother described how he had screamed and been trembling with fear. The general practitioner asked about the duration and origin of the symptoms. The boy's mother explained that they had been building up over several months, but there was no specific incident that had seemed to trigger the fear. The doctor told the parents that he was confident something could be done about this fear, which amounted to a phobia, and he referred the family to the health visitor attached to the practice.

continued overleaf

At a practice meeting four weeks later, the health visitor described her successful intervention with the family. Initially, the parents were helped to devise a graded hierarchy of exposure to cats. This consisted of looking at pictures of cats together, and then getting James' brother and sister to pretend to be cats. They had progressed to looking at cats through a glass window of their home, and then more closely through the local pet shop window. The health visitor outlined the plans, which were eventually to encourage James to enter the same room as someone holding a cat, moving on to stroking the cat while someone else held it, with the aim of finally holding a cat himself. The health visitor also reported that there was no indication of the origin or underlying cause of James' cat phobia.

Referral

Many local services include clinical psychologists or clinical nurse specialists, who are well trained to deal with anxiety disorders. The combination of individual and family work necessary to help some cases to improve may be too much for primary care.

Box 28.2:   Practice points about anxiety

- The symptoms may be psychological, physiological and behavioural.
- Anxiety may be generalised or specific. Specific anxiety includes phobias (of objects or situations) and panic attacks.
- Assessment should include a detailed enquiry about physical sensations, thoughts and feared consequences.
- The treatment of choice is behavioural, and is carried out mainly by parents. It involves facing up to feared situations, and overcoming the surges in anxiety that this will produce.
- Medication can sometimes be valuable for symptomatic relief.

Book for parents

Mental Health Foundation (2000) *The Anxious Child*. Mental Health Foundation, London. A small booklet that gives convenient basic information, available from the Mental Health Foundation, 20/21 Cornwall Terrace, London NW1 4QL (tel 020 7535 7400; fax 020 7535 7474); e-mail mhf@mhf.org.uk; website www.mhf.org.uk.

CHAPTER TWENTY NINE

School refusal

Introduction

Definitions

School refusal can be defined as *a child's avoidance of school which is known to his parents*. It is almost always linked to *anxiety*, although this may only be apparent when attempts are made to get the child to school. For this reason, it is sometimes called *school phobia*, but this implies that the anxiety is all related to school, whereas it may be at least partially home based. In contrast, *truancy* is *the wilful avoidance of school without parental knowledge*, and is far less likely to present in primary care. Usually the child leaves home as if to go to school but does not go there, or attends only for registration and then wanders, with others. In broad terms, school refusal is associated with disorders of emotion, and truancy is linked with disorders of conduct.

It is the role of the *educational welfare officers* or *educational social workers* (similar job, but different names in different areas) to ensure satisfactory attendance at all of the schools to which they are attached. They therefore have the important task of supporting the parents of children who are having difficulty in attending. In some areas, the school educational psychologist may also be involved. Referral to child mental health services may be made directly from these professionals or the school, or via the general practitioner.

Presentation

The way in which school refusal presents in primary care is often with physical symptoms such as nausea, abdominal pains, headaches or diarrhoea. These can be regarded as an expression of the child's distress at being forced to go to school, and they usually subside either once the child is sure that he has got off school for the day – or on Friday evening! The general practitioner has a very important role in the management of school refusal in assessing the severity of these symptoms, investigating and referring as necessary (but minimally) and, when appropriate, reinforcing the efforts of other professionals and the child's parents to get him back to school.

Hybrid conditions occur, including elements of both truancy and school refusal. For instance, children in families where there is a negative attitude to school attendance may have particular difficulties – multiple children in the same family may fail to attend, and sometimes multiple families on the same housing estate.

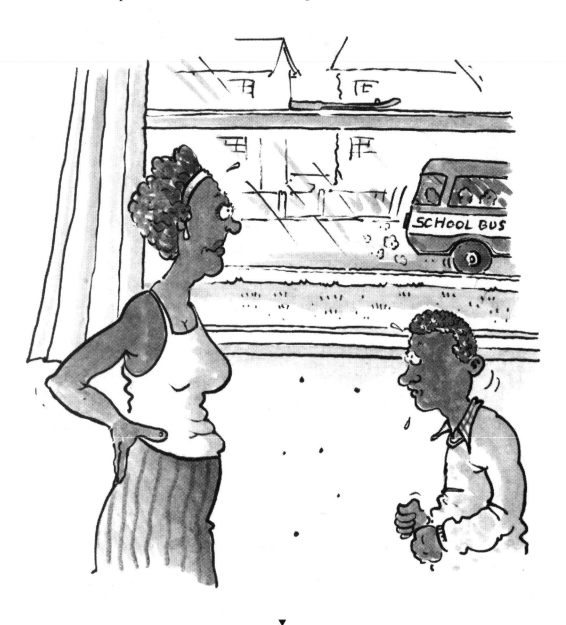

▼

Prevalence

Minor forms of school refusal are common, and are likely to involve the general practitioner in assessing anxiety or physical symptoms. Complete refusal to attend school is rarer, and is likely to involve referral to child mental health services. The prevalence is similar in girls and boys. The condition may occur at any age, but is said to peak at times of school transition (ages 5 and 11 years), and in the penultimate GCSE years (14–15 years).

Assessment

It is important to take a history of the pattern of school attendance, associated somatic symptoms and expressed anxiety, if any. Enquire specifically about the autonomic symptoms of anxiety (e.g. fast breathing, racing heart, feeling sick, butterflies in the tummy, diarrhoea, sweating, shaking, pins and needles). The timing of the symptoms is particularly important. Are they worse during the morning, especially on Mondays? Are they better later on in the day, especially on Fridays? Are they better at weekends?

A history of *separation anxiety* is important. Were there difficulties separating at nursery school/primary school/going to stay with friends? Is this problem long-standing, or has it developed recently? Is the child having any academic difficulties at school? What is the current pattern of friendships (social isolation, or close friendships at school and outside school)? A withdrawal from friends or a lessening of interest in previously enjoyed activities may indicate a *depressive disorder* (*see* Chapter 33).

A frequent *family pattern* in school refusal is an overprotective mother who responds with significant anxiety to each of her child's symptoms, and an absent or uninvolved father. In extreme cases, the mother may have agoraphobia, and may need one of the children (often the youngest) to stay at home to help her to get out of the house.

A brief individual interview with the child is more likely to elicit *sources of anxiety*, but many of the same questions can be asked in the presence of parents. Bullying at school is possibly the single most important possibility (*see* Chapter 24). A direct question such as 'Is anyone at school calling you names, or doing anything nasty to you?' should suffice. The journey to school can also be highly aversive for some children, as severe bullying can occur on the school bus. A knowledge of the family can give clues to the child's anxieties about what might happen when he is not at home. Have there been any deaths or illnesses in the extended family recently? Has either parent been unwell? Try screening questions for depression, such as 'Do you think you're unhappy at the moment?' or 'What do you enjoy doing at the moment?'. This can lead on to a question either about a reduction in interest or social activities, or about what the child does when he is not at school, which may sometimes be inadvertently very rewarding.

Management

Establish with the parents *that they want their child to return to school*. If they do not, then there is little point in your proceeding further. For instance, if they think he is too ill, irrespective of your opinion that he is not, then a paediatric referral may be necessary to give adequate reassurance. If the parents believe that attending school is doing their child no good, then either they will have to teach their child at home, or they will have to answer to the educational welfare service, who may decide to use court proceedings.

If the parents request *home tuition*, refuse this. Home tuition should be used only as a last resort, and is an admission of defeat. The child is unlikely to return to school once there is a home tutor, and this isolates him even further from his peer group. It is also important that the parents collaborate with each other and keep in constant contact with the school.

The aim is *to get the child back to school* as soon as possible. This should be done using graded exposure, which involves the following steps.

1 Clarify the child's anxieties.
2 Deal with these as far as possible. For example, ask the parents to insist that the school should put a stop to the bullying, or ask them to have a discussion with the child about the deaths and illnesses in the family.
3 Ask the parents to negotiate with the school the smallest possible first step. This might be merely a trip to the school premises out of school hours without going in, or an hour spent in the special needs room.
4 Encourage the parents to support the child in this. Warn them that this or subsequent steps may increase the child's anxiety and either worsen their physical symptoms or lead to anger and aggression.
5 Enable the parents to negotiate with the school and the child what the next steps should be, and if one step proves to be too large, break it down into much smaller components. It is important to pay attention to practical details, such as what happens in school if a particular step is too taxing. There must be a face-saving alternative to having to run out of school, such as going to a particular teacher.
6 Praise the parents and the child for any small success, and ensure that the parents also praise the child effusively.

Referral

Many parents can adopt this plan with the minimum of support and guidance. An incipient school attendance problem can be dealt with at an early stage, when it is easiest to resolve. Pitfalls include prolonged attention to physical symptoms, which in some cases can allow a pattern of school refusal to become established, as for example in chronic fatigue syndrome (*see* Chapter 36). Paediatric referral may be necessary at an early stage for parents who will not accept a general practitioner's reassurance.

Some parents may find it difficult to collaborate effectively with each other or with the school. An energetic educational welfare officer should be able to broker agreements. If your knowledge of the family dynamics suggests that parental authority will be difficult to establish, or that the extent of anxiety or depression is going to make return to school very difficult, then a referral should be made at an early stage to your local child and adolescent mental health service.

Case study 29.1

Tracy was a nine-year-old girl who had had difficulty in making friends at her new school since her family had moved house one year earlier. She had developed a flu-like illness in February, and had been off school for several weeks feeling ill. Her mother brought her to the health centre to ask what was wrong. A diagnosis of viral illness was made, and symptomatic treatment was advised.

The symptoms persisted into the Easter term, and Tracy was missing about three days of school every week. Her mother was concerned about a serious underlying illness, while her father was insistent that she should just get back to school. Her general practitioner took a careful history which revealed that Tracy perked up at weekends. He conducted a full examination, and sent off a urine and stool culture, a full blood count and erythrocyte sedimentation rate. Reviewing the results two weeks later, he reassured both parents firmly, and discussed a gradual return to school.

The parents were able to agree with a very amenable teacher at school that Tracy could come in for as little of the school day as she felt able to. She gradually progressed, over the course of several months, from one lesson a day to half days and then full days. Her father helped her to keep a diary of her progress on the family computer. Her mother drove her in to school, so that she did not have to cope with the school bus. Once Tracy could manage afternoons, her mother also visited her over lunch, which they had in the car together, as it turned out that the social pressures of lunchtime were too much for her. Once she was attending school full-time, she was able to experiment with journeys on the school bus and lunchtime with the friends she was now making.

Tracy could easily have developed both chronic fatigue syndrome and an established school refusal problem. With early intervention, and parents who were able to work very effectively both with each other and with the school, neither of these labels were necessary, and Tracy was able to return to a normal developmental pathway.

Prognosis

The prognosis is better in younger children, and in those who have been out of school for only a short time. Behavioural treatments of the type described above are effective in about 90% of primary school children with a short history. After illnesses and holidays the child may experience some apprehension about returning to school, but if the parents are warned about this and take prompt action the problem need not recur.

Secondary school children fare worse, particularly if they have been out of school for more than a few weeks before treatment is attempted. After the age of 14 years the success rate is very low, and alternative educational placements are often necessary.

Box 29.1:   Practice points for school refusal

- Establish whether the parents accept the need to get their child to school.
- Decide which is the best agency to take the lead in helping them – primary care, the educational welfare service, or the local child and family mental health service.
- If another agency takes the lead, the general practitioner's role may be restricted to deciding whether the child has a genuine medical reason for staying off school.
- If the general practitioner takes the lead, which is advisable in mild early cases, they should urge the parents to link up with the school, both to sort out any sources of anxiety at school, and then to construct a return to school in small manageable steps.
- Ensure that the parents are receiving enough continuing support to carry the plan through, and revise it as necessary.

CHAPTER THIRTY

Recurrent abdominal pain

Introduction

Recurrent abdominal pain is a common problem affecting around 10% of school-age children.[1] Boys and girls are affected to a similar extent, and there is no clear social class link. Approximately 10% of cases of recurrent abdominal pain have a clear organic cause. The remaining 90% are of unknown aetiology. These are often considered to be psychogenic, but it may be that we shall have a clearer understanding of physiological causes in the future. Hospital admissions due to non-specific abdominal pain are 40% more frequent during school terms,[2] suggesting that at least sometimes there are important emotional factors involved.

Abdominal pain associated with pallor, anorexia, nausea or vomiting may be caused by abdominal migraine, even in the absence of headaches.[3] There is often a family history of migraine. A similar condition used to be referred to as the 'periodic syndrome', consisting of a combination of recurrent abdominal pain, headaches, vomiting and fever. Some studies suggest that many cases of recurrent abdominal pain may be an early expression of migraine,[4] although other work has focused on the similarities between recurrent abdominal pain and adult irritable bowel syndrome.[5]

Generally accepted organic causes of recurrent pain include urinary tract infections, mesenteric adenitis, constipation, peptic ulcers and inflammatory bowel disease.

The long-term outlook for children with recurrent abdominal pain is interesting. Follow-up studies of these children that were conducted in the 1970s suggest that up to half of them may continue to suffer from abdominal pain as adults.[6] This is more likely to be the case if their parents suffer from abdominal pain, which suggests a possible genetic component.

Assessment

A careful history and examination are essential. These should give enough information to indicate whether further investigations or referral are necessary. Table 30.1 lists some differentiating features.

Table 30.1: Differentiating between organic and non-organic causes of abdominal pain

Indicators of organic causes	Indicators of non-organic causes
Acute onset	Vague onset
Continuous	Intermittent/recurrent
Well localised	Poorly localised
May radiate to the back	Central without radiation
One pain only	Pain occurs elsewhere in the body
Peripheral (Apley's law)	The child points at or near the umbilicus
Wakes the child at night	The child is not woken by the pain
Diminishes appetite	The child eats well
Fever	Fever was said to be a non-organic component of the periodic syndrome, but this is now disputed
Vomiting	Vomiting may be self-induced or due to anxiety
Urinary or bowel symptoms	No other symptoms of organic disorder
No relation to school day	Only occurs on school mornings
No evidence of emotional distress	Evidence of anxiety, tension or low mood

History

Determine the nature of the pain as shown in Table 30.1. Enquire about triggers, focusing on possible dietary causes, as well as life events and other potential causes of stress. It may be useful to ask about pain in other family members, especially in childhood, and about migraine and irritable bowel syndrome. Direct questioning about bowel habit may reveal a history of constipation or alternating constipation and diarrhoea. Consider asking the parent and child what they think may be causing the pain. If you suspect stressors within the family, it may be worth interviewing the child alone.

Examination

It is important to examine the child carefully, if only to reassure both the child and their parent that the problem has been taken seriously. Height and weight should be plotted on a centile chart. Deviation from a previous growth curve is a significant pointer to organic disease. Examine the abdomen to exclude localised tenderness, guarding or constipation. It is also worth examining the eardrums, chest and genitalia (children may refer pain originating elsewhere to the abdomen, and sexual abuse comes into the differential diagnosis of abdominal pain as it does for every other child psychiatric disorder).

Investigations

Investigations should be kept to a minimum, as an endless search for possible causes reinforces in the mind of the child and their parents that there must be a serious cause that no one can pinpoint. Tests that are appropriate in primary care include a full blood count, erythrocyte sedimentation rate, urinary microscopy and urinary culture. If you have the option of arranging an abdominal ultrasound examination, then this may be well worth the effort, as both parents and children often find normal imaging tests very reassuring. Stool cultures may be helpful to exclude *Giardia lamblia*, or if there is a history of foreign travel, but are probably not worthwhile unless there are clear bowel symptoms. Constipation can be assessed by a plain abdominal X-ray, but an X-ray before and 72 hours after the ingestion of radio-opaque markers is more sensitive and specific (Professor David Candy, personal communication), and this should perhaps be left to a specialist.

If the parents accept that there is an emotional or behavioural cause, then an 'ABC' diary (*see* p. 74) – or a very thorough history – may be helpful in identifying triggers and inadvertent rewards or secondary gain. A dietary record may be useful for identifying trigger foods.

Management and referral

If no findings are suggestive of organic causes after this degree of history, examination and investigations, you have a choice between paediatric referral and reassurance. Your knowledge of the family should guide you in this decision. If the parents are not likely to be reassured without a specialist opinion, then you will have to arrange one. If you decide to reassure them, remember:

- this will work better *after* you have taken everything seriously
- to explain everything to the parent *and* the child
- the pain is not caused by a serious illness. Lack of a serious cause does not mean lack of a cause. It is common not to be able to find the cause
- although it is frustrating not to know what is causing the pain, it is important to move on and find ways of dealing with the pain
- the pain is real and not imaginary ('it really hurts'). The analogy to tension headaches or irritable bowel syndrome in adults may help parents to understand this. The child will need no convincing
- stress makes the pain worse – 'things that make you worried or upset' will be easier for the child to understand. Avoidable stressors should be removed. The child will need help, preferably from the parents, in dealing with unavoidable stresses (e.g. starting a new school)
- the parents may try simple measures such as tummy rubs or hot-water bottles. Most will have already tried paracetamol without success. Warn the parents that giving too much attention to the pain may 'keep it alive', whereas ignoring it may help it to subside. Explain to the child that the pain may not feel so bad if they get involved in some activity that they enjoy
- abdominal migraine is a possible cause. One study reported improvement with pizotifen.[7] This may be worth a trial if there are suggestive associated symptoms, as described above.

Other problems may coexist with recurrent abdominal pain. School refusal (*see* Chapter 29) is potentially one of the most serious, and should be addressed as soon as possible. It is also worth considering whether the child is trying to communicate something with the pain that is difficult to express in other ways (e.g. a fear of bullies at school or abuse in the home). There may also be family anxieties that need to be clarified. For instance, perhaps a relative died of cancer after having initially been diagnosed with psychogenic pain. If this type of underlying anxiety is not addressed, it may prevent the pain from resolving.

Failure to provide reassurance is an indication for referral to a paediatrician, rather than for performing further investigations.

Case study 30.1

Terry, aged nine, was brought to the health centre by his mother, Michelle, who told the general practitioner that Terry had been experiencing stomach pains for two to three months. These had not responded to paracetamol or mebeverine, which had been prescribed by another doctor in the practice one month previously. Michelle was wondering why the pains had not gone away, and was worried that they might be due to something serious.

On enquiry, the general practitioner found that the pain had come on gradually and that it came and went. It did seem to be worse on school days and Sunday evenings, but Michelle had not kept Terry away from school for more than a couple of days. Terry denied that there were any problems at school, and he specifically denied that he was being bullied. Michelle commented that Terry had always been good at his schoolwork, but these days often seemed frustrated when doing his homework. Terry was never woken by the pain, he was eating well and he seemed to be growing normally. He was active and had no other symptoms such as vomiting or a change in bowel habit.

The doctor's examination was unremarkable. No masses or enlarged organs would be felt in the abdomen, and urinalysis was normal. Terry was approximately on the 50th centile for both height and weight.

The doctor went through the features of Terry's pain that suggested it was not serious in origin. He emphasised that Terry was eating normally and growing normally (both good signs). He mentioned that it was not unusual for children of this age to suffer from stomach pains from time to time, which usually went away again after a few months. He arranged for Terry to have a full blood count taken at the surgery and an abdominal ultrasound examination at the local district general hospital. However, he stressed that the tests were highly likely to produce normal results, and that he was only doing these in order to confirm that Terry did not have a serious problem.

At follow-up four weeks later, the doctor confirmed that the blood test and ultrasound examination were both normal. He suggested that Michelle should talk to Terry's teachers about how well he was getting on at school and whether he was finding the work demanding. The doctor also suggested that it would be wise to explore with the school whether there was any possibility that Terry was being bullied, despite his denial of this.

Box 30.1:   Practice points for recurrent abdominal pain

- Care in the history and examination are essential:

    to distinguish an organic from a non-organic cause
    to convince the child and parent that you are taking them seriously.

- Limit the number of investigations in order to be most effective in reassuring.
- Reassurance does not mean dismissing the pain.
- If you cannot reassure the child and their parents, refer to a paediatrician.

References

1   Apley J and Naish N (1958) Recurrent abdominal pain: a field study of 1000 school children. *Arch Dis Child.* **33**: 165–70.

2   Williams N, Jackson D, Lambert PC and Johnstone JM (1999) Incidence of non-specific abdominal pain in children during school term: population survey based on discharge diagnosis. *BMJ.* **318**:1455.

3   Abu-Arafeh IA and Russell G (1995) Prevalence and clinical features of abdominal migraine compared with those of migraine headache. *Arch Dis Child.* **72**: 413–17.

4   Mavromichalis I, Zaramboiukas T and Giala MM (1995) Migraine of gastrointestinal origin. *Eur J Paediatrics.* **154**: 406–10.

5   Hyams JS, Treem WR, Justinich CJ, Davis P, Shoup M and Burke G (1995) Characterisation of symptoms in children with recurrent abdominal pain: resemblance to irritable bowel syndrome. *J Pediatr Gastroenterol Nutrition.* **20**: 209–14.

6   Apley J and Hale B (1973) Children with recurrent abdominal pain: how do they grow up? *BMJ.* **3**: 7–9.

7   Symon DN and Russell G (1995) Double-blind placebo-controlled trial of pizotifen syrup in the treatment of abdominal migraine. *Arch Dis Child.* **72**: 48–50.

CHAPTER THIRTY ONE

Physical presentations of emotional distress

Introduction

Up to 5% of children who consult general practitioners have a primary mental health problem.[1] Associated psychosocial factors relevant to the presenting problem are noted in about 20% of schoolchildren.[2,3] Different terminology is used to describe these conditions, so some definitions may be helpful.

Psychosomatic presentations

A broad definition might be any physical presentation to which the doctor feels that psychological or social factors are contributing in a significant way (e.g. stress-induced asthma). A narrower definition is used to describe the way in which some physical symptoms are especially likely to represent the somatisation of emotional distress (e.g. headache or abdominal pain). *See* Box 1.1 on p. 4.

Hysterical, conversion or dissociative disorders

Hysteria has been defined as the presence of physical symptoms in the absence of disease, or a condition where the disease is present but insufficient to explain the symptom. An alternative way to view hysteria is as *abnormal illness behaviour*. By taking on the sick role, the child may be gaining a number of advantages (e.g. adult attention, permission not to attend school, or an excuse for not achieving as much as expected).

The term 'hysteria' has gone out of favour because it has been used in so many senses. The concept of '*conversion disorder*' derives from the Freudian idea that an internal conflict, usually unconscious, manifests externally as (or 'converts' to) a physical symptom. This symptom cannot be explained by known pathological mechanisms. The absence of a physical explanation is a dangerous criterion to use on its own. Long-term follow-up studies have shown that up to 50% of so-called 'hysterical disorders' turn out to be a rare condition that the clinician had not considered.[4] *Dissociation* implies a lack of integration of awareness, and the term 'dissociation disorder' is sometimes used synonymously with 'conversion disorder'. In both cases there must be a temporal link with stressful events, problems or needs, as well as unexplained symptoms.

Assessment

Examples of ways in which emotional distress may present as physical symptoms include the following:

- tension headaches
- recurrent abdominal pain (*see* Chapter 30).
- asthma attacks brought on by anxiety or associated with hyperventilation
- diarrhoea related to anxiety
- palpitations (and many other autonomic nervous symptoms that can occur as an expression of anxiety) (*see* Chapter 28)
- pseudo-convulsions. These often occur in children who already have epilepsy, and so are familiar with fits and professional reactions to them
- deficit symptoms – aphasia, loss of vision, loss of hearing, loss of sensation in a non-dermatomal distribution, or limb weakness. It is debatable whether chronic fatigue should be included here
- active symptoms – pain in a non-dermatomal distribution, or abnormal movements
- the child is excessively disabled in relation to the objective effects of the disease. Occasionally a child will be suffering from a genuine physical illness, but the symptoms will persist when the organic cause has resolved. Sometimes disabling symptoms seem to have started with a minor physical illness such as a cold.

A clear history is invaluable. Examination may reveal inconsistencies, either with anatomy or over time. It is important to convince the child and their parents that you are taking them seriously, but the details are probably best left to specialists. Investigations should be kept to a minimum.

If you want to suggest this type of diagnosis in a referral letter, you should have some kind of hypothesis about why the child needs to adopt the sick role. Consider also '*secondary gain*'. This term also derives from Freudian ideas. The primary gain is not having to deal consciously with whatever conflicts are being converted into physical symptoms. The secondary gain refers to the unexpected rewards of this. This may include parents giving the child more attention, not having to go to school, not having to compete, getting a lot of doctors interested in one, and so on. Family factors may also be relevant. Many children find that their parents will only agree with each other when a child is ill. Such factors can be regarded as maintaining causes.

Management and referral

If the family acknowledges the possibility that there is a psychological cause for the problem, treatment is much easier. In any case, it is important to stress to the family that although no organic cause can be found, the symptom is genuine and the child's experience is real. Be vigilant about saying that you believe in the symptoms even if you do not – the child will not be willing to return to you if he thinks that you do not believe him. Explaining that having such symptoms may be very stressful, and that in some children stress or psychological upsets can make physical symptoms worse, can often improve co-operation of the child and their family with professionals.

The difficulty for many children is how to relinquish the symptoms *without loss of face*. One particularly successful face-saving treatment may be a course of physiotherapy.

Suggestion can be helpful with these children. A good prognosis should be given at an early stage, with the advice that recovery should occur quickly. It is important to follow these children up closely and to monitor their progress.

Referral to a paediatrician should be made early on if the situation is at all complicated. For simpler problems, referral should be considered if the symptoms do not improve appreciably within about four to six weeks. It is wisest to leave any referral to a child psychologist or psychiatrist to be decided by the paediatrician.

Case study 31.1

Sophie, aged 13 years, was well known as an asthma patient. Sometimes the attacks seemed to come on because she was anxious, and she gave a history suggestive of hyperventilation. On one occasion, she went direct to Accident and Emergency, and was discharged with a diagnosis of hyperventilation, since her chest was entirely clear. She was admitted to hospital the next day very ill with diabetic ketoacidosis.

Case study 31.2

Clarissa, aged ten years, was taken to Accident and Emergency unable to walk. The casualty officer could find no (other) neurological abnormalities on examination. He decided she must be hysterical,[31.1] and sent her home. When she was eventually admitted to the paediatric ward, she thought that no one was going to believe her. Investigations were all normal, although it was thought that she might have had a mild form of Guillain–Barré disease (the cerebrospinal fluid protein level was at the upper limit of normal, some time after what sounded like an acute viral infection). Clarissa found it difficult to trust professionals. Despite intensive physiotherapy, it took her over a year to get better. Some of this time was spent on a children's psychiatric in-patient unit. Much later it emerged that she had been sexually abused by a friend of her elder brother's.

Box 31.1:   Practice points for the physical presentations of emotional distress

- Keep an open mind about whether symptoms are 'organic' or 'non-organic' – the distinction is of less use to families than to doctors.
- Believe in the distress, and convince the child that you believe in their symptoms.
- Try to find a way for the child to return to normal functioning (e.g. physiotherapy).
- Refer the child to a paediatrician if:

    there is doubt about the diagnosis
    the family requires a specialist opinion
    it looks as if the problem may become intractable.

Note

31.1   One of the reasons why this term has gone out of favour is the pejorative way it has been used, particularly to describe females!

References

1   Garralda ME and Bailey D (1986) Children with psychiatric disorders in primary care. *J Child Psychol Psychiatry.* **27**: 611–24.

2   Bailey V, Graham P and Boniface D (1978) How much child psychiatry does a general practitioner do? *J R Coll Gen Pract.* **28**: 621–6.

3   Garralda ME (1994) Primary care psychiatry. In: M Rutter, E Taylor and L Hersov (eds) *Child and Adolescent Psychiatry.* Blackwell Scientific Publications, Oxford.

4   Marsden CD (1986) Hysteria: a neurologist's view. *Psychol Med.* **16**: 277–88.

CHAPTER THIRTY TWO

Tics and Tourette's syndrome

Introduction

Why bother?

Children with tics are often regarded as anxious or naughty. While they may be both, it seems that both tics and Tourette's syndrome are significantly under-diagnosed, and teasing or bullying often result. Although many children need no specific treatment, recognition of the condition can help the child and their parents to deal with the consequences more effectively, particularly by removing blame.

Definitions

A tic is a sudden, purposeless, repetitive stereotyped movement or phonic production. *Simple tics* are single movements. Examples include eye-blinking (the commonest type), shoulder-shrugging, head-flicking, nose-wrinkling and grimacing. Vocal tics include grunts, barks, spits, sniffs, throat-clearing, coughs or words (swear words occur in less than one-third of cases). *Complex tics* are sequences of movements, or include movements and vocalisations together. The combination of multiple motor tics with one or more vocal tics is called *Gilles de la Tourette's syndrome*, or *Tourette's syndrome* for short. This may include complex behaviours, such as touching, licking, pirouetting or smelling, which may be very difficult to distinguish from obsessions.

Causation

Tics used to be regarded as a manifestation of anxiety. Although anxiety or tension may worsen tics, they are just as likely to disappear during an absorbing activity, and come flooding back when the child relaxes. Tics can be suppressed for a time at will, but are essentially involuntary, or partly voluntary in response to a premonitory urge. There is often a family history of tics, and a basis which is at least partly biological is now generally accepted. It is probably easiest to think of Tourette's syndrome as being due to some impairment of the movement-control centres of the brain, such as the basal ganglia, but this must be an oversimplification.

Presentation

The mean age of onset of Tourette's syndrome is 7 years (range 2–21 years), usually with motor tics such as blinking. Tics are more common in boys than in girls. The tics characteristically wax and wane in frequency and severity over hours, days, weeks, months and years, with no obvious pattern. Tourette's syndrome starts to improve in late adolescence or early adulthood, and continues to improve with age.

Prevalence

Tourette's syndrome used to be regarded as very rare. However, recent community studies have suggested otherwise. One study found that secondary school pupils had a rate of 3% for Tourette's disorder and 18% for tics.[1] The prevalence is even higher in pupils with special needs, especially those with emotional and behavioural disorders. The diagnosis is usually missed (probably because it is not considered). Tourette's syndrome is associated with a number of other disorders, including attention-deficit hyperactivity disorder, obsessive-compulsive disorder, oppositional defiant disorder, self-injurious behaviour, failure to inhibit aggression, and anxiety and depression.[2] These associations may partly explain its high prevalence in the special needs population.

Assessment

It is unlikely that a short meeting in the health centre will reveal much direct evidence of tics. It is easy for you to blink and miss the one tic that is noticed by the parent. Children often do not notice their own tics. A careful history is therefore essential. Parents may not know what you mean by the term 'tics', so you should demonstrate this (which may break the ice). The history can be supplemented by diary-keeping (e.g. with the Yale Global Tic Severity Scale,[3] which simply lists, in diary form, the different types of motor and phonic tic, together with associated symptoms). Teachers' accounts can be helpful, but tics occur less often in the classroom, and in any case teachers may not notice them even if they do occur. It is more important to ask about any effects of the tics in school, particularly teasing by other pupils, or getting into trouble with the class teacher (usually for making noises). If obsessions or compulsions occur, it is worth asking for details, as the differential diagnosis includes obsessive-compulsive disorder and Asperger's disorder (*see* Chapter 27, on obsessive-compulsive disorder).

No investigations are necessary.

Management

If you feel able to make the diagnosis yourself, this will help the family to avoid a long wait to see a specialist, who may not necessarily have any greater knowledge of Tourette's syndrome than you do.

You should emphasise to the parents the difficulty that the child has in controlling the involuntary movements and noises, and ensure that they impress this upon the child's teachers. Otherwise the child may be regarded as merely anxious or naughty.

Psychological treatments were in vogue for a while, but there was never any definite evidence that they worked.[32.1] They are time-consuming and only partially effective, so should probably be reserved for children with severe forms of the disorder and whose parents refuse medication.

Medication should be held in reserve for as long as possible. It is only partially effective, and all of the medications in common usage have significant side-effects. The number of different preparations that are used demonstrates that there is no one best treatment, and it is impossible to tell in advance which medication will suit a particular child. Because there is so much variability in the symptoms, it is often difficult to tell whether a particular medication is effective. Monitoring with diaries will provide more objective evidence of benefit than simple parental reports, but can be very time-consuming for the parents.

It is probably safest to start with small doses of clonidine, particularly in younger children, in order to avoid the possible extra-pyramidal side-effects of antipsychotics. Clonidine is particularly useful with comorbid attention-deficit hyperactivity disorder. However, it probably reduces tic severity by one-third, compared to a figure of two-thirds with antipsychotics.[4] First choices in view of current knowledge would probably be sulpiride or risperidone, but these can cause drowsiness and increased appetite (*see* Chapter 39). Although haloperidol and pimozide have been shown to be effective in numerous trials, we prefer not to recommend these because of their side-effects. The general principle is to start with the lowest possible dose, and to work gradually upwards, reducing the dose if side-effects become troublesome.

Referral

It is curious that, by tradition, children with suspected Tourette's syndrome seem to be referred to child psychiatrists rather than to paediatric neurologists, whereas adults are referred to neurologists. This may be because of the comorbid mental health problems that are so common, particularly attention-deficit hyperactivity disorder and obsessive-compulsive symptoms. However, what is needed initially is a medical diagnosis and consideration of medication, which might be provided more effectively and rapidly by an interested paediatrician. Specialist psychological input may require referral to the local child mental health team, or to a more specialist team. There seems to be little point in referring to a team in which no one has an interest in tic disorders, since in our experience this results in under-diagnosis and unnecessary distress for both children and parents.

Case study 32.1

Roger, aged nine years, was brought to the surgery by his mother Tracey, who said that his teacher was complaining about his making noises in class. These mainly consisted of sniffing, coughing and throat-clearing. Roger said that he did not have a cold and he never coughed up any sputum. There was no history of asthma or nocturnal cough. The general practitioner examined his chest and ear, nose and throat system, which were unremark-able. He suddenly remembered having read an article about Tourette's syndrome, and asked whether Roger had any tics or twitches. Roger and his mother looked blank. The general practitioner then imitated an eye blink and a shoulder twitch. Tracey smiled and said that Roger used to blink his eyes a lot, but was not doing it so much now. On further enquiry, it seemed that Roger also turned his head to one side on occasion, and felt compelled to touch the side of his desk at school exactly seven times each lesson. The general practitioner asked Roger whether he was ever bullied or teased, and Roger said that he had been called 'weirdo' once or twice, but that he had ignored it and it had stopped. The general practitioner then explained that he thought Roger probably had a mild form of Tourette's syndrome, and he asked whether Tracey would like a referral. She said that she did not want to visit a child psychiatrist, and also that she was not at all keen on medication for the condition. She agreed that the doctor could telephone Roger's class teacher to explain that the noises in class were due to a medical condition, and that they would be difficult for Roger to control.

Roger came to the health centre six months later about something else. His tics were about the same, although they fluctuated a great deal, but he was not getting into trouble with his teacher, who had quickly dealt with a recurrence of teasing.

Box 32.1:   Practice points about tics and Tourette's syndrome

- Tics are common, especially in children at special schools, and they often go undiagnosed.
- The diagnosis of Tourette's syndrome is made by considering the possibility and asking the right questions. Occasionally, tics will be observed.
- Making the diagnosis of involuntary movements will provide enough help for most children. A few may require medication.
- Refer the child if there is any doubt about the diagnosis, or if there are problems with medication.

Note

32.1 Clinical experience in the Tourette's clinic at the Hospital for Sick Children at Great Ormond Street suggests that habit reversal, massed practice, relaxation and guided imagery can all achieve some degree of success.

References

1   Mason A, Banerjee S, Eapen V, Zeitlin H and Robertson MM (1998) The prevalence of Tourette syndrome in a mainstream school population. *Dev Med Child Neurol.* **40**: 292–6.

2   Robertson MM (2000) Tourette syndrome, associated conditions and the complexities of treatment. *Brain.* **123**: 425–62.

3   Leckman JF, Riddle MA, Hardin MT, Ort SI, Swartz KL and Stevenson J (1989) The Yale Global Tic Severity Scale: initial testing of a clinician-rated scale of tic severity. *J Am Acad Child Adolesc Psychiatry.* **28**: 566–73.

4   Goodman R and Scott S (1997) *Child Psychiatry.* Blackwell Science, Oxford.

PART 5

Problems that present mainly in adolescence

Depression

Introduction

The term *depression* can be used to refer to a *mood*, *symptom* or *syndrome*. Low *moods* are common understandable reactions to unhappy experiences. Depressive *symptoms* (e.g. sad mood, tearfulness, loss of interest, social withdrawal) are also common in children with unhappy life experiences, but may be part of a *syndrome*. This seldom occurs under the age of six years, and is uncommon in pre-pubertal children, but its incidence increases dramatically with puberty, becoming more common in girls than in boys. This is the main reason why adolescent girls present with mental health problems more often than adolescent boys.

Depression affects at least 2% of children under 12 years of age and 5% of teenagers. Epidemiological studies show that much of this depression is under-recognised. It may masquerade as bad behaviour, particularly in boys. Poor functioning at school, in social situations or within the family may be apparent, whereas the underlying mood changes may not be.

The depressive syndrome

The syndrome of depression is a pervasive mood disorder associated with significant suffering or impairment of functioning. In adolescents, the presentation is usually atypical. For instance, there may be hypersomnolence rather than insomnia, and bouts of low mood rather than a continuous low mood. Parents and professionals are often fooled by superficial euthymia, and may find it difficult to distinguish a mood disorder from ordinary moodiness. Young people often conceal from their parents the severity of their low mood and any suicidal thoughts.

Symptoms that are comparable to those in adults

These include the following:

- low mood
- loss of interest

- lack of enjoyment in anything
- social withdrawal
- irritability
- low self-esteem
- guilt
- tearfulness
- physical symptoms (e.g. pains in head, abdomen or chest).

Symptoms that are more likely to occur in adolescents or children

These include the following:

- running away from home
- separation anxiety – which may present as school refusal
- decline in school work
- antisocial behaviour, especially in boys
- initial and middle insomnia are more common than early-morning wakening
- requiring excessive amounts of sleep (even for a teenager!)
- eating more may be a sign of depression as well as eating less
- complaints of boredom.

Symptoms that vary with age

These include the following.

- Sadness and helplessness are prominent in six- to eight-year-olds.
- Eight- to eleven-year-olds report feeling unloved and unfairly treated.
- Guilt and despair are more noticeable after the age of 11 years.
- Suicidal ideation varies with age. Under 11 years, children are more likely to think of jumping out of windows or running in front of cars, whereas adolescents are more likely to think of taking an overdose. Either age group may think of hanging themselves. The younger the child, the lower the likelihood of completed suicide.

Presentation

This is often:

- with somatic symptoms
- combined with anxiety.

Assessment

Diagnostic questions

To determine whether a young person is depressed, the ideal approach is to see her on her own as well as seeing her parents. The parents may be largely unaware of how their teenager feels inside.

Ask open questions first, followed by more specific ones. In general, screening questions are very similar to those for adults, as the following examples demonstrate.

- 'Have you been feeling as happy as usual/sadder than usual/down in the dumps recently?'
- 'What sort of things do you enjoy doing at the moment?'
- 'How have you been getting on with your friends recently?'
- 'How have you been getting on with your family recently?'
- 'Do you think you've been getting cross more than usual recently?'
- 'Are you crying a lot?'
- 'How do you feel about yourself at the moment?'

Do not be afraid to ask about suicidal ideas or intent – there is no evidence that this affects the risk of suicidal actions. On the contrary, the young person may be relieved to be able to share such ideas and feelings. A general question about feeling like dying can be followed by a more specific question about concrete plans.

Ask specifically and in detail about sleep and appetite.

- 'What time do you go to bed?'
- 'What time do you get off to sleep?'
- 'What happens in between?'
- 'Do you wake up after you have gone to sleep? How many times? How long does it take you to get back to sleep?'
- 'What do you feel like when you wake up? Are you refreshed or exhausted?'
- 'Have you been eating more or less than usual recently?'

The time pattern of adolescent depression is different from that for adults. Mood is characteristically very variable and less pervasive than in adults. A depressed adolescent may be in the depths of despair one moment, and enjoying a social outing with friends an hour later. The fact that she can still enjoy certain aspects of her life does not exclude a depressive disorder. In adults, diagnostic criteria demand a duration of symptoms of at least two weeks. In adolescents, it is probably wiser to wait until mood and other changes have persisted for four weeks before making a diagnosis.

You will find that many of these questions may be met with a shrug of the shoulders, a 'Don't know ...' or no answer at all. This seems to be more common in boys, who are probably less likely to go to see a professional anyway, and in whom depression tends to be under-diagnosed. Faced with this difficulty, you may either arrange to see the young person again, or make a referral. However, such recalcitrance suggests that the young person may not accept a referral.

Try to reach a decision as to whether the constellation of depressive symptoms is present and is affecting the young person's functioning. The differential diagnosis includes sadness appropriate to circumstances, anxiety, and overuse of recreational drugs or alcohol, although all of these may coexist with a depressive disorder.

Contributory factors

As in the case of young people who harm themselves, there may be concealed contributory factors, such as past sexual abuse or rape, family relationship difficulties, or bullying at school. It is particularly important to enquire about losses, some of which may not be obvious. For instance, the death of a pet may be a major life event for a young person, as may moving house and school, friends or close relatives moving away, or grandparents dying. Biological contributory factors may also be important, as depression has a strong genetic component (shared in some families with alcoholism).

Treatment

A useful starting point is to explain to the parents, with the consent of the young person and in her presence, how she is feeling. This can lead on to a discussion of the nature of depression, perhaps backed up by a factsheet[1] or a readable book.[2]

Treatment should be tailored to the individual child, young person or family, and may include social, psychological and pharmacological components.

Social interventions

These may include addressing any sources of distress (e.g. bullying), and removing opportunities for self-harm (e.g. paracetamol lying around the house). Practical help with examination stress or social activities may be relatively easy to organise.

Psychological interventions

Talking about feelings and sources of worry can be helpful, whoever the listener is. Many young people prefer to talk to friends rather than to a professional. Alternatives include sympathetic staff at school, youth workers, other trusted adults from within or outside the family, or a practice counsellor or primary child mental health worker. Trials of cognitive–behavioural therapy[3] and interpersonal therapy (which focuses on relationships, role conflict and grief), both in adolescents, have shown benefit, but these treatments may not be available in primary care or even in local clinics. In practice, sympathetic listening may be enough to help recovery, particularly if it is combined with attention to social factors and practical problem-solving.

Pharmacological interventions

It may not be best practice to confine treatment to antidepressants, but they can be a useful adjunct to social or psychological treatments, particularly in the presence of biological symptoms. Merely discussing the possibility of using antidepressants emphasises the severity of the condition, which can help the parents' efforts to understand their child, and may also help the teenager to feel understood.

The first choice for the drug treatment of depression should now be selective serotonin reuptake inhibitors, because they are safer in overdose, and depressed adolescents are at high risk of impulsive overdose. Fluoxetine has not only been shown to be effective in a randomised controlled trial,[5] but it also has advantages over other selective serotonin reuptake inhibitors for adolescents. Its long half-life means that it does not matter too much if a dose is missed, and withdrawal effects on stopping do not occur (as they do for instance with paroxetine and venlafaxine). For young people with marked sleep disturbance, the newer and more specific mirtazapine is less stimulating, and the benefits on sleep start immediately (*see* Chapter 39).

An interesting clinical observation is that low doses of tricyclic antidepressants can be effective, perhaps because of the beneficial effects on sleep and anxiety, but this has not been confirmed by research. In contrast, St John's Wort (the active ingredient of which is probably hypericin) has now been shown in several trials to be effective in adults, probably for mild depression.[6] There is no reason not to regard it as safe and effective for adolescents. The difficulty is that there is no universal agreement on the correct dose or exact preparation, and it is not yet prescribable, so that families have to pay for it over the counter.

Case study 33.1

Melanie Johnson, aged 15 years, was brought by her mother Sarah to Dr Helen Carruthers' afternoon surgery. Sarah encouraged Melanie to tell the doctor about problems she was having with poor concentration and struggling to keep up with her schoolwork in recent weeks. Melanie was rather hesitant, and the general practitioner sensed that she might prefer to talk to her on her own. Mrs Johnson agreed to wait in the waiting-room, and once alone the doctor stressed to Melanie that anything she said to her would be treated in confidence.

Melanie confirmed that she was having problems with her schoolwork, which was unusual for her. She did find it difficult to concentrate. Melanie thought that it might be because she had split up with her fairly long-standing boyfriend a couple of months

continued overleaf

previously. She was feeling really quite unhappy and had lost interest in her usual social life with her friends during this period. On enquiry, she admitted that she had been tearful most days, had trouble getting to sleep and was waking in the early hours of the morning. She had not been drinking alcohol, but she smoked cannabis once or twice a week. In reply to the question whether she had ever felt so bad she thought life was not worth living, Melanie confessed that she had fleetingly thought of taking an overdose, but she had not collected any pills together or made any definite plans.

The doctor then asked whether Melanie had anyone she could talk to about her problems. She was finding it very difficult to talk to her mother, and they kept having rows about her relationship with her ex-boyfriend (who was 18 years old) and her poor performance at school. She did not want her mother to know that she and her boyfriend had been having sex together. Her grandmother on her mother's side, who had been a significant support for both Melanie and Sarah, had died six months earlier. She believed that her stepfather was trying hard to help her, too, but she had never really got on with him. Her father had recently moved further away from home, and she could now only see him during the school holidays.

The doctor agreed that she would not tell Melanie's mother about her sexual activity or her use of cannabis. She asked her mother to rejoin them, and she explained to both Melanie and Sarah that this problem was one of depression, probably due to the loss of Melanie's father, grandmother and boyfriend, coupled with the academic stress of school life. She explained that Melanie had enough symptoms to justify treatment with a course of antidepressants. Sarah raised the issue of whether these would be addictive, and the doctor explained that they were not addictive, but needed to be taken for several months in order to restore levels of chemicals in the brain that had become run down during the depression. Melanie and Sarah agreed to think about antidepressants and to come to see the doctor again the following week armed with questions they might like to ask her.

Over the course of several appointments the doctor initiated a course of antidepressants, namely 20 mg of fluoxetine every morning. In the absence of a practice counsellor, and because of the long waiting-list for appointments with the local child mental health service (which did not prioritise depressed adolescents), the doctor decided she would see Melanie herself, fortnightly after school, in extended appointments for support. She also arranged for Melanie's mother to see one of her partners within the practice, who eventually prescribed antidepressants for her, too, and arranged for her to see a CRUSE counsellor about her bereavement.

After six weeks it was clear that the antidepressants were helping both mother and daughter. Melanie had resumed regular contact with her best friend and felt she could now talk more easily to her mother. The doctor continued to see Melanie at intervals until six months had passed, when the antidepressants were stopped. Six weeks later at a follow-up check she was still managing well.

Referral

Should all depressed adolescents be referred to a specialist service? This depends on the configuration of local services. For instance, in some areas the school health service (community paediatricians and school nurses) may be able to offer diagnosis and treatment that addresses at least the school-based issues. Some areas now have child mental health workers who will be able to manage a proportion of depressed adolescents. Some practice counsellors are willing to see adolescents. Such tier 2 services can be used as a way of selecting patients for referral to tier 3 services (*see* Chapter 2 on referral).

Guidelines for referral

Clear suicidal intent, indicated by well-formulated plans and a stated wish to die, indicates a need for urgent referral. A severe depressive episode, with marked impairment of functioning and biological symptoms, will also require specialist assessment and treatment.

Prognosis

Depression tends to recover quickly in response to treatment, and the milder cases resolve even without treatment. However, in the longer term the majority of those who have a more severe episode will relapse after recovery (70% will have another episode within the next five years).

Box 33.1:   Practice points for the management of depression

- Children and adolescents may develop a depressive disorder that shares many similarities with the adult equivalent.
- Assessment should include an exploration of contributing factors and mood changes.
- Ask specifically about suicidal ideas and intent.
- Treatment should ideally include a combination of social, psychological and pharmacological components.

References

1   Royal College of Psychiatrists (1999) *Depression in Children and Young People: How to Recognise and Help*. Factsheet No. 33. Available from the Royal College of Psychiatrists, 17 Belgrave Square, London SW1X 8PG (tel 020 7235 2351 ext 146; fax 020 7245 1231) e-mail booksales@ rcpsych.ac.uk; website http://www.rcpsych.ac.uk/pub/pubsfs.htm.

2   Graham P and Hughes C (1995) *So Young, So Sad, So Listen*. Gaskell, London. This book is very easy to read and packed with useful information.

3 Harrington R, Whittaker J and Shoebridge P (1998) Psychological treatment of depression in children and adolescents. A review of treatment research. *Br J Psychiatry*. **173**: 291–8.

4 Mufson L, Weissman MM, Moreau D and Garfinkel R (1999) Efficacy of interpersonal psychotherapy for depressed adolescents. *Arch Gen Psychiatry*. **56**: 573–9.

5 Emslie GJ, Rush J, Weinberg WA *et al.* (1997) A double-blind, randomized, placebo-controlled trial of fluoxetine in children and adolescents with depression. *Arch Gen Psychiatry*. **54**: 1031–7.

6 Maidment I (2000) The use of St John's Wort in the treatment of depression. *Psychiatr Bull*. **24**: 232–4.

CHAPTER THIRTY FOUR

Overdose and other self-harm

Definition and prevalence

Deliberate self-harm is rare in childhood, but becomes more common among teenagers, especially girls. However, boys should be taken particularly seriously because of the higher risk of completed suicide, and the greater secrecy involved (the ratio of girls to boys ranges from 3:2 in community samples to 7:1 in clinic samples). Depression is less likely to be present in self-harming adolescents (approximately 40%) than in self-harming adults (approximately 80%).

Self-harm in adolescence most commonly takes the form of overdosing or self-cutting. Any tablets taken are usually those that are most readily available in the household, such as paracetamol, other analgesics or antidepressants. Attempted hanging is rarer, but far more serious, as it can easily prove fatal, irrespective of intent. Other forms of attempted suicide, such as self-shooting and carbon monoxide poisoning, are even rarer in children and adolescents, because of lack of access to the means of death.

Cutting is the form of self-harm that is least likely to lead to completed suicide. It ranges in adolescents from one or two attempts at scratching an arm, which is extremely common, to widespread blood-letting on various parts of the body, sometimes involving words (e.g. 'misery' or 'let me die'). Deep cutting, which damages tendons and blood vessels, seems to be less common in adolescents than in young adults. Self-cutting is particularly likely to become a habit. There seems to be a physiological effect of drawing blood, in that anxiety and dysphoria are markedly reduced. This provides positive reinforcement, so the behaviour continues, and is also often copied by others.

Self-harm cannot be regarded as psychologically normal, but thoughts about the possibility of killing oneself have been found to be so common in community surveys of teenagers that they are at least statistically normal. One American study found that:

- 27% of 14- to 17-year-olds thought about suicide in a 12-month period
- 16% made a specific plan
- 8% made an attempt
- 2% received medical attention.

Such thoughts and actions are less common below the age of 11 years, but they do still occur. Thoughts may be about hanging, knifing or jumping out of windows, and actions may include running away from home, which can be seen as the equivalent of an overdose (unless it is to escape from abuse). Suicidal thoughts and self-harming acts become more common with increasing age, peaking in the mid-twenties. Self-harm appears to be more common in families of lower socio-economic status. A family history of self-harm, friendship with other teenagers who are self-harming, and modelling on pop stars who have killed themselves may also increase the risk.

Non-fatal acts of self-harm (sometimes referred to as parasuicide) are important for the following reasons:

- Around 15–25% make further suicidal attempts. Risk factors for repetition include male gender, conduct disorder, excessive alcohol use, hopelessness and living in local authority care.
- Around 1–2% will later succeed in killing themselves.
- The first act of self-harm is a golden opportunity for secondary prevention – that is, the prevention of subsequent self-harm or suicide.[1] Changes in the attitudes and beliefs of family members are more likely when anxiety levels are high. (Primary prevention – that is, the restriction of opportunities for suicide – has proved difficult. Recently, analgesics have become available in maximum pack sizes of 25 tablets, which should make it slightly more difficult to obtain a lethal dose.)
- Self-harming can usefully be regarded as a form of communication. The communication has been described as *'a message in a bottle'*, since it is not always easy to decipher exactly what is intended (consciously or unconsciously).[2] If at least some of the communication can be heard, and if the content can be expressed in some other way, then the self-harm need not recur. Teenagers are less likely to repeat an act of self-harm if they feel understood by those around them.

Referral

Best practice is that all children and adolescents who have harmed themselves should be admitted to hospital, although local policies and cut-off ages vary. Should the large number of teenagers who make specific plans without carrying them out (16% according to the above study) receive professional attention? In practice, most of these cases do not come into contact with professionals, so the question only arises in connection with those who present for help, usually with a problem other than their suicidal ideas. The presenting problem should be evaluated for each adolescent, but the presence of specific plans for suicide increases the seriousness of the situation, and usually indicates that referral should at least be discussed.

Most adolescents tell someone soon after taking an overdose, and this is an appropriate time to refer them to the casualty department, from where there should be standard arrangements for admission, usually to a paediatric ward. Admission is necessary for at least three reasons:

*   to minimise the medical complications. For instance, in the case of paracetamol ingestion, blood levels and administration of an antidote (acetylcysteine) may be required
*   to allow a full psychosocial assessment to be made, including the assessment of suicidal intent and the possibility of depressive disorder
*   to impress upon the whole family the seriousness of the event.

It is important to remember that there need not be a correlation between the medical and psychological seriousness of the episode. For instance, a girl may have taken only five paracetamol tablets, yet still be genuinely wishing to die, or significantly depressed.

When should an adolescent *not* be referred for specialist help? The decision to refer is straightforward if there is any question of life being endangered, irrespective of whether the teenager gives consent. In some cases it may be necessary to insist that the parents take the situation seriously. There is research evidence that general practitioners have a unique role in the prevention of suicide, as many young people consult during the three months before suicide (37% according to one study).[3] However, there are two groups who may be managed exclusively in primary care.

1   Some teenagers decide not to tell anyone, even after quite serious overdoses. This situation is more common in boys. Some will eventually reveal what has happened, long after any medical consequences have subsided. The general practitioner may be involved at this stage. A specialist opinion should still be discussed, but if the teenager refuses this, and is sufficiently mature to make this decision, then there is little point in making the referral.
2   Self-cutting is often kept secret, and many cutters do not want referral. Those on the left-hand side of Table 34.1 probably do not require referral.

Table 34.1:   Indicators of severity in an adolescent who cuts herself

Does not require referral	Referral should be discussed
Superficial cutting, leading to little bleeding, and scars that heal quickly	Deep scars, some of which require stitching
Nothing to indicate abuse	A known history of sexual abuse or rape, or promiscuous sexual activity
No other self-harm	Associated with overdosing
No history of bingeing, vomiting or distorted body image	Associated with an eating disorder
A sensible attitude to experimentation with drugs and alcohol	Use of drugs or alcohol that is potentially dangerous
Mood changes are transient	Persistent depression or anxiety

Assessment

A screening instrument: PATHOS

This consists of the following five questions.

- 'Have you had **Problems** for longer than one month?'
- 'Were you **Alone** in the house when you overdosed?'
- 'Did you plan the overdose for more than **Three** hours?'
- 'Are you feeling **HOpeless** about the future – that things will not get much better?'
- 'Were you feeling **Sad** for most of the time before the overdose?'.

The higher the score out of five, the more the overdose is cause for concern, since higher scores correlate with suicidal intent and depression.

This screening assessment can be supplemented by a history of events leading up to and following the episode. It is particularly important to enquire about the intent at the time of the act of self-harm, and about any persisting intent. Some teenagers will say that they just wanted to go to sleep, or that they wanted to escape from an impossible situation. Others will say that they momentarily wanted to die. A continuing desire to die is of more concern. Prolonged attempts to conceal the overdose from others are more worrying than telling the nearest person available immediately. Sometimes the choice of who is told gives important clues to the teenager's relationships. For instance, a girl who takes an overdose at midnight but waits until the next morning at school before telling a friend is likely to be experiencing difficulties with her parents.

It is also important to assess drug and alcohol intake, and whether there is a depressive disorder. In addition, there should be some enquiry about abuse, which should be open enough to include a variety of forms of abuse, and should *not* specify any abuser. Most teenagers, when seen on their own, do not object to a direct question about abuse, although they may not answer it truthfully, or they may not regard what has happened to them as fitting into whatever category you describe. For instance, you could say 'Some teenagers who take an overdose (or cut themselves) have been bullied or sexually abused or raped. Have any of these happened to you?'.

The meaning of the act

Interpreting the episode of self-harm as an attempt to communicate something that cannot be communicated in any other way suggests several possibilities.

- The topic may be difficult to talk about.
- Some feelings are very difficult for anyone to describe.
- The teenager has difficulty putting her feelings into words, and tends to keep things to herself.

- The teenager does not find it easy to talk to the people in immediate contact with her (i.e. family, friends and teachers).

Relatives often respond by treating the episode as trivial, manipulative, devious or attention-seeking. These are *not* helpful ways of viewing it, even though there may be some truth in some of these opinions.

Questions specific to cutting

Uncovering the feelings behind the act of cutting is seldom easy. One approach is to ask about the feelings that follow the act. Invariably, the response is about a sense of relief or release of some anxiety, anger, tension or other emotion that is difficult to bear. It may then be possible to explore the basis for these feelings in present or past experiences (such as pressure of examinations, or abuse). Although this may be too time-consuming for primary care, it is often even more difficult in a specialist service, which can generate much resentment about having to see a mental health professional. It is important to remain neutral in the face of the scars from cutting – disgust will not endear you to the adolescent.

Treatment

The single most helpful thing a professional can do after an overdose is to encourage communication between the adolescent in crisis and important others around her. These may include her family, boyfriend, other friends and schoolteachers. She may need encouragement to explain what is worrying her. In some cases, it is impossible to decipher the 'message within the bottle', but this does not necessarily matter, so long as channels of communication are opened up to render a further overdose unnecessary.

If the parents are angry or ashamed about their daughter's action, it is important to reframe these emotions as evidence of concern, construing them in a positive light. For instance, you could say (to the adolescent in her parents' presence) 'It is clear that your parents are very worried about you. They are quite right to be concerned. It shows how much they care about you'.

It is essential to have an interview with the adolescent on her own, in order to explore the meaning of the episode and the degree of suicidal intent (of which parents are usually unaware). With her permission, a version of this can be told to the family. In many cases this may be sufficient to enable the family to understand the 'message in the bottle'. It may sometimes be necessary to talk to other agencies, such as the school in cases of academic pressure or bullying, or Social Services in cases of abuse.

In the special case of self-cutting, the shame of the teenager and their parents can sometimes be reduced by informing them that this is common, infectious and (in the absence of the risk factors on the right-hand side of Table 34.1 above) seldom dangerous. It may be unsightly and significantly upsetting for others. It may also help to explain that the habit is very difficult to stop, because the physiological effect provides such relief. Cutting can be a way of dealing with feelings that would otherwise lead to an overdose.[4]

Treatment is more likely to be successful if it is started when the teenager first presents, rather than when the behaviour has become a chronic pattern.

Case study 34.1

The doctor had not seen Emma, aged 15 years, for three years. Before he called for her to come through from the waiting-room, he noted from her records that she had been to see one of his partners one month previously, complaining of feeling tense, but had apparently refused to sit down and talk, had become upset when pressed to do so, and had left the surgery in a hurry before the partner had been able to assess her problem properly.

On the present occasion, Emma's mother Jo accompanied her into the doctor's surgery, and whilst Jo sat in the patient's chair, Emma declined to sit down and remained standing in the corner by the door, looking very anxious and wary. Jo told the doctor that she was very worried about Emma, who had been cutting herself on the forearms. Jo and Emma had had a big argument the day before, when Jo had caught sight of Emma's arms, which she had kept covered all summer. She had told her mother she had also taken an overdose of 20 paracetamol tablets a month ago. Jo still seemed angry, but was also very concerned about Emma, worried that she was going to hurt herself seriously, and she thought that her daughter ought to see a psychiatrist. Emma told the doctor she was all right really, just a bit tense, and that she would not agree to see a psychiatrist.

The doctor asked Jo to step outside for a moment so that he could talk to Emma alone. Emma refused his gentle request that she sit down, so the consultation continued with her standing by the door. She told the doctor that cutting released some of the tension she was feeling. This seemed to be related to feeling upset that her parents were splitting up. Her father had moved out during the summer, and he had asked Emma to go and live with him and his new partner. Jo had forbidden Emma to have any contact with her father, and was seeing a solicitor about a divorce. Emma said that several of her friends had also been cutting themselves, usually at school. She had taken the tablets after leaving the surgery on the previous occasion, and thought at the time that she wanted to kill herself. Now she no longer felt suicidal, and she denied any plans to take pills again.

The doctor secured Emma's permission to share what she had told him with her mother. He explained that cutting was quite common, that it was used to relieve tension, and that if Emma was willing to talk more about how she was feeling then this would probably reduce the cutting. The doctor reassured Jo as much as he could that in his opinion Emma was not suicidal now, and that she should not be pressurised into seeing a psychiatrist. Jo appeared to accept that she needed to talk more with Emma about the split with her husband and about what was going to happen in the future. The doctor asked Emma to come back and see him in a double appointment the next day, together with her mother.

Later that week, at the regular practice meeting, the doctor raised the issue of Emma's previous consultation with his partner the month before. The partner was concerned that Emma had taken an overdose very soon after seeing him, and with the benefit of hindsight thought that he should not have tried to insist that she must sit down, as this insistence had probably precipitated her flight in a panic.

Box 34.1:   Practice points about overdose and other self-harm

- An overdose is a form of communication.
- Even if you cannot interpret the message that is being sent, enhancing communication between the adolescent and important others will help.
- Hospital admission is advisable immediately after an adolescent's overdose or attempted suicide.
- Superficial self-cutting in isolation is of far less concern.
- Questioning needs to explore the meaning of the act, as well as possible suicidal risk or depression.

References

1   Hill P (1994) Adolescents. In: R Williams and HG Morgan (eds) *Suicide Prevention: The Challenge Confronted.* HMSO, London.

2   Kingsbury SJ (1993) Parasuicide in adolescence: a message in a bottle. *ACPP Rev Newsletter.* **15**: 253–9.

3   Appleby L, Amos T, Doyle U, Tomenson B and Woodman M (1996) General practitioners and young suicides: a preventive role for primary care. *Br J Psychiatry.* **168**: 330–3.

4   Solomon Y and Farrand J (1996) 'Why don't you do it properly?'. Young women who self-injure. *J Adolesc.* **19**: 111–19.

CHAPTER THIRTY FIVE

Eating disorders

Introduction and definitions

Eating disorders in childhood and adolescence can be classified as follows.

Selective eating (or meal refusal)

This can be defined as adherence to a limited range of foods or a refusal to eat at meal-times, or both.

Anorexia nervosa

This can be defined as follows:

1 determined food avoidance
2 weight loss, or a failure to maintain the steady weight gain expected for the young person's age
3 preoccupation with weight and shape, often with a distorted body image.

Bulimia nervosa

This can be defined as follows:

1 recurrent binges, where a binge is defined as a large amount of food eaten in a short time, accompanied by a sense of lack of control
2 recurrent compensatory behaviour, such as self-induced vomiting, laxative abuse, fasting or exercise
3 self-evaluation is unduly influenced by body weight and shape.

Obesity

This can be defined as excessive weight in relation to age and height.

Food avoidance emotional disorder

This term refers to emotional disorders in which food avoidance is prominent, such as certain cases of depression, obsessive-compulsive disorder or school refusal, but which do not fulfil the diagnostic criteria for anorexia nervosa.

Functional dysphagia

This is a rare condition in which the history is of a traumatic episode of choking or difficulty in swallowing, followed by food avoidance that is usually selective, and that may lead to weight loss.

Pervasive refusal syndrome

This condition is very rare. It affects girls aged 8–14 years, who not only stop eating, but also stop drinking, walking, talking or caring for themselves.

The last three conditions are listed here because they may be confused with anorexia nervosa. As they are rare, they will not be discussed further.

The continuum from normal to abnormal

Worship of thinness is part of our culture. Dieting is very common, and often ineffective. In some children and teenagers, dieting becomes an obsession and seems to develop a power of its own. Doing without food is regarded as virtuous. In individuals with anorexia nervosa, starvation becomes an addiction. In those with bulimia nervosa, binge-eating becomes a habit which is very difficult to give up. This may result in the individual becoming overweight or underweight, or maintaining a normal weight, depending on the balance between the binges and the compensatory behaviour. Such behaviours as self-induced vomiting, laxative abuse and excessive exercise also occur in anorexia nervosa, and the two conditions have many features in common (*see* Figure 35.1). For instance, anorexia may often develop into bulimia, and it seems that many of the symptoms may serve the function of getting rid of feelings, as well as avoiding fatness or food.

Epidemiology and differential diagnosis

Eating disorders are mainly reported in cultures where food is plentiful and thinness is valued. There is an association with higher social class, but it is not certain how much of this is due to higher referral rates.

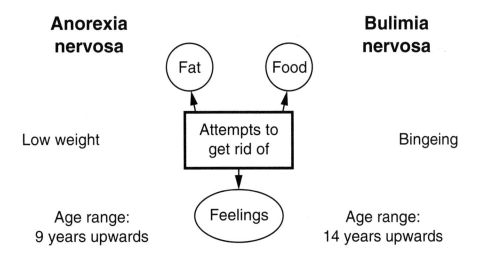

Figure 35.1:   Similarities and differences between anorexia nervosa and bulimia nervosa.

Selective eating

This is very common in pre-school children, and may start at an early age (for a discussion of selective eating and meal refusal in babies and toddlers, *see* Chapter 18). Some children continue into primary and even secondary school with excessive faddiness, causing consternation to their families. However, most children develop a wider tolerance of foods by adolescence, and there seems to be no increased risk of other eating disorders.

Some mothers of children who display selective eating may have past or present eating disorders. Very commonly the mother has exaggerated views about how much food a small child needs, or about the importance of feeding – especially the view that the rejection of her food by the child is equivalent to rejection of her.

Most children who display selective eating are physically normal. However, some have chewing difficulties due to oral–motor dysfunction. This may occur in neurological disorders that affect the cranial nerves, and in cleft palate. In very persistent cases in older children it is worth questioning whether there is an underlying cause such as obsessive-compulsive disorder or autistic spectrum disorder.

Anorexia nervosa

This can begin in children as young as eight years. The prevalence is 0.1–0.2% in adolescent populations, and less than this before puberty (but apparently increasing). Although only 5–10% of adolescent and young adult cases occur in males, 20–30% of childhood cases are boys. The importance of anorexia nervosa that starts before puberty is that it can permanently impair growth and ovarian development.

Typical features of anorexia nervosa in children and adolescents are as follows. The onset may be associated with an episode of dieting (perhaps in response to being called fat), or an anti-food pact with a friend, or following an illness such as a viral infection. It is difficult to break the diet, even for a previously favourite food, such as ice-cream. There may be denial of hunger, and deception, such as flushing a packed school lunch down the toilet. Mealtimes may be accompanied by anxiety. The anorexic girl may be obsessed with food. She may cook for the whole family, while insisting on eating only in isolation, or she may develop ritualistic eating habits, such as cutting food into tiny pieces. She is often also obsessed with exercise (e.g. running rather than walking, standing rather than sitting, or waking rather than allowing sleep). However thin she is, she still regards herself as fat. Perfectionism and high levels of achievement in all areas of school are common, but not invariable.

The differential diagnosis of anorexia nervosa includes the following.

- *Depressive disorder*. Social withdrawal, irritability and sleep disturbance occur in both depression and anorexia nervosa, and the distinction may sometimes be difficult, but the attitude to food and body image is crucial.
- *Medical illness*. Medical disorders that can sometimes be mistaken for anorexia nervosa include Crohn's disease, diabetes mellitus, hyperthyroidism, renal failure and malignancy, especially mid-brain tumours. Investigations should include a full blood count, erythrocyte sedimentation rate, urea, electrolytes, glucose and liver function tests.
- *Drug use*. Recreational drugs that cause weight loss include amphetamines and ecstasy.

Bulimia nervosa

This does not seem to start before puberty, and seldom before the age of 14 years. The peak age of onset is probably in late adolescence, although binge-eating and vomiting are usually kept secret for years, and most cases present in their twenties. The prevalence in the age range 15–30 years is 1–3% in females, and about one-tenth of this in males.

Obesity

This condition is very common, the exact prevalence varying both according to the definition used, and between countries. Genetic factors probably play at least as important a part as cultural and other environmental factors. There is some evidence of continuity between childhood and adult obesity, but this is not inevitable. Many overweight children become thinner during the adolescent growth spurt, particularly if they end up tall (which can be predicted from their parents' heights, as explained on standard growth charts).

Management of eating disorders in primary care

Selective eating

Monitor the child's weight and linear growth. If these are satisfactory, the growth chart can be used to allay the parents' anxiety. If there is significant doubt that the child is receiving an appropriate balance of nutrients, refer them to a paediatric dietitian. If the child's growth chart is not satisfactory, or the parents' anxiety cannot be allayed, then refer the child to a paediatrician, who may in turn refer them on to the local child and family service.

Relaxation of parental pressure to eat a wide range of foods often results in the child gradually experimenting more widely of their own accord. Even if it does not, the parents can usually come to accept the situation. Established food fads do not respond well to psychological treatments (Bryan Lask, personal communication), and it is probably not a good use of resources to attempt to treat selective eating in primary school children. When the child is old enough to want to alter the situation himself, perhaps by 13 or 14 years of age, treatment is more likely to work.

Case study 35.1

A nine-year-old boy was eating nothing but yeast extract (Marmite), bread, margarine and milk. A full dietary assessment revealed that his dietary intake was adequate in quality and quantity, and his growth chart was satisfactory. No further management was indicated.

Anorexia nervosa

It is essential to plot height and weight on a growth chart. The ideal weight should be calculated as the weight on the same centile as the height, and can serve as a target for weight gain. The key figure to calculate is the ratio of actual weight to ideal weight, expressed as a percentage. If the weight is less than 70% of the ideal value, then specialist referral is urgently required. A weight below 85% of the ideal value is worrying, particularly if it is associated with cessation of periods or continuing weight loss.

Static weight and impaired height increase in children have the same significance as weight loss in adolescents and adults (previous measurements can be obtained from the child's records; often the school nurse will have such data). In long-standing cases, interpretation of the growth chart should take growth retardation into account. The ideal height will be on the same centile as premorbid height.

A reasonable management plan in primary care, before referral, or while waiting for a specialist appointment, could include the following.

- *Increasing parental anxiety.* It may seem natural to want to reassure the parents, but in the face of a potentially life-threatening condition they need to be worried. They need to make every effort to be in charge of their child (rather than vice versa), and it is essential that they work together in this. The earlier the process starts, the easier it is to succeed. Do not attempt to suggest ways of making their daughter eat – they should be able to sort this out for themselves (e.g. by using rewards and sanctions, such as provision or prohibition of a favourite activity).

- *Engage the young person by externalising the problem.* Describe the disorder as something that takes people over – it is making the young person do things she does not really want to do ('Let's fight the anorexia monster together').
- *Dietary management.* This may include keeping a diary of food intake, setting a target weight, and weekly or fortnightly weighing in order to monitor progress. A rough guideline to aim for is one pound or half a kilogram per week, or somewhat less if the body weight is above 80%. A valuable benchmark of success is the return of menstruation. Referral to a dietitian can be very useful both to assess current calorie intake, and for advice on a sensible eating regime. If the young person or their parents do not want a psychiatric referral, it can be useful to say that you will only insist on this if the weight continues to fall.

Case study 35.2

A 14-year-old girl was brought to her general practitioner by her mother, with a four-month history of loss of weight, and decreasing oral intake. The growth chart showed a height on the 75th centile, and a weight on the 25th centile. Her weight was calculated to be 79% of the ideal weight. She said that she had been teased by someone at school about her weight, and several friends were on diets, of whom she was the most successful. She admitted to still thinking that she was too fat, and to doing press-ups in her room every evening, but she did not admit to bingeing, vomiting or using laxatives. Her periods had started a year before, but then stopped two months ago. She had no boyfriend. School records subsequently showed that her weight had been on the 90th centile two years before.

The general practitioner explained to the girl that she was being overtaken by ideas about dieting that were making her go too far. She was becoming dangerously thin, and if she continued to lose weight she would probably have to go to hospital, and she would certainly have to see a child psychiatrist. The mother was not happy about this, but was suitably concerned, and agreed to bring her husband to an evening appointment two weeks later.

The general practitioner sent the girl to the local dietitian, who judged her oral intake to be 900 calories per day. She suggested this should be 2000 calories per day, and advised her on what a healthy diet should be.

The general practitioner saw the parents on their own and explained his concern that their daughter was developing anorexia nervosa. He went on to describe the implications of this if weight loss continued, and the life-threatening nature of the disorder if it was allowed to become severe. He invited them to think of ways in which they could be firm about encouraging their daughter to eat. The parents brainstormed this problem and generated a number of possible solutions.

Fortnightly weights showed an initial weight gain, which then slowed down. Appointments with the dietitian were reduced in frequency from fortnightly to monthly, and reviews by the general practitioner were reduced from monthly to two-monthly. Six months later, the girl's periods returned, but she still thought that she was too fat for at least part of the time, despite being on the 50th centile for weight (83% of the 75th centile).

> **Box 35.1:   Summary points about anorexia nervosa in children and adolescents**
>
> • Attitudes to food and fatness are more extreme than in other causes of weight loss.
> • Anorexia nervosa can begin in children as young as eight. It may present with failure to follow centiles, rather than actual weight loss.
> • The parents need to be in control of their child's tendency to eat too little. The earlier this happens in the course of the disease, the better the prognosis.
> • Successful management can be relatively straightforward if the condition is recognised early enough.
> • Whether the child is to be referred or not, calculate the percentage of ideal weight (plot height and weight on a growth chart, determine the ideal weight as weight on the same centile as height, and divide actual weight by ideal weight).

Bulimia nervosa

Young people often do not present for help with teenage symptoms of bingeing and vomiting until they are no longer teenagers. They are often unwilling to let their parents (or anyone else) know the extent of their symptoms, and are ambivalent about seeking help. This makes any form of treatment problematic, particularly family therapy. Individual therapy has been shown to be successful in clinical trials, but can be time-consuming. It either focuses on food and the thoughts and feelings associated with it, as in cognitive–behavioural therapy, or else it focuses on relationships and their links to feelings, without any discussion of food.

The only treatment modality that is practicable in primary care is medication. High-dose fluoxetine (60 mg per day, in a single morning dose) has been shown to be effective in controlling symptoms, but is not a long-term cure.

Advice about medical complications can also be useful. Vomiting or laxative use can be life-threatening if it is frequent enough for the serum potassium concentration to fall below normal. If you suspect this, electrolytes should be measured. Teenagers are often impressed by stories of rotting tooth enamel, and a visit to the dentist should be encouraged.

For a teenager who genuinely wants help, and is likely to be able to persist with it, referral should be made to a specialist service.

Obesity

Obese children are usually fat because their intake of calories exceeds their calorie expenditure. Although genetic factors may be relevant, and family eating habits are invariably so, endocrine causes are rare. One of the conditions that predisposes to the most severe obesity is the Prader–Willi syndrome, which should be diagnosed in the early years of life because of dysmorphic features and floppiness. Other syndromes are probably even rarer. Low self-esteem and other psychological problems are common, but it is not easy to tell whether they are the cause or the consequence of the obesity.

Recommended treatment for childhood obesity includes the following components:[1]

- a balanced healthy diet. Reductions in calorie intake can be achieved by eliminating takeaway and ready prepared foods, which tend to be particularly energy dense, and by limiting portion sizes. Limiting eating to mealtimes, and avoiding high-fat snacks such as crisps and biscuits, as well as high-sugar drinks, may also help
- an equal emphasis on exercise
- a goal of gradual weight loss of about 0.5 kg per week
- parental support
- behaviour therapy for both the child and their parents to help them to achieve the diet and exercise goals.

In many cases, this treatment may be best organised by a paediatric dietitian. However, in the long term, primary care professionals have a major role to play in helping to shape a family's attitudes to food.

Reference

1   Frühbeck G (2000) Childhood obesity: time for action, not complacency. *BMJ.* **320**: 328–9.

Acknowledgements

We are indebted to Dr Rebecca Park, Research Associate and Honorary Consultant in Child and Adolescent Psychiatry, Section of Developmental Psychiatry, University of Cambridge, for comments on an earlier draft of this chapter.

Further information for young people and their parents

The Eating Disorders Association, Sackville Place, 44 Magdalen Street, Norwich NR3 1JU (tel 01603 619090; fax 01603 664915; helpline 01603 765050 4.00–6.00 p.m. Monday to Friday). Recorded messages about anorexia and bulimia can be heard by dialling 0891 615466.

Mental Health Foundation (2000) *All About Anorexia Nervosa* and *All About Bulimia Nervosa*. Mental Health Foundation, London. Two small booklets that provide convenient basic information, available from the Mental Health Foundation, 20/21 Cornwall Terrace, London NW1 4QL (tel 020 7535 7400; fax 020 7535 7474; e-mail mhf@mhf.org.uk); website www.mhf.org.uk.

Royal College of Psychiatrists (1999) *Worries About Weight*. Mental Health and Growing Up Factsheets. No. 27. Royal College of Psychiatrists, London; website http://www.rcpsych.ac.uk/pub/pubsfs.htm. Available from the Royal College of Psychiatrists, 17 Belgrave Square, London SW1X 8PG (tel 020 7235 2351, ext 146; fax 020 7245 1231; e-mail booksales@rcpsych.ac.uk).

Schmidt U and Treasure J (1993) *Getting Better Bit(e) by Bit(e)*. Psychology Press. This book may be helpful for older adolescents as well as adults with bulimia.

Treasure J (1997) *Anorexia Nervosa*. Psychology Press. This book answers some of the questions that are asked by sufferers, their families and friends.

CHAPTER THIRTY SIX

Chronic fatigue syndrome

Introduction and definitions

Chronic fatigue syndrome is the current preferred name for a condition of uncertain aetiology and debated status, which undoubtedly poses significant challenges to afflicted children, not least in terms of missed schooling. Other names that have been used include neurasthenia, myalgic encephalomyelitis and post-viral fatigue syndrome. The first of these has gone out of fashion, and the second and third imply causal factors which have not been established, although infections (e.g. Epstein–Barr virus) may be part of the initiating process in a certain proportion of cases. Many parents prefer the abbreviation *'ME'*, disliking the term 'chronic fatigue syndrome'. In such cases it is probably wise to adopt the family's terminology in the interests of engagement.

Research definitions developed by a group of UK clinicians[1] and a group of American clinicians[2] have been adapted for use in children by three Royal Colleges.[3] These are listed in Box 36.1.

Box 36.1: Definition of chronic fatigue syndrome in children

Persistent or relapsing chronic fatigue:
- present for three months for at least 50% of the time
- clinically evaluated so that known medical conditions are excluded
- not the result of ongoing exertion
- both mental and physical activity are affected
- results in a substantial reduction in previous levels of activity (occupational, educational, social or personal).

Some of the following may be present, not pre-dating the fatigue:
- muscle pain
- impairment of short-term memory or concentration (on self-report)

continued overleaf

- sore throat
- tender cervical or axillary lymph nodes
- multiple joint pain without joint swelling or redness
- headaches of a new type, pattern or severity
- unrefreshing sleep
- post-exertional malaise lasting for more than 24 hours
- symptoms of anxiety or depression
- poor school attendance.

Debate over whether the disease is physical or psychological is unhelpful. Most children and their parents find it easier, at any rate initially, to think of the illness as purely physical. It is best not to confront this view and risk alienating the family, who may in time come to appreciate the stresses and other psychosocial factors that have possibly contributed to the illness. A very simple model of the illness is that there is some as yet unidentified physiological disturbance that is maintained by a rest–exertion cycle. When the child rests, this leads to more difficulty in their subsequently being active, yet when they over-exert, this also leads to more exhaustion. Either way, the state of fatigue continues.

Assessment

The history and examination should be directed at establishing the diagnosis and evaluating the alternatives. Possible differential diagnoses may include occult inflammatory bowel disease, thyroid disorders, eating disorders, substance misuse and depression.

Depression is interesting in relation to chronic fatigue syndrome, as it shares many of the same diagnostic features, which can sometimes make it extremely difficult to decide whether a young person has one (and if so which) or both conditions. Moreover, the dismissive and unhelpful attitude of healthcare professionals to many sufferers from chronic fatigue may lead to a sense of isolation, demoralisation and hopelessness. In some cases this may provide an adequate explanation for the associated depressive symptomatology.[4] There may also be symptoms of anxiety that are reported as somatic symptoms.

A limited number of physical investigations is indicated[3] (see Box 36.2). These should be completed quickly, as an extended period of investigation will reinforce the patient's tendency to believe that they have a disease that is not understood by doctors, and it will also delay the setting up of an appropriate treatment plan. Although tests for infectious mononucleosis are useful, extended investigation for many other possible viral infections may be expensive and counter-productive. For instance, such extensive tests may reinforce the view that there is some serious underlying but ill-understood disease process. (It must be emphasised that glandular fever is one possible precursor to chronic fatigue syndrome, rather than a differential diagnosis.)

Box 36.2:   Investigations for chronic fatigue syndrome

Full blood count and erythrocyte sedimentation rate
Liver function tests and urea and electrolytes
Monospot, Paul–Bunnell or Epstein–Barr IgM test
Thyroid-stimulating hormone and free thyroxine
Creatine kinase
Urine protein and sugar

Management

The Royal Colleges jointly recommend management in primary care whenever possible.
Professionals involved with education, such as the school nurse, the class teacher in primary school or the head of year in secondary school, may be needed to help to negotiate attendance details. Engagement with the child and family is an essential first step, and may be hindered by the involvement of too many specialists. A confrontation between individuals with differing attitudes to the disease should be avoided, and the family's terminology should be adopted. The Joint Report recommends monitoring progress at least weekly,[3] but this is not always necessary, and it may be unrealistic.

Management options depend on the stage at which the disease presents. The most effective time at which to intervene is *before* the symptoms have reached a chronic, self-perpetuating phase. Thus the exhaustion that is seen in the early stages of something that might develop into chronic fatigue syndrome should be treated with firm attempts to keep the child active, and to maintain school attendance.

If a rapid return to normal activities cannot be enforced, then a more gradual programme will be necessary. This may involve very small goals of slight increases (such as 5% each week) in physical activity, mental exertion and social participation. Examples might include walking a little further each week, reading slightly more each day, or engaging in more social activities each month. Out-patient visits to a paediatric physiotherapist can be very helpful in encouraging this behavioural approach, without threatening the belief that the condition is mainly somatic. School attendance may need to be mornings only (or even single lessons only) initially. However, home tuition is likely to prolong the illness. If it is unavoidable, the home tutor should be engaged in the task of helping the child to return gradually to school. Parents need to be encouraged to strike a balance between the need for rest and the need to keep on increasing activity levels, however slowly. Graded exercise programmes have been shown to be effective, whereas prolonged rest has been found to worsen fatigue.[5] There will inevitably be setbacks whenever the child has an intercurrent infection, and it is helpful to predict this.

Medication is of no proven benefit. Clinical experience suggests that antidepressants are usually ineffective. It is possible that low-dose tricyclic antidepressants (amitriptyline or dothiepin) may help mild degrees of initial or middle insomnia (*see* Chapter 39), but they are unlikely to rectify a completely distorted sleep–wake cycle.

Cognitive–behavioural therapy is of proven benefit in adults, at least when provided by highly trained therapists in specialist centres. Although we know of no trials that have demonstrated its effectiveness in adolescents, it is likely to be as effective as the regrading programme described above (which it subsumes). Challenging negative or distorted cognitions may help to support the behavioural programme. For instance, a young person who is hopeless about getting better can be asked to consider how many years he thinks it will take before he is well enough to engage in a particular activity he would like to do. He can then be asked how he thinks he might shorten the time between now and then.

Crucial to the success of a graded exercise and school attendance programme, with or without cognitive elements, is involving the parents in helping their child to carry it out. It is also important to monitor for signs of anxiety and depression. General practitioners have been reported to be in a unique position to encourage the family to progress, because they usually have a closer knowledge of individual family members than do specialists.[6]

If you take on the management of the disease in primary care, an explanation of both the disease and the vicious cycles involved is reported to be essential.[7] This should include an explanation of the way that too much rest causes muscle wasting, which exacerbates exhaustion, and too little activity leads to sleep rhythm disturbance, which makes a proper daytime routine very difficult to achieve. It is also important to encourage optimism.

Referral

Parents and children are likely to prefer to see a paediatrician rather than a psychologist or psychiatrist. This makes it difficult to refer them for specialist psychological treatment. It is worth ensuring before referral that the specialist to whom you refer is sympathetic to the diagnosis. The preferred model of specialist treatment is by a paediatric team that includes psychological or psychiatric input.[8] This may not be available in all districts, and may not be acceptable to all families even if it is. Referral for a paediatric assessment should always be possible, but it may be preferable to manage the case mainly or exclusively in primary care. At the other end of the spectrum of severity, some cases may require admission to a specialised unit.

Case study 36.1

Jeremy Jones, a 14-year-old boy, was brought to see the doctor by his parents, who informed the general practitioner in no uncertain terms that they would not go back to see the child psychologist. Jeremy had been suffering from symptoms of severe fatigue for several months, and such was the severity of the condition that he could not get out of bed until midday, and was missing whole days of school because of complete exhaustion. The general practitioner had previously referred him to a paediatrician, who saw him twice and then referred him to a psychologist. The family fell out with the psychologist and refused to go back, as they were convinced that Jeremy had a physical problem, not a mental one.

continued opposite

The general practitioner agreed to support the family, as they were not keen on referral to yet another specialist. The doctor did not argue whether chronic fatigue syndrome was a physical or mental health problem, but was optimistic about it, emphasising that the condition usually improved and that they should make plans to increase Jeremy's level of activity over time. However, he warned them not to attempt to rush the increase in activity. The general practitioner set the initial goal that Jeremy would start to get up slightly earlier each day, keeping a diary of the length of time he spent in bed.

The general practitioner saw the family in follow-up appointments every three weeks over the next few months. In discussion they set small goals for Jeremy that he would be able to achieve in terms of increasing his exercise level and his attendance at school, monitored in his diary. His initial successes were rather few and far between, and there were a number of setbacks apparently related to viral infections. The general practitioner saw the family regularly and encouraged them to continue the strategy.

Over the course of two years, a steady improvement was achieved, and by the start of his first GCSE year, Jeremy was attending school full-time.

Box 36.3:   Practice points for chronic fatigue syndrome

- Treat as if it were an organic disease (in view of the current state of knowledge, a 'don't know' attitude is safest).
- Be optimistic – behavioural and cognitive treatments have been shown to work.
- Agree a plan for increasing activity with achievable goals.
- Monitor progress in terms of activity levels and improvement in physical and psychological symptoms.
- Use paradox – instruct the family not to go too fast.

Acknowledgements

We are indebted to Jo Richards, Research Fellow in Child and Adolescent Psychiatry, for her help with this chapter.

References

1   Sharpe MC, Archard LC, Banatvala JC *et al.* (1991) Chronic fatigue syndrome: guidelines for research. *J R Soc Med.* **84**: 118–21.

2   Fukuda K, Straus SE, Hickie I *et al.* (1994) The chronic fatigue syndrome: a comprehensive approach to its definition and study. *Ann Intern Med.* **121**: 953–9.

3   Royal Colleges of Physicians, Psychiatrists and General Practitioners (1996) *Chronic Fatigue Syndrome: Report of a Joint Working Group.* Royal Colleges of Physicians, Psychiatrists and General Practitioners, London.

4   Richards J (2000) Chronic fatigue syndrome in children and adolescents. *Clin Child Psychol Psychiatry.* **5**: 31–51.

5   Reid S, Chalder T, Cleare A, Hotopf M and Wessely S (2000) Chronic fatigue syndrome. *BMJ.* **320**: 292–6.

6   Graham H (1990) Family interventions in general practice: a case of chronic fatigue. *J Fam Therapy.* **13**: 225–30.

7   Wright JB and Beverley DW (1998) Chronic fatigue syndrome. *Arch Dis Child.* **79**: 368–74.

8   Vereker MI (1992) Chronic fatigue syndrome: a joint paediatric–psychiatric approach. *Arch Dis Child.* **67**: 550–5.

CHAPTER THIRTY SEVEN

Substance misuse

Introduction

Prevalence

Many young people experiment with drugs on a one-off basis, either infrequently or more regularly. Reported rates in the UK vary tremendously, both geographically and over time. The use of cigarettes and alcohol is ubiquitous. Many older schoolchildren try some illegal substance, usually cannabis[37.1] or ecstasy, at some stage, but only a small proportion are regular users.

Other substances used include solvents, other hallucinogens (e.g. LSD), amphetamines, opiates (including heroin and cocaine) and drugs that should be available only on prescription (e.g. benzodiazepines and antidepressants). Patterns of use change frequently, and may be very different in different parts of the country.

Age

The average age at which adolescents start experimenting with drugs is 12–15 years.

Sex differences

Girls are less likely to use drugs and start using them later than boys, but the gender gap is rapidly decreasing.

When do you need to worry?

Experimental use is not a cause for concern unless there are medical complications. More habitual use becomes a problem if there is a sustained effect on functioning – for instance, in the 15-year-old boy who does not go to school, hangs out with older boys and resorts to frequent theft to pay for the habit. Psychological dependence may develop, but may not be recognised by the young person as a problem.

It is unusual for a teenager to present for help with drug use as the identified problem. Those that attend a primary care setting are likely to be there because their parents are worried about them, and because of some other problem that may or may not be related to the drug use (e.g. school difficulties, depression, anxiety, psychosomatic complaints or inappropriate sexual behaviour). Affective symptoms are more common in girls, while conduct problems, including truancy and delinquency, are more common in boys. Drug use is likely to be concealed (especially in the presence of parents) or minimised.

A routine enquiry should always be made of any teenager (preferably on his own) about drug use, without necessarily expecting to receive a truthful answer. Try not to tell the parents if you can avoid doing so, as the teenager may then tell you more next time.

Box 37.1:   Clues to excessive use of drugs

These are often non-specific, but may include the following.
- A change in attitude and behaviour, such as lying, stealing or loss of previous interests.
- A noticeable change in the pattern of mood, which may be 'up and down' or persistent.
- A sudden deterioration of physical health. Frequent or persistent headaches, sore throat and a runny nose may indicate solvent inhalation, which may also cause pimples around the mouth and nose, and red eyes. Amphetamines may cause a dramatic loss of weight as well as sleeplessness. Ecstacy may also cause health problems, sometimes because of contaminants in the drug.
- Drug users are more likely to have casual sex and less likely to use condoms, and are therefore more at risk of sexually transmitted diseases, including human immunodeficiency virus. This is also a risk for the small minority of teenagers who inject drugs, if they share needles.

Most adolescents survive a period of drug experimentation relatively unscathed, and do not present to primary care services for any related problems. Only a small number of those who experiment with drugs progress to addiction. Those who progress to regular drug usage are individuals who have more social opportunity (especially peer group pressure), whose personality predisposes them, or whose personal circumstances lead them to seek a means of escape.

Management

There is a limited amount that can be done for adolescents who are using drugs excessively. They very seldom want to do anything about their drug use, regarding it as anything but a problem, and viewing adults who define it as a problem as having misguided attitudes or simply being envious.

A reasonable aim for primary care is 'harm minimisation' – that is, to minimise the risks of current usage, to ensure that adequate information is available and to prevent experimental usage from progressing to problem usage. If it is the parents who are most concerned, it is important to have a supply of drugs leaflets (*see* list at the end of this chapter) to give away, and to provide telephone numbers of advice lines if parents want them.

The young person may require different types of information, such as contact details of local voluntary agencies or sources of free contraceptive advice. Pointing out the medical dangers of the drugs is likely to be of only limited effectiveness.

Referral

Since most drugs counselling agencies require some degree of self-motivation, it is only worth making a referral if you can come to some agreement that the consequences of drug use (even if these are merely the hassle from parents), are undesirable. In any case, not many areas have adequate drug services for young people, and some services do not cater for the needs of those under 16 years of age.

Box 37.2:   Practice points about drug use

- Drug use may be a factor for any teenager who presents to primary care, but it is not usually the presenting problem.
- Teenagers are unlikely to regard their drug use as a problem.
- The majority of teenagers steer clear of addictive drugs.
- Sometimes discussion of the facts about drugs in a neutral way may lead to more rational choices, or at least safer behaviour with the same choices.

Note

37.1   The available medical evidence suggests that moderate use of cannabis is significantly safer than use of alcohol or cigarettes.

Sources of information and help

National Drugs Helpline. Free, confidential and open 24 hours a day (tel 0800 776600).

Institute for the Study of Drug Dependence and **Standing Committee on Drug Abuse**, Waterbridge House, 32–36 Loman Street, London SE1 9EO (tel 020 7928 1211). Can tell you about local drug advice agencies in your area. They also produce a wealth of publications.

Lifeline, 101–103 Oldham Street, Manchester M4 1LW (tel 0161 839 2054).

Re-Solv, 30A High Street, Stone, Staffordshire ST15 8AW (tel 01785 817885).

Booklets

Health Education Authority (1998) *A Parent's Guide to Drugs and Alcohol*. Health Education Authority, London.

Health Education Authority (1997) *Drugs: The Facts*. Health Education Authority, London.
Both available from the Health Education Authority, Trevelyan House, 30 Great Peter Street, London SW1P 2HW; website www.hea.org.uk.

D-mag Drugs Info 1998. Published by the Institute for the Study of Drug Dependence, 32 Loman Street, London SE1 0EE (tel 020 7928 1211; fax 020 7928 1771).

(Multiple copies of these booklets are available by telephoning 01304 614731, or from HEA Customer Services, Marston Book Services, PO Box 269, Abingdon, Oxon OX14 4YN; tel 01235 465565; fax 01235 465556).

Tacade: Educating for Health (1996) *Check Out the Facts*. Manchester (tel 0161 745 8925).

Ives R (1992) *Solvents – a Parent's Guide: the Signs; the Dangers; What to Do*. Department of Health and HMSO, London.

DTSK (1994) *Drugs and Solvents: The Things You Should Know*. Available free from BAPS, Health Education Publication Unit, DSS Distribution Centre, Heywood Stores, Manchester Road, Heywood, Lancashire OL10 2PZ (tel 0800 555777).

Royal College of Psychiatrists (1999) *Drug and Alcohol Misuse* (Mental Health and Growing Up Factsheet No. 34) and *Alcohol and Drugs: What Parents Need to Know* (Mental Health and Growing Up Factsheet No. 35). Available from Royal College of Psychiatrists, 17 Belgrave Square, London SW1X 8PG (tel 020 7235 2351 ext 146; fax 020 7245 1231; e-mail booksales@rcpsych.ac.uk; website http://www.rcpsych.ac.uk/pub/pubsfs.htm.

PART 6

Detailed treatment options

CHAPTER THIRTY EIGHT

Behavioural techniques for use by enthusiastic professionals in primary care

Introduction

Techniques that can be taught to parents of pre-school children include play, praise, tangible rewards, commands, ignoring, distraction, holding and consequences.[1-3] When teaching these techniques to parents, it is important to establish a collaborative relationship.[4] Parents are experts on their own children, and on what techniques will and will not work with them. It is important to respect this. Parents may often be reminded of their own childhood by discussion of parenting issues. They may well cast you in the role of a parent, and possibly see you as like one or both of their own parents. A useful guideline is to try to treat the parents you are helping in the same way that you hope they will treat their children – that is, positively and with respect. (*See* Figure 6.1 on p. 72.)

Play

Professionals may assume that all parents intuitively know how to play with their children. However, this is emphatically not the case. Many parents fail to find time to play with their children, and others have had no experience as children themselves of adults spending individual time with them, so are inhibited by their inbuilt ideas about parenting. Playing with a child for ten minutes each day is sufficient. The benefits of play include not only developing a more positive relationship between parent and child, but also developing the child's skills in the following areas:

- creativity and imagination
- vocabulary and general knowledge

- conflict resolution
- problem-solving skills
- the appreciation of values.

Qualities of play

These include the following.

Following the child's lead

It is essential to allow the child to dictate the choice and pace of activity. Play may be the only time during the day when the child is in charge. He will savour this opportunity, and it may make it easier for him to accept the parent being in charge at other times. Some parents find it difficult initially to find an activity that interests the child. Once the child has realised that he has a wide choice, and is in control, this will be easier. If parents are playing a competitive game, it may be best to let the child set some of the rules, rather than getting into a power struggle.

Allowing the child time

It is very tempting to take over or rush the child. However, this is not the best way to foster independence or self-esteem.

The value of attention

It is not essential to talk or join in the game, although this may help. Focusing and maintaining attention on the child is essential. The parents must not watch television or read the paper while playing.

Descriptive commenting

This very un-British activity involves giving feedback to the child on what he is doing. This is surprisingly difficult to do in a neutral way. It is tempting to ask questions, or even to give a string of commands. It may help to think of this as like 'sportscasting'. Providing a running commentary on children's activities gives them a sense of self-worth, and provides a foundation for labelled praise (*see* below).

Understanding the developmental level of the child

Developmentally appropriate toys or games should be available. Toys that are too young for the child or games that are too difficult for them will not hold their attention. It is important to follow the cues given by the child as to what is or is not suitable.

Fostering the child's imagination

For play to be successful, the child's imagination should be respected, even if this means using a toy in a different way from what an adult would expect (e.g. using a building construction kit to make a giraffe, or using saucepans as drums). Imaginary companions are commonly involved in play. Make-believe is an important part of growing up, and play that involves fantasy can start as early as 18 months, progressing steadily into middle childhood, before it begins to disappear. It helps children to develop a variety of cognitive, emotional and social skills. Fantasy helps children to think symbolically, and to distinguish between what is real and what is not. Role play can foster understanding of others' feelings. Examples of 'pretend' play include using chairs and tables to represent houses and palaces, dressing up in old clothes, or using dolls or puppets to represent imaginary or real people.

Ignoring whining and yelling

Try to get on with the play, rather than getting drawn into disciplinary wrangles.

Preparing the child for the end of play

It is important for the parent's sake, and sometimes also for the other children's, to limit the amount of time spent playing. Ten minutes a day is enough to make a difference. Children are likely to complain when the play has to stop. However, this will be less of a problem if a warning is given a few minutes before the end of play.

Praise

Many children appreciate a parent watching them in silence while they play. Comments and praise about what the child is doing may add to the benefit for the child, but questions and commands are less helpful in the context of play. In other contexts it is helpful for the child to receive positive reinforcement for whatever he is doing right, and for any efforts in the right direction. One of the most powerful means of positive reinforcement is praise, which may have both verbal and non-verbal components. This improves the child's self-esteem, and helps him to feel more positive towards his caregivers.

Effective praising techniques

These include the following.

Selecting positive aspects of behaviour to attend to, rather than negatives ones

For instance, you might say 'I like the way you are playing quietly over there.' This is surprisingly difficult, particularly with children who have become highly skilled at gaining attention by riling their parents.

Labelled praise

This means specifying exactly what you are praising. It is much more effective to say 'You've really made a good effort to eat up everything on your plate' than just to mutter vaguely 'Good boy'.

The following *non-verbal signals* can be used to enhance the effect of praise:

- tone of voice
- eye contact
- facial expression
- body position
- hugs or cuddles.

Praising immediately (within five to ten seconds)

If parents leave too long a gap before giving praise (depending on the age of the child), the child will not link the praise with what they have done, so it will not be an effective positive reinforcement (this applies to *any* form of positive reinforcement).

Praising steps in the right direction

It is important to do this, rather than waiting for perfect results, or a complete task, before giving praise. This may also involve praising unsuccessful efforts – for instance, 'That's a really good try'.

Tangible reward systems

Unexpected rewards

These can be used to reward behaviour that parents want to happen more often. This means being on the look-out for desirable behaviour, and thinking up appropriate rewards that are readily available. For instance, a child may tidy up his toys without being asked. A suitable positive reinforcement in this case might be to read him a favourite story for ten minutes, straight away, or to have his a favourite dish for the next meal.

The 'when/then' rule

This means making a reward contingent on a behaviour. It is important that the reward is given after the behaviour, rather than before it (for instance, 'When you've tidied your toys away, *then* you can have a lolly from the freezer.'

The use of charts, stars, stickers and point systems

These all require planning. Ask the parents to write a list of all the behaviours they would like to see more and all the behaviours they would like to see less. The second list may well be longer than the first, so some help may be needed to think of positive behaviours that can be encouraged. One of these may be the best one to start with. Define the behaviour carefully, so that it is clear what the child is expected to do. Then decide on a tangible reward. This could be a star or sticker on a chart (*see* Box 38.1), points that are written down, or poker chips that are collected. There is usually a cash-in value when enough stars or points are accumulated.

For a successful reward programme, it is important to remember the following guidelines.

- Warn the parents that such programmes are very hard work, and require attention to detail and perseverance.
- The child should be involved in planning the programme. This includes the choice of the most exciting type of token (e.g. a particular brand of sticker), the choice of what the tokens can be traded in for (e.g. going out to a friend's house, renting a video or going to the cinema), and the precise behaviours to be rewarded (e.g. going to bed before a certain time, or doing one of a certain range of household chores).
- The tokens should be easily attainable at first, but the tasks should then gradually become more difficult. It is best if the child can earn at least one reward each day.
- The tokens and rewards should gradually be replaced by social approval.
- The rewards should be inexpensive. The programme should be phased out after two to three months, and not continued indefinitely, although new programmes can be started.
- The programme should initially be simple, involving only one or two behaviours.
- Tokens, stickers or stars should be given immediately after the desired behaviour (not before, and not too long afterwards). The child's behaviour must be closely monitored to make sure that it is exactly what was wanted.
- Tokens, stickers or stars should not be removed for bad behaviour, as doing this is likely to make the child lose interest in the programme.
- If the child has difficulty in completing the set tasks, encourage the parent to be positive towards the child, just as you should adopt a positive attitude towards the parent. The child should be led to expect success, and if this proves too difficult, the tasks that are being set should be made easier.
- The reward programme should be constantly monitored, and adapted to make it as effective as possible for the child concerned.

Box 38.1:   An example of a sticker chart for bedtime and morning routines

Behaviour	Sun/ Mon	Mon/ Tues	Tues/ Wed	Wed/ Thurs	Thurs/ Fri	Fri/ Sat	Sat/ Sun
In bed by 8.30 p.m.							
Lights out by 9 p.m.							
Up by 7 a.m.							
Dressed by 8 a.m.							
Total stickers							

Rewards:

Daily

2 stickers: a special snack on the way to school

3 stickers: an extra bedtime story

Weekly

10 stickers: a favourite comic

15 stickers: a new audiotape

Case study 38.1

The doctor's first consultation on a busy Monday morning was not an easy one. Mr and Mrs Evans described the absolute failure of their first week's attempts at using a star chart to change their son Mike's behaviour. Mike was four years old and, although he went to bed with no protests at 7 p.m., had developed the habit of getting out of bed several times during the late evening and coming downstairs, demanding a drink. It would then be very difficult to persuade him to go back to bed. Unless he was cuddled for an hour or so, he would throw a tantrum – behaviour that was proving less and less acceptable to his parents. The doctor had suggested using a star chart to reward Mike for not getting out of bed in the evening, but the promise of a star in the morning on putting him to bed had only worked for one night, after which the behaviour had returned to its previous pattern, despite all his parents' pleadings and threats. There seemed to be no way that Mike was going to earn the five stars needed to gain the promised bag of sweets. Meanwhile his parents were obviously very frustrated and upset. The doctor agreed to discuss Mike's problem with the health visitor.

The health visitor listened with some amusement to the doctor's description of what he had asked the Evans to do. She pointed out that star charts would only work in certain circumstances. First, especially with a younger child, the initial reward had to be given immediately after the child had behaved in a desirable way. The change in behaviour had to be easily achievable at the start. To begin with, she suggested that Mike needed to be given a star on his chart for going back to bed promptly when asked to do so. If he earned three stars, then he should be rewarded with something he chose himself if possible – something a little unusual that he really wanted, rather than a bag of sweets, which he was probably quite used to being given in any case. She suggested that he should be allowed to choose the particular

continued opposite

type of chart and stickers to be used. Once he had received one or two rewards, the demands placed on him could be increased and his behaviour modified for longer. At each stage, he should be able to answer clearly when asked what he had to do in order to get a star. Most importantly, his parents should not show their frustration or anger if he failed to comply at first, as this would make the situation worse.

Two weeks later, the doctor was able to report a much happier situation to the health visitor. Giving Mike a Batman sticker each time he went straight back to bed after his drink had met with some initial success. He earned three stickers in the first two nights, and had been rewarded with the promised trip to an airport perimeter fence to watch the aeroplanes taking off and landing. Mike's parents were moving on to asking him to go straight back to bed without a drink, for which he would earn two stickers each time. Once he collected ten of these, his father was going to take him on a special trip to fly his kite. His parents were much happier and could see how using this system of reward might eventually work to prevent Mike getting out of bed altogether.

Comments

The number of target behaviours in the chart, and the type and timing of rewards, will need to be adjusted to the individual child. Some children need to be rewarded straight away, while others can hold on to the idea of a reward for a whole day or a whole week. It is essential to adapt any tangible reward programme to the individual circumstances of both parent and child.

Effective commands

An *effective command* should be simple, developmentally appropriate, and mean something definite. Demands such as 'Be good!' or 'Show me some respect!' are too vague, and do not specify to the child what he has to do. 'Please would you do what I say before I have finished counting to five' is more specific, but would have to be simplified for a young child (probably by breaking the statement down into small parts). Commands should also be positive and polite, and should use 'do' in preference to 'don't' and 'stop' (for instance 'Please pick up that sweet paper'). Commands that specify what should *not* be done are likely to encourage just that behaviour (for instance 'Stop fighting').

Unclear commands are less effective. For instance, 'Your clothes are all over the floor of the bedroom' is not really a command at all, but a critical comment, which is likely to breed resentment rather than co-operative action. A better approach would be 'Could you please put those clothes into the clothes cupboard?'

Parents often shower their children with *multiple commands*. A child may get caught in a bewildering muddle of things he is expected to do, so it is hardly surprising that he does not achieve most of them. It is much more effective to give only one command at a time. Some commands are smothered in a flurry of explanations or questions. Many children will argue with the explanation, so that the original command is forgotten. Help parents to think about what they are asking, and to prune commands to only those that are necessary, with the minimum of explanation and no questions.

This process may be helped by asking both parents to decide on a short list of essential *household rules*. These could be posted on the refrigerator so that everyone (including baby-sitters) knows what the rules are.

Children should be given an opportunity to comply with any command. It is essential to '*catch them being good*', and to praise compliance as soon as it appears, even if it is only partial (for example 'Thank you for putting your trousers away so neatly', even though the other clothes have not been touched).

Alternatives to straight commands include a '*when/then' command* – for instance, 'When you have put the sweet papers in the bin, then you can go out and play with your friend' (*see* section on tangible reward systems above). This gives the child the option of not complying, but the phrasing anticipates compliance. A slightly different type of instruction is an '*if/then' warning*, which specifies an undesirable consequence for non-compliance – for instance, 'If you don't close the door when you go outside, then you will have to go to time out' or 'If you don't eat your food during the mealtime, then you won't be able to eat it later' (*see* sections on time out and logical consequences below).

A command is more likely to be effective if the child is prepared for it. Interrupting an engrossing activity with an unwelcome instruction is unlikely to achieve much except aggravation. A *warning* could prepare the child. For instance, to a child who is busy building something with blocks, a parent could say 'In two more minutes, it will be time to put the blocks away'. For children to whom 'two minutes' means nothing, a timer could be used. Warnings can be even more effective if they take into account children's wishes – for instance 'When that television programme is finished, please come to the table for dinner'.

For children to whom more than one adult gives commands, it is important that *each supports the other*. This means being aware of the commands issued by the other adult, reinforcing compliance with these, and not issuing counter-commands.

Children will ignore commands if there is no *follow-through*. For compliance, there should be reinforcement in the form of praise or some other reward. For non-compliance, parents should either impose a time out or a consequence (*see* below), after first issuing a warning statement such as 'If you don't put the sweet papers away, you will have to go to time out'.

Ignoring and distraction

Some parents believe that ignoring is not a useful form of discipline. The truth is that it is both a very powerful technique and difficult to carry out. Many children would rather be screamed at than ignored. As shouting or any other form of attention is likely to maintain unwanted behaviours, those behaviours that are not dangerous can often be eliminated if they are systematically ignored, especially if positive attention for desirable behaviour is given instead. Behaviours that can successfully be ignored in pre-school children include the following:

- whining
- temper tantrums
- protests when prohibited from doing or having something
- swearing
- facial grimaces
- minor squabbles between children
- nose-picking
- nail-biting
- brief crying in the middle of the night
- minor squabbles between children
- messy eating
- faddy eating.

Ignoring means avoiding all verbal and non-verbal communication with the child, and moving away so as to avoid physical contact. It is best for the parent to avert their gaze from the child, at an angle of 90–180°, so as to avoid inadvertent facial expressions which, either through annoyance or amusement, would have a reinforcing effect. The parent should not express any anger, and should maintain a neutral facial expression, the aim being to make the child think that she is not affected at all by his behaviour. It is probably a good idea for the parent to explain the use of ignoring to the child, but this should be done in advance, when the child is calm and receptive, not while they are doing something that requires ignoring.

Distraction works well in combination with ignoring. This can take two forms – either the parent distracting the child on to an alternative activity, or the parent distracting herself so as not to give any attention to the child. The best time to introduce a distraction for a child is when he has started to calm down.

Tell the parents about the expected *'extinction burst'* – the rule is that the ignored behaviour will get worse before it gets better. Warn them not to give in. For instance, consider the example of a four-year-old girl who wants to go outside, and who argues with her mother about this for several minutes. Her mother decides to issue a firm command – 'I am afraid you cannot go outside at the moment, and that is final' – and then ignores her daughter's protests. The girl escalates her demands in an effort to get what she wants. Provided that the mother persists in ignoring the arguments, the girl will eventually stop, but not before she has become significantly more obnoxious and tried to prolong things beyond the limit of her mother's patience. If the mother gives in, she will be negatively reinforcing the girl's arguing, whining and non-compliance. This is one reason why ignoring is so difficult to carry out.

Another difficulty that some parents have with ignoring is that they feel it is *not punishing the child enough*. In fact, it is more effective than punishment because it maintains a positive relationship with the child, and shows him that you are not affected by his actions or feelings. However, it is important not to maintain ignoring over such a long period that it becomes a punishment or an expression of anger. It is most effective when followed immediately by giving positive attention for a desired behaviour, preferably within five seconds of this appearing.

It is tempting for the parent to *leave the room* in order to ignore more effectively. At times this can be very successful. However, the difficulty with this approach is not being available to witness the return of behaviours that can be positively reinforced. It can also make some children anxious. In more extreme cases, ignoring can be *abusive* – for instance, threatening to leave or abandon the child, which is counter-productive, as it is a threat that cannot be carried out, and it makes the child feel insecure.

Ignoring can be effective in the presence of siblings if it involves differential praise. For instance, at a mealtime the child who is eating quietly should be praised while the child who is throwing food around should be ignored. However, with other behaviours *attention from siblings or others* (e.g. in a bus or supermarket) can make ignoring impossible. It is also inadvisable for destructive behaviours, lying, stealing, non-compliance or forgetting chores.

Time out

Time out is a shorthand for 'time out from positive social reinforcement'. The principle is that bad behaviour is often maintained by any form of social attention, which is rewarding for the child. The behaviour should stop if the attention is removed from the child, either by ignoring, or by all of the other people in the room leaving it, or by removing the child from the room to an environment in which they do not receive any attention. Like many of the other techniques described in this chapter, time out requires attention to detail. It is likely to be most successful if started when the child is young (two to five years of age), and if there is a positive relationship between the child and the parent. This is why play and praise should be taught first.

The choice of a *location* for time out is crucial. A home visit may be particularly helpful for providing an idea of the possibilities of a particular house or flat. Time out can be achieved successfully with a chair, on the stairs, or in a room. The chair must be in the corner of a room or in a hall, provided that this is well away from family activities and not in view of the television. Half-way up the stairs can be suitably unstimulating. Some children will not stay on a chair or on a step of the stairs, and for them a room is needed, either as a back-up or as the first option. The room should preferably be dull and boring, but safe enough for the child to be left alone in it. Families with little space may need to use the child's own bedroom for time out. There are two disadvantages to this. First, if the child is able to play with or destroy toys or games, these will have to be removed, and secondly, if the child finds the experience too aversive, this may make bedtimes more difficult.

From the list of unwanted behaviours, help the parent to *select one or two behaviours* with which to start time out. Behaviours that cannot be ignored, such as hitting, being destructive and non-compliance, are a suitable choice. Other behaviours can be added after several weeks. The parent should describe to the child what time out will be like in advance of using it and at a time when the child is calm and receptive (i.e. not in the heat of a disciplinary exchange).

The *length* of time out is another important consideration. A rough guideline is that the duration should be one minute for each year of the child's age. Durations of longer than five minutes are no more effective. It can be helpful to set a kitchen timer. Most psychological researchers in the field suggest that the child should be quiet before being let out, but in practice this is not essential. There is some debate about the maximum duration of time out. Our experience is that some parents will make time out into an abusive experience for their children, and that the technique is not working if it has to be continued for longer than about 30 minutes. The child needs to get the message that being quiet will cause time out to stop, and that even a brief period of calm may be sufficient for this. If this does not happen, then alternatives should be tried (*see* below). If time out works, then it will not need to be used very often, and it can be administered for brief periods of five minutes or so, followed immediately by an opportunity for the child to be successful and reap praise.

Time out can be used automatically for infringements of household rules (e.g. hitting), or after a *warning*, for non-compliance. This will be of the 'if/then' sort: 'If you don't pick that chewing-gum up off the floor, then you'll go to time out'. The warning can be followed by a pause of about five seconds, which can be marked in the first few weeks by counting down from 5 to 1.

Children may *refuse to go to time out*. Parents should be advised to *take* children aged five or under to time out, gently but firmly. A child of six years or older should have one minute added on to time out for each refusal to go, up to a maximum of ten minutes. At that point a warning should be given to go to time out or lose a privilege. This might be not watching a favourite television programme, or having no access to a favourite toy for a day.

During time out, most children will at first try to *argue* or wriggle their way out of it. It is important to sustain the child in the time-out setting without becoming involved in an argument, which is of course just another form of gratifying attention. (The parent should, if possible, avoid all interaction during time out.) Advise the parent to return the child gently to time out, stating the rule only once more: 'You have to stay on your chair/in your room for five minutes – you can then come out when you're quiet.' If the child gets off the chair repeatedly, then a room must be used. If possible, the door to the room should be left ajar, or the child may become anxious. If the child repeatedly tries to leave the room, the parent will have to shut the door. For children who repeatedly try to open the door, the parent will either have to lock the door, or hold it shut, while avoiding all other forms of attention. You will have to decide which is the most suitable approach for the family involved, allowing for their potential for abuse. Loss of privilege can also be used as a sanction – for example, 'If you come out again before the time is up, I will put the television away until tomorrow'.

Once time out is over, the parents must be calm and positive. If the time out was for non-compliance, the parent should repeat the original command. If the child complies, the parent should simply praise their compliance – for example, 'Well done for picking up the chewing-gum'. If not, then the entire sequence of time out will need to be repeated (*see* Figure 38.1), although in practice children seldom need repeated time outs.

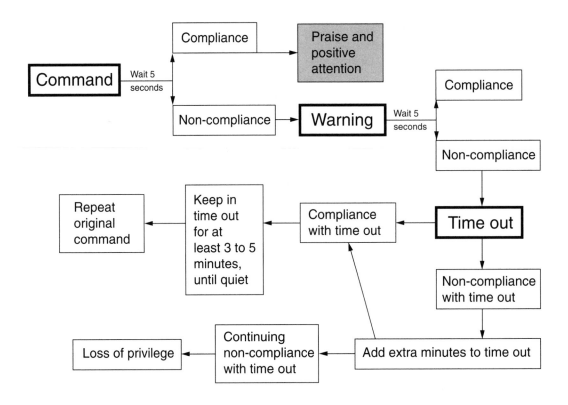

Figure 38.1:   Sequence of actions in time out.

It is important to follow through consistently, otherwise some children may use time out as a way to get out of chores. If the time out was for an infringement of household rules (e.g. hitting), the parent must set aside angry feelings and temptations to criticise, and find something to praise as soon as possible. For instance, saying (angrily) 'I wish you would play quietly with your sister; you're such a pain when you fight', although it may be honest, is rubbing the child's nose in what he has done, giving him a self-image of being 'a pain', and impressing upon him that he is likely to do it again. It would be more effective to say 'Please try again; I know you can do it', but the parent may need a considerable amout of professional support to be able to say this.

Parents need specific coaching to *edit out criticisms* and expressions of anger and upset, however understandable these may be. Shouting 'I'm fed up with you messing up the carpet. You make so much extra work. Go to time out at once!' reflects what every parent must have felt at some time, but is likely to result in the child refusing to go to time out, or trading insults with his parent, which could lead to an escalating argument. Explain to the parents that there is some mental work they will need to do called 'editing', which involves setting aside the negative comments they feel like making and instead showing their calm side in order to be assertive. You could call it 'acting'. The parent in the above example might convert their statement to an internal dialogue only, and say

'I warned you that you would have to go to time out if you didn't pick the chewing-gum off the carpet. Now you will have to go. Get on to the time-out chair'.

Children have a variety of ways of *trying to evade the isolation of time out*. Some children make a lot of mess. It is best to avoid this if possible by tidying away in advance from the time-out space anything that can be used to make a mess. Failing this, the child should be expected to tidy any mess he makes, possibly with some parental help, and forfeit a token amount of pocket-money for any breakages. Other children threaten to vomit, or say that they need to use the lavatory. It is wisest to call such children's bluff, as it is extremely unlikely that any significant harm will come from this. Another ploy for getting out of time out is to threaten not to love the parent any more. Most parents are unaffected by this, but some may give in in order to reassure their child, in which case they will need professional support and rehearsal to show no reaction to this threat.

Parents sometimes say that they think *smacking* is more effective than time out, because it stops the behaviour more quickly and punishes the child more effectively. It may be morally correct to say that on no account should children be smacked, but this will merely inhibit the parent from being honest with you about the times she has smacked. (If you think that the smacking is sufficiently frequent and severe to constitute a child protection issue, then you may have to contact Social Services.) It is probably more effective to discuss smacking and time out as two alternative strategies, and to list the advantages and disadvantages of each, leaving the parents to make up their own minds. Our experience is that, in general, smacking is ineffective. Many children are undeterred by parental threats such as 'Do you want a smack?'. Some parents insist that smacking or threats of physical punishment are effective, although many admit that the main benefit is in relieving their own anger. Although smacking may have some advantages for the parent in the short term, it has long-term disadvantages. One is that children learn by modelling that aggression is the way to solve problems and cope with frustration. A second drawback is that children may learn to conceal their actions from their parents, and misbehave more elsewhere than at home. A third problem is that children may receive the message from smacking, and from the emotions that go with it, that they are unloved and unlovable, and they may then live up to this self-image (this may also happen if the parents issue insults or threats of rejection).

Be sure to safeguard against time out being used in an *abusive* way. We have already mentioned the danger of its being used for too long. Too frequent use can also be dangerous. Even if it is not actually abusive, the use of many time outs in a day is likely to breed resentment, or to make children feel that they cannot do anything right. Ideally, time out should not be used in a punitive way, but merely as a means of coping with an otherwise out-of-control situation. Most children dislike time out, but some will learn to take themselves to their room, on their own initiative, in order to calm down.

Time out can be used *in public* – for instance, outside a supermarket, or by saying 'If you don't stop whining/shouting/having a tantrum, then you'll have a time out when you get home'. Of course, this will only be effective if it is followed through at home.

Parents may themselves need time out, if they are feeling particularly stressed or angry. Professionals who are helping parents to deal with children's behaviour problems may find that much of their time has to be given to meeting the parents' needs, or encouraging the parents to find ways of meeting them, on a variety of levels (e.g. practical, social and emotional).

When teaching some of these techniques it is helpful to use *role play*. Initially this could involve the parent as the parent and the trainer as the child. It is better if the therapist does not role-play the parent, as this can be deskilling for the parent. Once the parent understands the technique, you should help her to explain the technique to her child, playing it through as if it were a game. Although the therapist could play the child while the child plays the parent, it is better not to let the parent play the child in this context, as the child may then think that the parent is in some way subordinate to them (and, for instance, that they could be put in time out). If you can get two or three parents together, or even a group, you can involve several of the parents in a role play, with one or more of them playing parents and one or more playing children.

Problem-solving

Many parents of children with behaviour problems have deficits in problem-solving skills, and this is known to be a significant factor in adolescent conduct disorder. Problem-solving tuition can be undertaken for both parents and young children[2] (given time), using the following five steps:

- Define the problem. 'What am I supposed to do?'
- Brainstorm solutions. 'What are some plans?'
- Evaluate consequences. 'What is the best plan?'
- Implementation. 'Am I using my plan?'
- Evaluate the outcome and revise the plan. 'How did I do?'

Younger children may have difficulty with the last two steps, but are capable of considering several alternative solutions, and of understanding that some are better than others.

Parents can be helped to teach children problem-solving with the use of stories, puppets and cartoons. First, parents can discuss hypothetical problems and go through the five steps. Secondly, they can apply the techniques to real-life problems. It is then important for the parent first to establish the child's view of the problem before coming to her own conclusions, then to help the child generate solutions (however daft they may be), to look at the consequences of the most promising two or three solutions, and finally to help the child to try out one or two of them. Parents may need support with their own feelings before they are able to help their child to think about his feelings and about the feelings of other people in the problem situation. The aim is to encourage the process of problem-solving, not necessarily to arrive at the best solution first time round.

For instance, a mother may feel devastated that her four-year-old son, Kevin, has been sent home early from a friend's house because he got into a fight. She will need to find out what happened, both from her son and from his friend's parent, and then discuss what could happen differently next time. She will need to start by trying to understand Kevin's point of view. Kevin's friend said that he did not think Kevin had any good videos, and Kevin over-reacted to this by hitting. What could he do next time someone says something that he doesn't like? Various solutions may be suggested during the discussion. Kevin could go home, say something nasty in return, steal one of his friend's videos, or kick him harder than before. Kevin's mother may explore his feelings further by asking 'How are you feeling about being sent home?', 'How did you feel when he said that about your videos?', and she can help Kevin to think about his friend's feelings by asking 'How do you think he felt when you hit him?', 'How can you tell if he is sad or happy?', 'What would happen if you said something nasty to him?', 'What would happen if you stole one of his videos?' and 'How can you make him be your friend?'. Eventually, Kevin may respond by saying that his friend asked to borrow a toy of his and, with a little help from his mother, he may come up with the idea of offering to swap this toy for one of his friend's videos.

Consequences

Natural and logical consequences are a useful behavioural technique for children aged five years or over, as they give children more responsibility and help them to develop decision-making skills, independence and the ability to learn from mistakes.

Natural consequences consist of leaving things to take their natural course – for example, allowing a child to get cold if she refuses to put her coat on, or letting a child remain in wet shoes for half an hour if he jumps in a puddle.

Logical consequences are designed by parents to fit the misbehaviour. Examples include felt-tip pens being removed for half an hour if they are used to draw on walls, or locking a bicycle up for 24 hours if it is used on a dangerous road.

The following *guidelines* need to be followed for consequences.

- Consequences should be appropriate for the age and level of understanding of the child concerned.
- The parents should be able to live with the consequences they have chosen, so that they can follow through with them. For example, there is little point in threatening to take the child to school in their pyjamas if they do not get dressed in time in the morning if this would be too embarrassing for the parent to do.
- Children should be warned in advance of consequences, and whenever possible involved in deciding what is appropriate. For instance, if children are fighting over which television programme to watch, a parent might give them a choice of taking turns to choose the programme, or taking turns not to watch television at all.
- Consequences should be applied immediately, and not for too long. Longer punishments are less effective, not more so.
- Consequences should be applied in a respectful and non-punitive way. For example, washing a child's mouth out with soap because he has been swearing is likely to make him feel degraded and angry.
- Consequences should be quickly followed by an opportunity to carry out the desired behaviour – for instance, once the bicycle or the felt-tip pens in the above example are returned.

Holding

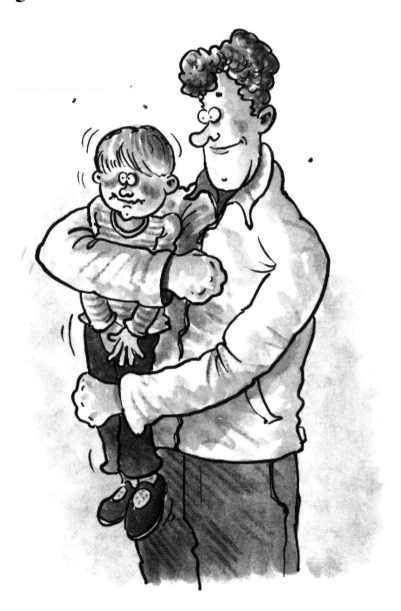

Figure 38.2:   A parent holding a young child. Note that the child should not be able to hurt the parent with either his arms or legs.

This can be used as an alternative to time out for some children. It is particularly useful for helping those aged five to eight years with out-of-control behaviour (e.g. a tantrum) to calm down. As with all of the behavioural techniques discussed in this chapter, it works better if carried out calmly and positively. It should also be used sparingly.

Holding consists of the parent restraining the child in a hug-like clasp in such a way that neither of them can be hurt. There are various ways of doing this, but the essential elements are to restrain the arms and legs without hurting the child. The parent's arms can be clasped around the child's chest and arms. The child's legs can be held in the same arm grip if he is small enough, otherwise they may need to be held within a scissor grasp from the parent's legs. It is probably best to have the child facing away from the parent's body, rather than towards it (some children bite).

Holding is not for the weak-hearted, as the position may have to be maintained for up to half an hour to give the child time to settle. The child should be told that he will be held until he has calmed down. This technique is not suitable for children who are too strong for the adult to manage.

Concerns have been expressed that on the one hand this behaviour could easily become abusive, and on the other children might enjoy the physical contact and find the experience rewarding. Although either possibility could be true in particular cases, most children dislike the experience but appear to benefit from it. In the short term it provides a welcome means for the child and the parent to regain control, and in the long term it allows children to develop a capacity to calm down on their own.

Practice points for parents

These can be used, for example, as refrigerator notes.

Box 38.2:   Play

- Aim to play with each child for ten minutes each day.
- Follow the child's lead.
- Allow the child to set the rules (e.g. about how toys are used, or the rules of a game).
- Watch silently, or select things the child is doing to praise.
- Warn the child a few minutes before the end of play.

Box 38.3: Commands

- Make sure that the child understands what you want him to do.
- Keep commands simple, and try to give only one command at a time.
- Be polite to your child and show him respect. He will then be more likely to display the same attitude towards you.
- Give praise or a reward immediately after your child has done what he was told.
- If he does not do as he is told after a warning, follow through with time out or a consequence.

Box 38.4: Praise

- Catch your child being good.
- Label what you like as you praise it.
- Give praise immediately.
- Use both words and signals (e.g. smiles, tone of voice, hugs or cuddles).
- Praise attempts to succeed as well as success.

Box 38.5: Rewards

- You can add a reward to your praise when you catch your child being good.
- You can promise a reward for a certain behaviour 'When ... then ...'.
- Give rewards immediately.
- Make sure that the child knows what the rewards are for.
- You can use stars, stickers, tokens or points as part of a reward programme.

Box 38.6: Ignoring

- Ignoring is not the same as doing nothing – it requires calmness and planning.
- Ignoring a behaviour for the first time will probably make it worse before it gets better.
- Try to distract your child on to something you would rather he did instead.
- Finish ignoring with praise for a desired behaviour, as soon as possible.
- With two or more children, try to pay attention to the one who is doing what you want, and ignore those who are misbehaving.

Box 38.7:   Time out

- Use time out for non-compliance or for behaviours that cannot be ignored.
- Do not use it too often.
- Plan in advance the space you will use for time out, and the duration.
- Give a warning, and then wait for five seconds.
- Instruct your child to go to the time-out space for five minutes, or however long you have decided he should remain there.
- If the child will not comply, use gentle physical force for younger children (two to five years), or add extra minutes for older children.
- Once your child is in time out, ignore arguments, and gently return him to his time-out space if he leaves it.
- Remember that if you get angry this will reward your child's misbehaviour.
- After time out is over, calmly repeat the original command.
- If your child will still not comply with this command, go through the whole sequence again.
- After time out, find an opportunity to praise your child as soon as possible.

Box 38.8:   Problem-solving

- Define the problem.
- Think of as many different solutions as possible.
- Choose one or two of these solutions.
- Evaluate the consequences, and then go back and choose a different solution if necessary.
- Use the solution you have chosen.
- Evaluate the success of this solution, and change it if necessary.

Box 38.9:   Consequences

- A natural consequence is what would happen naturally.
- A logical consequence fits the behaviour.
- Involve children in deciding consequences if possible.
- Apply consequences immediately and briefly.
- Find an opportunity to praise the child as soon as possible after the consequence is over.

References

1   Forehand RL and McMahon RJ (1981) *Helping the Noncompliant Child: A Clinician's Guide to Parent Training.* Guilford Press, New York.

2   Webster-Stratton C (1992) *The Incredible Years.* Umbrella Press, Toronto.

3   Barkley RA (1997) *Defiant Children: A Clinician's Manual for Parent Training.* Guilford Press, New York.

4   Webster-Stratton C and Herbert M (1994) *Troubled Families: Problem Children.* John Wiley & Sons, Chichester.

Reading materials and other information for parents

Although books are not suitable for everyone, some parents benefit greatly from reading self-help manuals.

Elliott M (1996) *501 Ways to be a Good Parent.* Hodder and Stoughton, London. A general compendium of advice about what to do, with less emphasis than in the other books listed on how to do it. It is humorous and very readable. The author is well known for her work on bullying for the charity **Kidscape**.

Hartley-Brewer E (1994) *Positive Parenting.* Mandarin Paperbacks, London. This book emphasises the need to build up a child's self-esteem. The author has run groups in schools, for which she has developed her own manual.

Phelan TW (1995) *1–2–3 Magic: Training Your Children to do What You Want.* Child Management Inc., Glen Ellyn, IL. This is a useful guide to effective commands and time out, with less emphasis on reinforcing wanted behaviours. There is also a videotape available from ADD Information Services, PO Box 340, Edgware, Middlesex HA8 9HL (tel 020 8905 2013).

Webster-Stratton C (1992) *The Incredible Years.* Umbrella Press, Toronto. This is a very useful adjunct to parent training groups, but it is difficult to obtain in the UK.

Other parents may need telephone or face-to-face contact.

A charitable organisation called **Parent Network** runs a group programme called **Parent-Link** at adult education centres throughout the country. The course teaches modules such as *Understanding Children* and an *Introduction to Family and Childcare*. Graduates of the programme can go on to run groups themselves. Details of local groups are available from the central office at 44–46 Caversham Road, London NW5 2DS (tel 020 7485 8535).

There are large numbers of other parenting group initiatives developing throughout the country (e.g. in Social Services family centres, schools and other settings). Two particularly well-established organisations which offer support for parents soon after childbirth in certain areas of the country are **Home Start**, 2 Salisbury Road, Leicester LE1 7OR (tel 0116 233 9955) and **Newpin**, Sutherland House, 35 Sutherland Square, Walworth, London SE17 3EE (tel 020 7703 6326).

Other charitable organisations, with confusingly similar names, include the following.

Exploring Parenthood, 4 Ivory Place, 20a Treadgold Street, London W11 4BP (tel 020 8960 1678; advice line 020 7221 6681, 11.00 a.m. to 4.00 p.m. Monday to Friday). This organisation offers support for any parent who is facing problems with their children, and provides advice, education, information and counselling.

Parentline, Endway House, The Endway, Hadleigh, Benfleet SS7 2AN (helpline 01702 559900; tel 01702 554782/0268 757077; fax 01702 554911). This is a national helpline for parents under stress. It is open from 9 a.m. to 6 p.m. every weekday, and from 1 p.m. to 6 p.m. on Saturdays.

Organisation for Parents Under Stress (Opus), Rayta House, 57 Hart Road, Thundersley, Essex S57 3PD (tel 01268 757077).

Parents Anonymous (tel 020 7263 8918).

CHAPTER THIRTY NINE

Formulary

For more detail, prescribers are advised to consult *Medicines for Children*.[1]

Sedatives

Promethazine hydrochloride (Phenergan)

Sedating antihistamine

Indication: night sedation in the context of a behavioural programme

Contraindications: neonates and premature infants; central nervous system depression; porphyria; hypersensitivity to phenothiazines. There have been reports of cot death in children under one year of age

Side-effects: paradoxical stimulation; nightmares; headache; antimuscarinic effects such as dry mouth and blurred vision. Children may be more susceptible than adults to side-effects

Dose at bedtime:

	1–2 mg/kg	
	1–2 years	10–20 mg
	2–5 years	15–25 mg
	5–12 years	20–25 mg
	12 years and above	25–50 mg

Trimeprazine tartrate (Vallergan)

Sedating antihistamine

Indication: night sedation in the context of a behavioural programme

Contraindications: hepatic or renal dysfunction; epilepsy; hypothyroidism

Side-effects: paradoxical stimulation; nightmares; nasal stuffiness; dry mouth; can cause morning drowsiness and restless irritability the next day

Dose at bedtime: 1.5–3 mg/kg

Chloral hydrate (Welldorm)[39.1]

Sedating antihistamine

Indication: night sedation, particularly for children with developmental difficulties (e.g. learning difficulties or autistic spectrum disorder)

Contraindications: cardiac disease; gastritis; respiratory insufficiency; porphyria

Side-effects: gastrointestinal irritation; abdominal distension; flatulence; rashes. Large doses can cause respiratory depression. Chloral is corrosive to skin and mucous membranes unless well diluted

Dose at bedtime: 30–50 mg/kg

Maximum single dose of 1 g below the age of 12 years

Triclofos Sodium

Chloral derivative

Indication, contraindications and side-effects: as for chloral hydrate, but reported to cause less gastrointestinal disturbance. In some children it appears to be less effective. Only available as liquid

Dose at bedtime: 30–50 mg/kg

Diazepam (Valium)

Benzodiazepine

Indication: can be used to suppress stage IV sleep for the short-term treatment of parasomnias such as night terrors and sleep-walking. Regular waking at a time just before these are expected to occur should be tried first

Contraindication: respiratory depression

Side-effects: drowsiness; confusion; ataxia; irritability; light-headedness; social inhibition. Dependence can occur with long-term use

Dose at bedtime: 1–5 mg

A short course of one week only is recommended

Zopiclone (Zimovane)

Non-benzodiazepine hypnotic
Indication: parasomnias; short-term night sedation in adolescents
Contraindications: hepatic and renal impairment; sleep apnoea or any other condition that affects respiration
Side-effects: unusual taste in mouth; light-headedness; nightmares; irritability the following day. Dependence has been reported
Dose at bedtime: 3.75 mg
                                    Recommended only for children aged 12 years or over

Medications for attention-deficit hyperactivity disorder (also *see* Chapter 22)

Methylphenidate hydrochloride (Ritalin[39.2] mg tablets, Equasym 5 mg, 10 mg and 20 mg tablets) [CONTROLLED DRUG]

Amphetamine derivative
Indication: attention-deficit hyperactivity disorder or attention-deficit disorder
Contraindications: psychosis; substance misuse; congenital heart disease. Can exacerbate tics and anxiety. Lowers seizure threshold
Side-effects: delayed onset of sleep; decreased appetite; increased metabolic rate; initial weight loss and subsequent failure to gain weight; headache; abdominal pain (usually transitory); tics; rebound hyperactivity in the evening; emotionality; a change of personality; an excessively calm state (which indicates an excessive dose, and usually responds to dose reduction); hallucinations. Dependence does not occur in children at the doses used to treat attention-deficit hyperactivity disorder. The tablets should not be prescribed to chaotic households. One of the main risks is that the tablets will be sold on the black market instead of being used therapeutically.
Dose: Titrate according to effects and side-effects
                                    Once a day to five times per day: standard is three times daily
                                    3–5 years   2.5–5 mg once or twice daily
                                    6–11 years   5–20 mg per dose; maximum 60 mg daily
                                    12–18 years   5–40 mg per dose; maximum 120 mg daily

Dexamphetamine sulphate (Dexedrine 5 mg tablets)
[CONTROLLED DRUG]

Amphetamine derivative
Indication: attention-deficit hyperactivity disorder or attention-deficit disorder
Contraindications and side effects: as for methylphenidate
Dose: Once a day to five times per day: standard is three times daily
                 3–5 years   1.25–5 mg once or twice daily
                 6–11 years   2.5–10 mg per dose; maximum 40 mg daily
                 12–18 years   5–20 mg per dose; maximum 80 mg daily

Imipramine can also be used for attention-deficit hyperactivity disorder, as a second-line treatment (*see* section on nocturnal enuresis below).

Clonidine (Dixarit 25 mg; Catapres 100 µg and 300 µg tablets and 250 µg modified-release capsules (Perlongets))

A central α_2 adrenergic agonist that reduces sympathetic outflow from the brain
Indications: attention-deficit hyperactivity disorder and tic disorder (*see* Chapter 32)
Contraindications and side-effects: drowsiness; nightmares; hypotension; depression
Dose: Titrate according to effects and side-effects. Monitor blood pressure.
1   As a single drug for attention-deficit hyperactivity disorder, usually in young children. Anecdotal evidence suggests that it may be worth trying in those with autistic spectrum disorder. Start at 25 µg 4-hourly up to three times a day and gradually increase the dose
2   As a single drug for tic disorder or Tourette's syndrome. More likely to be indicated in older children, so the dose may need to be proportionally higher, up to 100 µg three times a day
3   Three hours before bedtime to counteract the delayed sleep onset caused by stimulant medication (methylphenidate or dexamphetamine)
                 3–5 years   25–50 µg
                 6–11 years   25–200 µg
                 12–18 years   100–300 µg
    This non-simultaneous usage of clonidine is said to be safer than simultaneous use with stimulants (Professor Eric Taylor, personal communication)
4   Together with each dose of stimulant medication: 25–50 µg per dose. This usage is controversial, as some deaths have been reported in North America, with much ensuing debate in the literature;[2] there are alternative explanations in all cases. *Medicines for Children* recommends electrocardiographic monitoring for this combination

Medications for tics and Tourette's syndrome (also see Chapter 32)

Sulpiride

Antipsychotic
Indication: Tourette's syndrome
Contraindications: lowers seizure threshold. Plasma concentration is increased by propranolol
Side-effects: drowsiness; extra-pyramidal symptoms; increased appetite
Dose: Titrate according to effects and side-effects

| | 6–11 years | start with 50 mg at night; maximum 200 mg daily, in two divided doses |
| | 12–18 years | start with 100–200 mg twice daily; maximum 1.2 g daily |

Risperidone (Risperdal)

Antipsychotic
Indication: Tourette's syndrome; conduct disorder with or without attention-deficit hyperactivity disorder[3]
Contraindications and side-effects: as for sulpiride. Provide a small supply of an antidote to extra-pyramidal side-effects, such as procyclidine
Dose: Titrate according to effects and side-effects

| | 6–11 years | start with 0.5 mg at night; maximum 4 mg daily, in two divided doses |
| | 12–18 years | start with 0.5 mg 12-hourly; maximum 10 mg daily |

Antidepressants

There is a wide choice of antidepressants available. There is such a high risk of overdose in adolescents that treatment with full doses of tricyclic antidepressants is no longer justified, particularly since a controlled trial of fluoxetine in adolescents was published,[4] making selective serotonin reuptake inhibitors[39.3] the first-choice treatment. With the exception of citalopram, for which fatal overdose has been reported,[5] the selective serotonin reuptake inhibitors are safe in overdose. Related antidepressants with a slightly different range of receptor selectivity can also be useful, and are also safe in overdose. We mention our own selection here. For instance, we have found that paroxetine seems to be over-stimulating in children (although not in adults), and therefore we do not recommend this drug. A single daily dosage, and a dosage regime that requires no adjustment, both improve compliance.

Small doses of tricyclic antidepressants appear to be used widely for night sedation in adults, particularly if initial insomnia is associated with anxiety. Although we are unaware of any controlled trials (in adults or children), clinical experience suggests that this is remarkably effective, since the dose is very much lower than that recommended for depression. We are reluctant to recommend this practice in general, because adolescents can stockpile drugs, and subsequently take a large quantity all at once. However, we do think it deserves mention, and we include it here under the heading of amitriptyline. Dothiepin may be used more often, as it is more sedating.

Fluoxetine (Prozac)

Selective serotonin reuptake inhibitor
Indications: depression; obsessive-compulsive disorder; bulimia nervosa; anxiety disorders; panic disorder
Contraindications: hepatic or renal insufficiency. Lowers seizure threshold
Side-effects: nausea; gastrointestinal symptoms and reduction in appetite; rash (sometimes urticarial) which usually indicates that the drug should be stopped; headache; light-headedness or feeling 'spaced out'; restlessness. Like all antidepressants, it can precipitate mania. Diminished libido and anorgasmia may occur.
Dose: Morning dosage seems to avoid insomnia
                      20 mg daily for most indications and ages
                      For children under 12 years, 10 mg in 2.5 mL of liquid may be used
                      60 mg in morning for bulimia
                      The dose may be increased up to 60 mg daily in depression or obsessive-compulsive disorder

---

Sertraline (Lustral)

Selective serotonin reuptake inhibitor
Indications: depression; obsessive-compulsive disorder; anxiety disorders; panic disorder
Contraindications: as for fluoxetine
Side-effects: as for fluoxetine. Can be more sedative, and may cause raised transaminases and serum uric acid levels
Dose: 50 mg in morning
Can be increased up to 150 mg in morning

Citalopram (Cipramil)

Selective serotonin reuptake inhibitor
Indications: depression; panic disorder; anxiety disorder
Contraindications: as for fluoxetine
Side-effects: as for fluoxetine. There has been a single report from Sweden of six fatalities attributed to overdose with citalopram, and thought to be due to cardiac arrhythmias.[5] We are not aware of any confirmatory reports. However, this has made us cautious about using this drug as an antidepressant in adolescents, whose risk of overdose has to be regarded as high
Dose: 20 mg in morning
Can be increased up to 60 mg per day

Mirtazapine (Zispin)

A presynaptic α_2-antagonist, increasing central noradrenergic and serotonergic neurotransmission
Indications: depression, particularly where there is marked sleep disturbance (initial *and* middle insomnia)
Contraindications: as for fluoxetine
Side-effects: as for fluoxetine; can be more sedative, and may cause raised transaminases and serum uric acid levels; reversible fall in white blood cell count; weight gain
Dose: 15 mg at night for first week, then 30 mg at night
Can be increased up to 45 mg at night

Venlafaxine slow release (Efexor SL)

Serotonin and noradrenaline reuptake inhibitor
Indication: depression, particularly where there is intolerance or non-response to other antidepressants
Contraindications: as for fluoxetine; history of drug abuse; avoid abrupt withdrawal
Side-effects: nausea; headache; dry mouth; dizziness; return of symptoms upon withdrawal
Dose: 75 mg in morning
                                Can be increased to 150 mg daily

---

Amitriptyline (Tryptizol or Lentizol)

Tricyclic antidepressant
Indications: initial insomnia, particularly associated with anxiety. Can also be used for nocturnal enuresis
Contraindications: risk of overdose (i.e. adolescents with even mild depression) unless a parent can be relied upon to check supplies of tablets *and* compliance
Side-effects: as for imipramine, but can be more sedative: anticholinergic effects; postural hypotension; cardiac dysrhythmias; tremor; sweating; increased appetite and weight
Dose: 2–12 years   10–50 mg at night
                            12–18 years   50–150 mg at night

Anxiolytics

The selective serotonin reuptake inhibitors mentioned above are probably now the first choice for anxiety. Fluoxetine, sertraline and citalopram are all suitable. Propranolol is suitable for performance anxiety, and can help some children with continual anxiety. Other options include buspirone and alprazolam.

Propranolol (Inderal 10 mg, 40 mg and 80 mg tablets; also available as slow-release formulation and suspension)

Non-selective beta-adrenergic-blocking agent
Indications: performance anxiety; social phobia; generalised anxiety
Contraindications: asthma; hypotension. Care is needed if given with chlorpromazine, as blood levels of both are increased. Cimetidine and hydralazine also increase levels of beta-blocker
Side-effects: postural hypotension; bronchospasm; nightmares; sleep disturbance; mood changes; paraesthesia
Dose: 12–18 years   10–40 mg once to three times a day

Buspirone (Buspar)

An azaspirodecanedione, which is anxiolytic but not sedative, anticonvulsant or muscle-relaxant
Indications: anxiety; may take 3–6 weeks to start working
Contraindications: hepatic and renal impairment; epilepsy
Side-effects: nausea; dry mouth; vivid dreams; light-headedness; dizziness; headache
Dose: 2–12 years   5 mg two to three times daily
                                   12–18 years   5–15 mg two to three times daily

---

Alprazolam (Xanax)

Benzodiazepine
Indications: anxiety and panic disorder
Contraindication: respiratory depression
Side-effects: as for diazepam: drowsiness; confusion; ataxia; irritability; light-headedness; social inhibition. Dependence can occur with long-term use
Dose:
Anxiety   12–18 years   250–500 g three times a day
Panic disorder   12–18 years   500 g three times a day, increased stepwise every four days up to a maximum of 8 mg daily in divided doses

Not prescribable under the National Health Service: private prescription is required.

Drugs for the treatment of nocturnal enuresis

Tricyclic antidepressants have now been superseded by desmopressin. They may still have a place in the treatment of older children with responsible parents who have persisting nocturnal enuresis, a low risk of overdose, and who have not responded to any other treatment. Amitriptyline is mentioned above.

Imipramine

Tricyclic antidepressant

Indications: nocturnal enuresis; can also be used for attention-deficit hyper-activity disorder, in twice daily doses, with the same daily total as for enuresis, or slightly higher

Contraindications: porphyria; hepatic disease; cardiac impairment; presence of young children in chaotic household

Side-effects: anticholinergic effects; sedation; postural hypotension; cardiac dys-rhythmias; tremor; sweating; increased appetite and weight. *Toxicity in overdose.*

Dose: 7 years 25 mg, 8–11 years 25–50 mg, over 11 years 50–75 mg

Dose given at bedtime for a maximum of 3 months, including graded withdrawal

---

Desmopressin (DDAVP)

Vasopressin (antidiuretic hormone) analogue

Indication: nocturnal enuresis with normal urine-concentrating ability

Contraindications: renal impairment; psychogenic polydipsia. Disturbances of vision and hearing have been reported during prolonged therapy, and therefore these should be tested before commencing long-term treatment, and ideally at three-monthly intervals

Side-effects: frequent local reactions (e.g. pain, swelling); occasional gastro-intestinal disturbance or hypersensitivity reactions

Dose:

Intranasal: over five years 20–40 µg at night
Oral: over five years 200–400 µg at night

Withdraw for at least 1 week for reassessment every 3 months

Drugs used for the treatment of constipation

Lactulose (Duphalac)

Non-absorbable disaccharide, which acts as an osmotic laxative
Indication: constipation
Contraindications: intestinal obstruction; galactosaemia
Side-effects: abdominal discomfort and cramps; wind; diarrhoea
Dose:

Under 1 year	2.5 mL twice daily
1–5 years	5 mL twice daily
5–10 years	10 mL twice daily
10–18 years	15 mL twice daily

Docusate sodium (Dioctyl)

Stimulant laxative and softening agent
Indication: constipation
Contraindications: intestinal obstruction
Side-effects: abdominal discomfort and cramps; possible increased faecal overflow if there is faecal impaction in rectum
Dose:

Over 6 months	12.5 mg three times a day
2–12 years	12.5–25mg three times a day

Senna

Stimulant laxative
Indication: constipation
Contraindications: any abdominal symptoms; diabetics should have the tablets
Side-effects: griping may occur
Dose:
Syrup (7.5 mg/5 mL):

2–6 years	2.5–5 mL in morning
6–12 years	5–10 mL in morning
12–18 years	10–20 mL in morning

Tablets (7.5 mg):

6–12 years	1–2 tablets in morning
12–18 years	2–4 tablets in morning

Granules (one 5 ml teaspoon = 15 mg):

6–12 years	2.5–5 mL in morning
12–18 years	5–10 mL in morning

Sodium picosulphate (Laxoberal)

Stimulant laxative
Indication: constipation
Contraindications: undiagnosed abdominal pain, or where obstruction is suspected
Side-effects: occasional reports of mild abdominal discomfort
Dose:

	2–5 years	2.5 mL at night
	5–10 years	2.5–5 mL at night
	10–18 years	5–15 mL at night

Notes

39.1   Many drugs that are used in children are not licensed for the use or age range recommended in this book and in the above consensus publication.[1] Chloral hydrate is a good example of this. It is a very safe drug that we believe to be more effective than the other two antihistamines for night sedation, but it is not licensed in any of its preparations for this use.

39.2   Methylphenidate is licensed for children aged six years and above, and dexamphetamine is licensed for three-year-olds and above. This makes no particular sense. We have found that methylphenidate in very small doses is less likely to cause side-effects in under-fives. The availability of a 5 mg preparation makes it easier to give appropriately small doses, for instance starting at 2.5 mg.

39.3   Selective serotonin reuptake inhibitors are not licensed for use in children. They are nevertheless widely used in children down to about the age of eight years. We believe it is reasonable for general practitioners to prescribe antidepressants down to the age of 12 years.

References

1   Royal College of Paediatrics and Child Health (1999) *Medicines for Children*. Royal College of Paediatrics and Child Health, London; website www.bmbc.com/rcpch.

2   Wilens TE, Spencer TJ, Swanson JM, Connor DF and Cantwell D (1999) Combining methylphenidate and clonidine: a clinically sound medication option. *J Am Acad Child Adolesce Psychiatry.* **38**: 614–19.

3   Findling RL, McNamara NK, Branicky LA, Schlucter MD, Lemon E and Blumer JL (2000) A double-blind pilot study of risperidone in the treatment of conduct disorder. *J Am Acad Child Adolesc Psychiatry.* **39**: 509–16.

4   Emslie GJ, Rush J, Weinberg WA *et al.* (1997) A double-blind, randomized, placebo-controlled trial of fluoxetine in children and adolescents with depression. *Arch Gen Psychiatry.* **54**: 1031–7.

5   Ostrom M, Eriksson A, Thorson J and Spigset O (1996) Fatal overdose with citalopram (letter). *Lancet.* **348**: 339–40.

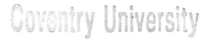

Index